Advances in the Management of Testosterone Deficiency

Frontiers of Hormone Research

Vol. 37

Series Editor

Ashley B. Grossman London

Advances in the Management of Testosterone Deficiency

Volume Editor

T. Hugh Jones Barnsley/Sheffield

29 figures, 1 in color, and 12 tables, 2009

KARGER Basel · Freiburg · Paris · London · New York · Bangalore · Bangkok · Shanghai · Singapore · Tokyo · Sydney

T. Hugh Jones
Robert Hague Centre for Diabetes and Endocrinology
Barnsley Hospital
NHS Foundation Trust
Barnsley, UK

and

Academic Unit of Diabetes, Endocrinology and Metabolism
The Medical School
University of Sheffield
Sheffield, UK

Library of Congress Cataloging-in-Publication Data

Advances in the management of testosterone deficiency / volume editor, T. Hugh Jones.
p. ; cm. – (Frontiers of hormone research, ISSN 0301-3073 ; v. 37)
Includes bibliographical references and indexes.
ISBN 978-3-8055-8622-1 (hard cover : alk. paper)
1. Hypogonadism. 2. Testosterone–Pathophysiology. I. Jones, T. Hugh (Thomas Hugh), 1954– II. Series.
[DNLM: 1. Testosterone–deficiency. W1 FR946F v.37 2008 / WJ 875 A244 2008]
RC898.A38 2009
616.6′5–dc22

2008023379

Bibliographic Indices. This publication is listed in bibliographic services, including Current Contents® and PubMed/MEDLINE.

www.karger.com
Printed in Switzerland on acid-free and non-aging paper (ISO 9706) by Reinhardt Druck, Basel
ISSN 0301–3073
ISBN 978–3–8055–8622–1

Contents

Foreword

For many years research on gonadal hormone replacement therapy has tended to concentrate on female hormones, particularly in terms of contraception and post-menopausal replacement. Testosterone replacement, when considered at all, was given to a small number of men in whom there was undoubted pituitary or testicular damage, and then most usually in terms of injectable testosterone esters which were relatively short-acting, and whose pharmacokinetics were highly unphysiological. However, the situation has changed dramatically over the last decade, as the forms of testosterone replacement have dramatically increased, and the indications for replacement have been greatly redefined. As clinicians, we are now in a situation where we can offer our patients a plethora of different types of replacement, and we customize their replacement according their preferences, lifestyle and personal requirements. We can also more carefully define who may or may not benefit from replacement, and discuss the long-term consequences in terms of risks and benefits. It is therefore very fitting that Hugh Jones has put together an outstanding team of authors to guide clinicians through the confused minefield of testosterone replacement treatments, their respective advantages and disadvantages, and the changes in indications for their use. As one whose research is at the leading edge of novel indications for testosterone replacement, Professor Jones is well placed to survey this growing field. I believe this is a valuable addition to our series, and one which will be of immense value to practising clinicians of many types, particularly andrologists and all those whose practice brings them into contact with hypogonadal men.

Ashley B. Grossman, London

Preface

There has been a considerable increase in the number of research publications related to different clinical aspects of testosterone deficiency in the male over recent years. However, male hypogonadism, the clinical syndrome of testosterone deficiency, still remains a poorly understood condition and clinically underrecognized by the medical profession. The aim of this book is to provide an update of current opinion on the management of hypogonadism based on recent advances from research studies as well as the clinical experience of the expert contributors.

Sir William Osler in 1892 wrote that: 'Medicine is a science of inconsistency and an art of probability.' This statement aptly portrays the challenges to the clinician in the diagnosis of hypogonadism, as the symptoms are non-specific, there are no clear cut-offs for the biochemical tests and some patients fail to respond to treatment. Recent publication of international guidelines on the diagnosis and management of hypogonadism and of late-onset hypogonadism has helped to raise awareness of the conditions and provide consensus views from groups of world experts.

To make the diagnosis of hypogonadism requires a good knowledge of the physiology of testosterone, clinical presentation and investigation, as well as the art of the clinician. The first part of this book aims to provide a clinical update on the current guidelines for the diagnosis and management of hypogonadism including advances in the biochemical assays for testosterone. It also addresses the potential clinical importance of differences in androgen receptor sensitivity as a result of genetic polymorphism. The clinical implication is that the testosterone replacement dose for an individual may be assessed using pharmacogenetic profiling. New modes of testosterone therapies, which allow physiological replacement, are addressed as well as issues regarding prostate safety.

Testosterone is not just a sex hormone but has important biological actions on many different tissues and organs. The second part of the book deals with recent advances in the knowledge of how testosterone deficiency can affect these systems and evidence as to whether or not testosterone replacement therapy can have specific clinical benefits on them. These specific areas include osteoporosis, frailty, cardiovascular disease, diabetes and the metabolic syndrome, other chronic diseases, the brain and erectile dysfunction.

The contributors to this book are all key opinion leaders and have been involved in active research in this clinical field. I wish to sincerely thank them for their excellent chapters. I hope that the reader will find the book informative and clinically useful. This in turn I would hope leads to a better understanding and awareness of hypogonadism, which can then be translated into clinical benefits for our patients.

T. Hugh Jones, Barnsley/Sheffield

Jones TH (ed): Advances in the Management of Testosterone Deficiency.
Front Horm Res. Basel, Karger, 2009, vol 37, pp 1–4

Introduction

In the past decade, several peer-reviewed studies have been reported in the medical literature, which have advanced our understanding of the management of male hypogonadism. However, many of these findings have not been put into routine clinical practice up to now. This book brings together key areas where our understanding and knowledge of hypogonadism have progressed. These include the diagnosis and management of hypogonadism and the role of testosterone deficiency in specific tissues and organ systems and its adverse effect on mortality.

Although male hypogonadism is an established clinical condition which can be treated, many men suffering from it are not diagnosed. There are several reasons for this, which include a lack of general clinical awareness, the non-specificity of its symptoms, biochemical tests which are not always easy to interpret, concerns over the safety of testosterone replacement therapy especially in older men, and the false perception that testosterone is a sex hormone which has no other specific health benefits. This is compounded by the fact that men in general see their doctors less often than women and are less likely to discuss their sex problems. Tiredness is a common symptom of hypogonadism which can be profound but there are not many medical practitioners who include the assessment of testosterone levels in the clinical workup of this symptom. Hypogonadism impairs well-being and quality of life and puts relationships and employment at risk. Guidelines for the diagnosis and management of hypogonadism [1] and late-onset hypogonadism [2] were published in 2006 to assist clinicians [Arver and Lehtihet, p. 5].

The diagnosis of hypogonadism in the presence of symptoms is dependent on the measurement and interpretation of the serum testosterone level. Total testosterone is widely used and threshold levels below which hypogonadism can be diagnosed (in the presence of symptoms) are provided in the published guidelines mentioned above. Levels in the lower-to-normal range can be consistent with the diagnosis of hypogonadism. The biologically active fractions of testosterone, free and bioavailable testosterone levels, in borderline cases can be helpful to the clinician when making the diagnosis. A working knowledge and current understanding of these tests is therefore important for the clinician to be able to interpret the values [Diver, p. 21].

One of the major recent advances has been new formulations of delivery with improved dosing schedules that allow replacement of testosterone to physiological levels [3]. These primarily include dermal gels, buccal tablets and depot injection therapy [Gooren, p. 32]. These formulations also allow therapies to be tailored to individual patient's preferences and needs.

There is evidence to support the notion that the level of tissue androgenization is not only dependent on the circulating testosterone level but also on the sensitivity of the androgen receptor. A polymorphism of the androgen receptor involving the number of CAG repeats in exon 1 is associated with differences in the biological actions of androgens [Zitzmann, p. 52]. These include effects on the prostate, spermatogenesis, bone density and psychological traits. Potentially further knowledge of this and other androgen receptor polymorphisms may lead to more accurate dosing of testosterone replacement therapy, i.e. pharmacogenetics.

Late-onset hypogonadism has now become the recognized terminology to describe symptomatic testosterone deficiency associated with aging. There is increasing evidence that its diagnosis and treatment is safe and improves well-being and quality of life [Gooren, p. 62]. There is also evidence that testosterone substitution has beneficial effects on specific conditions that are related to age which include frailty, osteoporosis, diabetes and cardiovascular disease. The importance of testosterone in normal bone turnover has been recognized for some time; however, testosterone levels are not always assayed in men with osteoporosis [Tuck and Francis, p. 123]. Frailty, including the risk of falls, is associated with low testosterone levels and studies are underway to determine if testosterone replacement therapy may be of clinical benefit [Srinivas-Shankar and Wu, p. 133]. Testosterone deficiency has significant adverse effects on cognition and is associated with the development of Alzheimer's disease. Only small studies have been conducted but they do signify that larger studies are indicated to investigate if there is a role for testosterone replacement therapy [Cherrier, p. 150].

Over the last 2 years, four population-based epidemiological studies have reported that low circulating testosterone levels are associated with an increase in mortality [4–7]. These studies have found the more positive link with all-cause mortality; however, in some studies there are specific correlations with death from respiratory disease, cardiovascular disease and cancer. A large follow-up study of men with locoregional prostate carcinoma has found that men treated with androgen suppression therapy have an increased hazard ratio for sudden cardiovascular death, myocardial infarction and diabetes [8]. The obvious question is whether or not these correlations with low testosterone levels are causative or a consequence of the disease process itself. Any inflammatory state results in an increase in the production of cytokines which are known to suppress the hypothalamic-pituitary axis. The associations and effects of testosterone deficiency in ageing, obesity and chronic disease must be taken in context with changes in other hormones such as growth hormone, glucocorticoids and cytokines.

To understand this in more detail, a wider knowledge of how testosterone deficiency affects these tissues is required. The major areas where such work has been performed are the metabolic syndrome and diabetes [Stanworth and Jones, p. 74] and coronary heart disease [Nettleship et al., p. 91]. Early evidence suggests that testosterone may have important beneficial effects in these conditions. Diabetes and the metabolic syndrome is associated with a high prevalence of hypogonadism, and testosterone substitution therapy can improve insulin resistance. Male gender is a major cardiovascular risk factor; however, there has been no adequate explanation for this phenomenon. There has been the perception that testosterone is bad for the heart and that the difference between sexes may also be that oestrogens are cardioprotective. There is recent evidence that testosterone deficiency is associated with the presence and degree of atherosclerosis and studies in animal models demonstrate that testosterone is atheroprotective. The role of testosterone substitution in chronic diseases including HIV, COPD and renal failure has been studied, albeit in small trials [Bhasin and Storer, p. 163]. Evidence has also been found that testosterone has a beneficial effect on the function of the immune system.

Erectile dysfunction is not only a symptom of hypogonadism but may be the first symptom of diabetes and/or cardiovascular disease. It has been stated that sexual health is a portal to men's health, particularly cardiovascular disease. In addition, we are only now beginning to understand the importance of the role of testosterone deficiency and its replacement in erectile dysfunction [Blute et al., p. 108].

One of the main concerns of testosterone replacement therapy has been whether or not it increases the risk of men developing prostate cancer. This concern is addressed by Morgentaler and Schulmann [p. 197] and their conclusion is that 'the available evidence strongly suggests that testosterone therapy is safe for the prostate'; however, 'it is strongly recommended that men undergoing testosterone therapy undergo regular monitoring for prostate cancer'. Testosterone therapy is contraindicated in men with heart failure but recent evidence using physiological testosterone substitution has shown that it has a beneficial effect in men with moderate chronic heart failure [Malkin et al., p. 183].

The current knowledge acquired from recent research on testosterone in several fields suggests that testosterone replacement may have significant benefits on quality of life and life expectancy. These findings underline the need for doctors to have an increased clinical awareness of hypogonadism and its diagnosis and treatment. However, larger and longer-term studies are needed to further evaluate these benefits and the safety of testosterone replacement therapy. Until further studies have become available for treating these novel indications, it is mandatory that the clinician first makes a sound diagnosis of hypogonadism before commencing testosterone therapy. In borderline cases where there is clinical suspicion as advised by the guidelines, a 3-month clinical trial of testosterone replacement therapy can be performed.

T. Hugh Jones, Barnsley/Sheffield

References

1 Bhasin S, Cunningham GR, Hayes FJ, et al: Testosterone therapy in adult men with androgen deficiency syndromes: an Endocrine Society Clinical Practise Guideline. J Clin Endocrinol Metab 2006;91:1995–2010.

2 Nieschlag E, Swerdloff R, Behre HM, et al: Investigation, treatment and monitoring of late-onset hypogonadism in males: ISA, ISSAM and EAU recommendations. J Androl 2006;27:135–137.

3 Nieschlag E, Behre HM, Bouchard P, et al: Testosterone replacement therapy: current trends and future directions. Hum Reprod Update 2004;10:409–419.

4 Shores MM, Matsumoto AM, Sloan KL, Kivlahan DR: Low serum testosterone and mortality in male veterans. Arch Intern Med 2006;166:1660–1665.

5 Araujo AB, Kupelian V, Page ST, et al: Sex steroids and all-cause mortality and cause-specific mortality in men. Arch Intern Med 2007;167:1252–1260.

6 Khaw K, Dowsett M, Folkerd E, et al: Endogenous testosterone and mortality due to all causes, cardiovascular disease, and cancer in men. European Prospective Investigation into Cancer in Norfolk (EPIC-Norfolk) prospective population study. Circulation 2007;116:2694–2701.

7 Laughlin GA, Barrett-Connor E, Bergstrom J: Low testosterone and mortality in older men. J Clin Endocrinol Metab 2008;93:68–75.

8 Keating NL, O'Malley J, Smith MR: Diabetes and cardiovascular disease during androgen deprivation therapy for prostate cancer. J Clin Oncol 2006;24:4448–4456.

Jones TH (ed): Advances in the Management of Testosterone Deficiency.
Front Horm Res. Basel, Karger, 2009, vol 37, pp 5–20

Current Guidelines for the Diagnosis of Testosterone Deficiency

Stefan Arver · Mikael Lehtihet

Centre for Andrology and Sexual Medicine, Department of Endocrinology, Metabolism and Diabetes, Karolinska University Hospital and Karolinska Institutet, Stockholm, Sweden

Abstract

Hypogonadism in males is a clinical syndrome complex which comprises symptoms with or without signs as well as biochemical evidence of testosterone deficiency. The diagnosis of hypogonadism thus includes both clinical history and examination as well as biochemical assessment of serum testosterone levels. Hypogonadal symptoms depend on the age at onset of hypogonadism, severity of the deficiency, its duration and sensitivity to androgen action. Prepubertal onset results in lack of virilization and pubertal development and produces features such as eunuchoid body proportions and undeveloped secondary sex characteristics. Development of hypogonadism in adult life is characterized by a loss of androgen-dependent functions such as reduction in muscle mass, a shift in body composition towards more adipose tissue, decreased sexual function with diminished libido, depressed mood, loss of psychological energy osteoporosis and several other possible symptoms. The majority of men who suffer from hypogonadism do not have classical endocrine disorders. These men present with concomitant disease such as metabolic syndrome or type 2 diabetes, chronic infections, inflammatory disease, COPD, or cardiovascular disease. All these conditions are associated with a high prevalence of hypogonadism. Pharmacological therapy with opiates and corticosteroids are also known to cause hypogonadism. Hypogonadal symptoms are precipitated at different testosterone levels. Total testosterone levels of less than 8 nmol/l highly support a diagnosis of hypogonadism whereas levels greater than 12 nmol/l are likely to be normal. The grey zone between 8 and 12 nmol/l requires further evaluation and assessment of free or non-sex hormone-binding globulin-bound (bioavailable) testosterone. A trial period of testosterone treatment may be required.

Testosterone Deficiency – Terminology

Hypogonadism is a clinical syndrome complex which comprises symptoms with or without signs as well as biochemical evidence of testosterone deficiency.

Male hypogonadism is classically related to relatively rare disorders of the hypothalamic-pituitary-gonadal axis. Thus the classical diagnosis of hypogonadism involves disorders such as Kallmann's syndrome, pituitary tumors (secondary hypogonadism) and Klinefelter's syndrome, and XX male syndrome (primary hypogonadism). It is however evident that hypogonadism is far more prevalent than these disorders and that men with symptoms related to testosterone deficiency are regularly seen in most clinical settings, though without being identified as potential candidates for testosterone replacement therapy. The classical underlying diseases causing hypogonadism are thus not responsible for the majority of testosterone deficiency in men. There is a need to make the diagnosis of hypogonadism less challenging and more familiar to physicians in a wide range of settings. Men with severe hypogonadism are easily diagnosed in a straightforward way, whilst men with less severe deficiency without a definite or clearly identifiable cause are more of a challenge. In these cases a combination of primary (testicular) and secondary (hypothalamic/pituitary) failure is often present.

The terminology regarding hypogonadism has not been very precise and in an effort to distinguish the more common forms of hypogonadism from the classical etiologies various nomenclatures have been put forward especially related to the increased prevalence of testosterone deficiency in elderly men, i.e. partial androgen deficiency in aging men, androgen deficiency in aging men and late-onset hypogonadism (LOH). These proposed names have also been prompted by the need to suppress the use of climacterium-related names (male climacterium, etc.) as they are misleading. In the current text the term testosterone deficiency or testosterone deficiency syndrome is used as a synonym for hypogonadism and includes the combination of low testosterone levels and the presence of clinical symptoms attributed to low testosterone levels. LOH has become a commonly used term and has been introduced to clearly identify hypogonadism occurring in aging men. The definition is similar to general hypogonadism but also includes the age aspect. In the recommendations for management of LOH [1] the definition reads: 'A clinical and biochemical syndrome associated with advancing age and characterized by typical symptoms and a deficiency in serum testosterone levels. It may result in significant detriment in the quality of life and adversely affect the function of multiple organs.' There is no clear definition of the age that defines advancing age, though taken from the context of the recommendations it may be interpreted as men over 60 years of age. The relevance of the age distinction is the increased prevalence of low testosterone levels in elderly men and that our knowledge and experience of risks and benefits of testosterone therapy in this group are limited. Most of our current knowledge and understanding of signs and symptoms of hypogonadism are based on experiences from clinical observations and substitution therapy in younger men. It remains to be clarified whether or not in the older men symptoms are precipitated by testosterone deficiency which do or do not regress with substitution therapy. An important contribution to this was the recent demonstration that the androgen-stimulated increment in lean body mass showed the same dose response relationship in young as well as elderly men [2]. Hypogonadism in aging men is often associated with obesity and/or concomitant medical disorders. The classification of hypogonadism into primary or secondary etiology is less clear. In many older men a low testosterone level occurs with LH levels within the normal range. This could be regarded as an insufficient hypothalamic or pituitary response to a low circulating testosterone level and thus a secondary hypogonadism. At the same time the testicular response to LH stimulation may be weakened indicating a primary component. These cases may be referred to as a state of mixed hypogonadism with both a primary and a secondary component.

It is well documented that testosterone replacement therapy in hypogonadal men improves muscle mass and strength, bone mineral density, mood, sexual function (libido and erectile function) as well as giving generally a feeling of increased energy. Identifying eligible men for testosterone therapy is based on a combination of serum testosterone measurements and clinical assessment of hypogonadal symptoms.

Symptoms and Signs of Testosterone Deficiency

The clinical presentation of hypogonadism depends on four main factors: (1) age at onset of androgen deficiency, (2) duration of androgen deficiency, (3) the profoundness of the deficiency and (4) genetic factors controlling androgen receptor responsiveness reflecting androgen receptor polymorphism and mutations.

Prepubertal onset results in lack of virilization, sustained height increase without closure of the epiphysis, lack of pubertal growth spurt, incomplete sexual development and aspermia. Adult onset results in a loss of the function of androgen-dependent pathways and symptoms and signs are often nonspecific and subject to the influence of comorbidity, age and other factors. Androgen deficiency-related symptoms and signs in the adult include reduced libido and reduced sexual activity, loss of spontaneous erections and erectile dysfunction, loss of body hair, reduced need to shave, reduced muscle mass and strength, and also flushes and sweating. Gynecomastia signifies a decease in testosterone levels as well as low-trauma fractures and very small testes (<5 ml). These symptoms are regarded as more specific to testosterone deficiency than other symptoms that are also reported to occur as a consequence of lowered testosterone levels. These symptoms include depressed mood and dysthymia, poor ability to concentrate and poor memory, decreased energy, initiative and self-confidence. Also irritability or aggressiveness is seen as a result of testosterone deficiency as well as a shift in body composition with increased body fat and BMI and diminished physical performance [3].

In the Endocrine Society Guidelines symptoms are separated into two groups, suggestive of hypogonadism (group A) and less specific symptoms (group B) [3] (table 1).

The selection of symptoms indicating androgen deficiency is based on clinical observations of hypogonadal men and from intervention studies with testosterone substitution therapy. There are no population-based symptom surveys relating symptoms to testosterone levels. There are few symptoms which are pathognomonic for hypogonadism, though lack of pubertal development (voice deepening, genital organ maturation, development of secondary hair and muscle accretion) is a strong indicator of hypogonadism in a person of postpubertal age. Whether loss of libido or spontaneous

Table 1. Classification of symptoms and signs of androgen deficiency according to the Endocrine Society's Clinical Guidelines

Group A: Symptoms and signs suggestive of androgen deficiency in men: incomplete sexual development, eunuchoidism, aspermia
Reduced sexual desire (libido) and activity
Decreased spontaneous erections
Breast discomfort, gynecomastia
Loss of body (axillar and pubic) hair, reduced shaving
Very small or shrinking testis (especially <5 ml)
Inability to father children, low or zero sperm counts
Height loss, low-trauma fracture, low bone mineral density
Reduced muscle mass and strength
Hot flushes, sweats
Group B: Symptoms and signs associated with androgen deficiency that are less specific than those in group A
Decreased energy, motivation, initiative, aggressiveness, self confidence
Feeling sad or blue, depressed mood, dysthymia
Poor concentration and memory
Sleep disturbance, increased sleepiness
Mild anemia (normochromic, normocytic, in the female range)
Increased body fat, body mass index
Diminished physical or work performance

erection is more suggestive than decreased energy or dysthymia of hypogonadism could be debated. The complete spectrum of symptoms potentially related to androgen deficiency needs to be assessed where hypogonadism is part of the differential diagnosis. Loss of body hair requires a long duration of hypogonadism and a beard may stay for decades in a severely hypogonadal man. Changes in hair growth and shaving frequency may be a more specific and sensitive indicator of testosterone deficiency.

The onset of symptoms seems to be related to prevailing testosterone levels [4]. There is evidence that the symptoms of hypogonadism are precipitated at different testosterone levels. This implies that there may be different thresholds for specific androgen-dependent pathways. Loss of libido and vigor becomes significant below a serum testosterone level of 15 nmol/l whilst erectile dysfunction and flushes are significantly related to a testosterone level below 8 nmol/l (see fig. 1 for further details).

Questionnaires and Interview Instruments for Hypogonadism Diagnosis

Questionnaires and a structured interview for the screening of male hypogonadism have been proposed and four different tools with some validation are currently available.

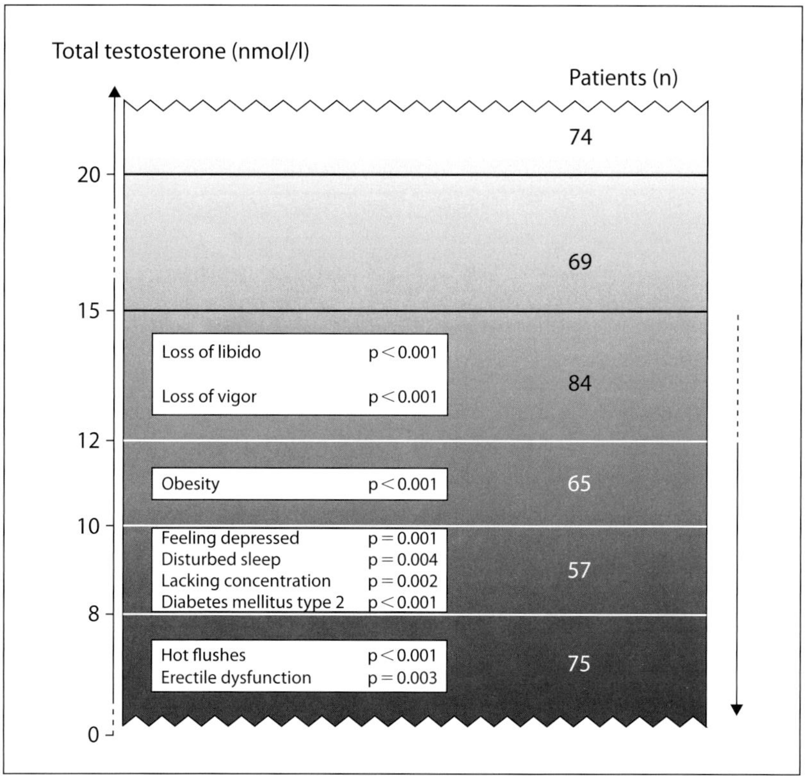

Fig. 1. Occurrence of symptoms in relation to testosterone levels [reproduced with permission, 4].

Table 2. Sensitivity and specificity of interview and screening questionnaires

	Sensitivity %	Specificity %
ADAM [7]	97	30
MMAS [8]	60	59
AMS [6]	83	39
Androtest [5]	68	65

ADAM = Androgen deficiency in aging men; MMAS = Massachusetts Male Aging Study.

Their limited specificity makes them unsuitable for general screening. The Androtest [5] has the best specificity at the cost of lower sensitivity (table 2) while the AMS [6] scale has met the widest use (fig. 2). These scales serve the purpose of strengthening the diagnostic criteria for hypogonadism and help in fulfilling the clinical requirement of symptoms in addition to low serum testosterone levels.

AMS Questionnaire

Which of the following symptoms apply to you at this time? Please, mark the appropriate box for each symptom. For symptoms that do not apply, please mark 'none'.

	Symptoms:	none	mild	moderate	severe	extremely severe
	Score =	1	2	3	4	5
1.	**Decline in your feeling of general well-being** (general state of health, subjective feeling)	☐	☐	☐	☐	☐
2.	**Joint pain and muscular ache** (lower back pain, joint pain, pain in a limb, general back ache)	☐	☐	☐	☐	☐
3.	**Excessive sweating** (unexpected/sudden episodes of sweating, hot flushes independent of strain)	☐	☐	☐	☐	☐
4.	**Sleep problems** (difficulty in falling asleep, difficulty in sleeping through, walking up early and feeling tired, poor sleep, sleeplessness)	☐	☐	☐	☐	☐
5.	**Increased need for sleep, often feeling tired**	☐	☐	☐	☐	☐
6.	**Irritability** (feeling aggressive, easily upset about little things, moody)	☐	☐	☐	☐	☐
7.	**Nervousness** (inner tension, restlessness, feeling fidgety)	☐	☐	☐	☐	☐
8.	**Anxiety** (feeling panicky)	☐	☐	☐	☐	☐
9.	**Physical exhaustion/lacking vitality** (general decrease in performance, reduced activity, lacking interest in leisure activities, feeling of getting less done, of achieving less, of having to force oneself to undertake activities)	☐	☐	☐	☐	☐
10.	**Decrease in muscular strength** (feeling of weakness)	☐	☐	☐	☐	☐
11.	**Depressive mood** (feeling down, sad, on the verge of tears, lack of drive, mood swings, feeling nothing is of any use)	☐	☐	☐	☐	☐
12.	**Feeling that you have passed your peak**	☐	☐	☐	☐	☐
13.	**Feeling burnt out, having hit rock-bottom**	☐	☐	☐	☐	☐
14.	**Decrease in beard growth**	☐	☐	☐	☐	☐
15.	**Decrease in ability/frequency to perform sexually**	☐	☐	☐	☐	☐
16.	**Decrease in the number of morning erections**	☐	☐	☐	☐	☐
17.	**Decrease in sexual desire/libido** (lacking pleasure in sex, lacking desire for sexual intercourse)	☐	☐	☐	☐	☐

Have you got any other major symptoms? **Yes** ☐ **No** ☐

If Yes, please describe: ______________________________

____

Fig. 2. AMS questionnaire [6].

Table 3. Androgen Deficiency in Aging Men (ADAM) questionnaire [7]

(1) Do you have a decrease in libido (sex drive)
(2) Do you have a lack of energy
(3) Do you have a decrease in strength and/or endurance
(4) Have you lost height?
(5) Have you noticed a decrease in enjoyment of life?
(6) Are you sad and/or grumpy
(7) Are your erections less strong?
(8) Have you noticed a recent deterioration in your ability to perform sports?
(9) Are you falling asleep after dinner?
(10) Has there been a recent deterioration in your work performance?

If you answered 'yes' to questions 1 or 7 or any 3 other questions, you may have low testosterone.

Symptoms related to comorbidities, psychological influence and age will influence and confound the diagnosis of hypogonadism. This is further compounded by the knowledge that there are no clear-cut levels where hypogonadal symptoms occur. All these factor significantly affect the overall assessment and decision making regarding a diagnosis of hypogonadism. It is becoming clear however that certain patient groups with specific comorbidities should have an increased awareness of hypogonadism as it is an additional factor afflicting the patients' physical and psychological status. Such conditions include but are not limited to metabolic syndrome, type 2 diabetes, cardiovascular disease, chronic obstructive pulmonary disease and depression.

Another valuable use of these questionnaires is the evaluation of treatment effects. Until we have access to instruments with higher specificity and sensitivity, preferably in the 90% range, they cannot be used for general screening in unselected patient populations (table 3).

The AMS evaluation is summarized in a total score and in subscales of psychological (Q 6, 7, 8, 11 and 13), sexual (Q 12, 14–17) and somatic (Q 1–5, 9, 10) subscales (fig. 2).

Measurement of Serum Testosterone

Measurement of serum testosterone is of key importance in the diagnosis of hypogonadism. Generally good testosterone assays are available at most hospital laboratories that reliably distinguish between low and normal testosterone levels in men. Total testosterone levels are affected by circadian variation, in some areas circannual variation and also by concomitant medical conditions and some medical treatments (opiates and glucocorticoids). Due to the circadian variation serum samples should be

ANDROTEST© is a structured interview for the screening of hypogonadism (total testosterone <10.4 nmol/l or 300 ng/dl in patients with sexual dysfunction). The test is applicable only to patients reporting at least one incidence of sexual intercourse during the past 3 months.

The interview is composed of 12 key items. The interviewer should ask the questions written in bold, using the exact words proposed. The further questions written in normal characters can be used to clarify the patient's answers if needed. The patient should be permitted to answer freely, using his own words.

The patient's answers are codified on a 0–3 scale by the interviewer, following detailed instructions reported after each item. For some of the items, the answers had a yes/no format.

The order in which the questions are presented should be observed, as alterations in this sequence could theoretically modify the patient's answers.

1) Age

After asking the patient how old he is, rank a progressive score as a function of patient's age at the time of the visit.

0 <40 years
1 40–49 years
2 50–59 years
3 >59 years

2) When did you undergo your sexual development (puberty)?

At what age did you undergo your sexual development? Did you experience puberty at the same time as your schoolmates? Did you notice that pubic hairs and the development of genitalia happened to you as well as to your schoolmates?

Rank 0 if patient reports a sexual development at the same time or before that of his schoolmates; 3 if patients reported a delayed puberty.

0 9–14 years (normal)
3 >14 years (delayed)

3) Have you ever had a pituitary disease?

Have you ever undergone surgery for pituitary disease? Have you ever been treated with medical therapy for pituitary disease?

The score will be 0 if patients did not report a pituitary disease, and 3 for an affirmative response.

0 No
3 Yes

4) Have you ever had a diagnosis of undescended testes (cryptorchidism)?

Have you ever undergone surgery for cryptorchidism? Have you ever been treated with medical therapy for cryptorchidism?

The score will be 0 if patients did not report a history of cryptorchidism (even monolateral), and 3 for an affirmative response.

0 No
3 Yes

5) Describe what happens during sexual intercourse: how often do you have lack of an erection?

The description of the problems refers to the last 3 months. Sometimes = <25%, quite often = 25–49%, often = 50–74%, and always = >75% of cases.

0 Sometimes
1 Quite often
2 Often
3 Always

Fig. 3. Androtest: structured interview with instructions [5].

6) Do you ever wake up with an erection?

How often has it happened in the last 3 months?

Rank 0 if patient reports spontaneous nocturnal/morning erection with the same frequency previously observed: 1 nocturnal/morning erections are present, but their frequency during the last 3 months is somewhat lower than that observed previously; 2 if the frequency of nocturnal/morning erections of the last 3 months is reduced by at least 50%; 3 if nocturnal/morning erections are not present.

0 Yes, regularly
1 Less frequently than in the past
2 Only occasionally
3 Never

7) How often have you practiced autoerotism (masturbation) in the last 3 months?

0 >8 times/month
1 3–7 times/month
2 1–2 times/month
3 Never

If the patient does not practice autoerotism (answer 3), the following question (#8) is not applicable. In this case rank 1 to question 8 and continue to question #9.

8) How do you feel during autoerotism?

After asking the question above, rank with the following score:

0 Well
1 With a little sense of guilt
2 With a big sense of guilt
3 With a very big sense of guilt

9) Have you had more or less desire to make love in the last 3 months?

Has your desire increased or reduced in comparison to the past?

Rank 0 when the patient's desire is unmodified or increased; 1 if desire is reduced.

0 Unmodified or increased desire
1 Reduced desire

10) Have you noticed a reduction of the quantity of the volume of ejaculate?

Rank 0 when the patient did not notice any modification of the volume of ejaculate; 1 when the patient has the feeling that the volume of ejaculate could be slightly reduced; 2 when the volume of ejaculate is markedly reduced; 3 when no ejaculation occurs.

0 No modification
1 Slightly reduced
2 Markedly reduced
3 Ejaculation absent

11) In the last 3 months has it been difficult to ejaculate (or to achieve climax) during sexual intercourse?

Are you able to ejaculate during sexual intercourse with penetration or only with manual or oral stimulation by your partner?

Rank 0 if patient did not report difficulties in ejaculating or, as in some rare cases, if ejaculation and climax could be obtained but only with autoerotism conducted in the absence of the partner or if it could not be obtained at all; 1 if ejaculation and climax were still possible, but only with great effort and after prolonged intercourse or if they were possible only with autoerotism, although in the presence of the partner, but not during coitus.

0 No
1 Yes

Fig. 3. (continued)

12) How much do you weigh and how tall are you?
After asking the patient his weigh and height the interviewer should rank a progressive score as a function of the calculation (body mass index = weight [kg]/height [m²]).
0 <25 kg/m²
1 25–29.9 kg/m²
2 30–34.9 kg/m²
3 >34.9 kg/m²

Fig. 3. (continued)

drawn between 7 and 10 in the morning after a normal night's sleep and without prior exposure to vigorous physical activity. Fasting samples are preferred as a glucose load suppresses testosterone levels. Low serum levels should be confirmed especially in men with borderline levels. In healthy young men as much as 15% of randomly taken serum testosterone samples show levels in the hypogonadal range [9].

Most testosterone in blood is bound to sex hormone-binding globulin (SHBG) and to albumin with only some 0.5–3% being unbound or free. The pool of albumin-bound testosterone is freely dissociated and participates in tissue interaction while the SHBG-bound fraction is tightly bound and considered not available for tissue interaction. Determination of non-SHBG-bound testosterone can be made in different ways. Ammonium precipitation (of the testosterone-SHBG complex) prior to testosterone measurement directly measures the non-SHBG-bound testosterone fraction [10]. Methods to calculate the available pool of testosterone, commonly referred to as non-SHBG-bound testosterone or bioavailable testosterone (Bio-T), are readily available even on the Internet (www.ISSAM.ch and www.him-link.com) and some laboratories also provide these calculated values. Free testosterone can only be measured with equilibrium dialysis and is only reliably available in a few research laboratories worldwide. Free testosterone assays based on analogue methods are readily available but should be avoided and are considered incorrect [11]. In clinical practice assessment of total testosterone is usually sufficient. In some cases SHBG levels may be exceedingly high or low and then estimation of the non-SHBG-bound fraction adds valuable information.

What to Measure: Total Testosterone, Free Testosterone or Bio-T?

The value of assessing Bio-T has been convincingly demonstrated in men with type 2 diabetes [12] where hypogonadal symptoms and sexual dysfunction were more closely related to non-SHBG-bound testosterone or calculated free testosterone levels (taking SHBG into consideration) than to total testosterone. Whether Bio-T is more discriminating in all circumstances than total testosterone remains to be elucidated. First-line analysis includes testosterone and SHBG assay; if the results show low levels of testosterone a repeat sample should be taken and then also include LH and

Table 4. Conditions with high and low SHBG levels

Conditions with high SHBG levels	Conditions with low SHBG levels
Aging	Obesity, hyperinsulinemia, metabolic syndrome, type 2 diabetes
Catabolic conditions (general disease, malnutrition, malabsorption, HIV infection)	Use of anabolic steroids, progestins and glucocorticoids
Medication (anticonvulsants and estrogen)	Hypothyroidism
Hepatic cirrhosis, hyperthyroidism, acromegaly	Nephrotic syndrome

prolactin. The latter will be helpful to distinguish primary from secondary hypogonadism and the eventual need for further endocrine evaluation (table 4).

General screening of testosterone levels is not indicated and should be limited to men who seek medical attention with symptoms suggestive of testosterone deficiency and to some groups of men with specific underlying disorders known to have a high prevalence of hypogonadism. These conditions include but are not limited to men with suspected pituitary tumor or disease in the pituitary-hypothalamic region, osteoporosis or low-trauma fracture, moderate to severe chronic obstructive disease, catabolic conditions with wasting (e.g. HIV infection) and men treated with medication that interferes with testosterone production or metabolism, such as glucocorticoids, opiates and ketoconazole.

Interpretation of Testosterone Assessment

There is no clear level of testosterone that unambiguously separates normal from hypogonadal men and there is no uniform threshold where symptoms start to occur [1, 3]. There is no level beyond which androgen therapy improves the health of all men. The interpretation of data thus relies on clinical assessment of symptoms and signs taking into account SHBG levels. Genotype differences also play a role in the evaluation of patients and may also be of importance in the management of androgen replacement therapy. Variation in CAG repeat length on exon 1 of the androgen receptor determines the transactivation activity of the receptor. Shorter CAG repeats code for a more active receptor while long CAG repeats code for a less active and thus less androgenic receptor. Clinical use of CAG repeat length determination may be a part of androgen evaluation but more data are needed. CAG repeat length may however be of direct value in the dose adjustment of testosterone therapy [13].

A practical approach [1] to clinical evaluation of testosterone determination is to recognize the different thresholds and the variability in androgen sensitivity and thus regard (1) levels below 8 nmol/l as suggestive of testosterone deficiency, (2) a level between 8 and 12 nmol/l as a grey zone, in which individuals may be testosterone deficient or replete and (3) levels >12 nmol/l as most likely normal and not related to any androgen-dependent symptoms [4]. A cutoff level of 10.4 nmol/l as put forward by the Endocrine Society recommendations could also be used though there are several studies on hypogonadal men that have used 12 nmol as the higher limit for inclusion. Moreover the lack of a defined hypogonadal level and the limitation of defining hypogonadism by biochemical testosterone assessment prompt for careful assessment and in the clinical situation we still need to rely on good clinical judgment and understanding the limitations of our supportive diagnostic tools. Although there are data that suggest that some androgen-dependent symptoms become significant even in the range up to 15 nmol/l, no recommendation so far have stretched the lower limit of normal testosterone to that level. Thus a normal male without symptoms of hypogonadism and a testosterone level of above 8 nmol/l is considered normal while a male with signs and symptoms and a testosterone level of 11 nmol/l is considered a likely candidate for androgen therapy. Note that the reference values are not age dependent and testosterone effects on body composition and muscle mass remain the same in young and elderly men [2]. Current guidelines do not support the use of age-adjusted reference ranges as there is no evidence suggesting that elderly men should have a reduced testosterone requirement [1, 3]. In the current recommendations issued by the International Society of Andrology (ISA), International Society for the Study of the Aging Male (ISSAM), European Academy of Andrology (EAA) and the European Urology Association (EUA) clear cutoff levels of testosterone are suggested.

Evaluation of Suspicious Secondary Hypogonadism

Hypogonadism has a complex and varied pathogenesis and a definitive etiological diagnosis is not always attainable. Most cases of clinical hypogonadism in middle age and elderly men have a combination of primary and secondary hypogonadism and mixed hypogonadism (tables 4, 5).

An important question is when to extend the investigation when a patient presents with hypogonadal symptoms and low testosterone levels in combination with low or normal gonadotropin levels, i.e. secondary hypogonadism. In secondary hypogonadism adequate stimulation of testicular Leydig cells by LH from the pituitary is lacking due to either hypothalamic or pituitary failure. Secondary hypogonadism or contribution by a relative gonadotropin deficiency becomes more prevalent as we age and a mixed etiology with both a primary and a secondary component seems to be overall the most common background to hypogonadism. In the vast majority of these cases there are no pituitary tumor or other underlying disease processes that need specific treatment, though it is important not to overlook the presence of treatable underlying disorders. Assessment of pituitary function and evaluation of the local topography in the pituitary and hypothalamic region with imaging (magnetic resonance

Table 5. Causes of mixed hypogonadism

Aging
Alcohol abuse
Diabetes mellitus/metabolic cluster syndrome
Drugs (glucocorticoids, opioids and ketoconazole)
Chronic infections (HIV) and autoimmune disease
Systemic disease (liver failure, uremia, sickle cell disease, hemochromatosis)

imaging, MRI) is clearly indicated if testosterone levels are very low, i.e. <5 nmol/l and LH levels below the mid-reference range according to the local laboratory [3, 14, 15]. If there is a suspicion of pituitary failure gonadotropin levels that are low, not present or lower than expected for the level of testosterone, which often is below 5 nmol/l, should raise the suspicion of hypothalamic or pituitary hypogonadism. The most frequent causes in adults are pituitary adenomas, both secreting and not secreting adenomas. Metastases in the pituitary and/or hypohyseal stalk, postoperative states and postradiotherapy of the area can cause secondary hypogonadism. Other causes are iron overload (hemochromatosis), sarcoidosis and other infiltration disorders. Idiopathic hypogonadotropic hypogonadism is a diagnosis made after exclusion of other causes of hypogonadotropic hypogonadism (fig. 4).

Diagnosis of Secondary Hypogonadism

Modern imaging techniques with MRI and computerized tomography have made the diagnosis of pituitary tumors much easier. Endocrine evaluation of the anterior pituitary function with LH, FSH, prolactin, TSH, ACTH, and GH and their corresponding peripheral hormones testosterone, cortisol, thyroid hormone and IGF should be assessed in order to clarify the extent of pituitary dysfunction and thus the need for substitution therapy. The reader is therefore referred to textbooks of internal medicine and endocrinology for further insight into hypothalamic and pituitary diseases.

Large pituitary adenomas may cause partial or complete hypopituitarism by impinging of neighboring structures (e.g. adjacent normal gland, pituitary stalk). Compression of the optic chiasm by mass effect is also associated with disturbance of vision. The chiasm is found at a variable distance above the diaphragma sella and in some subjects the distance is less than 10 mm. Approximately 90% of neuronal axons in the chiasma are responsible for central vision and it is not uncommon to find an early disturbance by visual examination (e.g. foggy vision). The most common visual disorder caused by large pituitary adenoma or other diseases causing mass effect in this area is bitemporal hemianopia or bilateral scotoma rather than hemianopia. If the

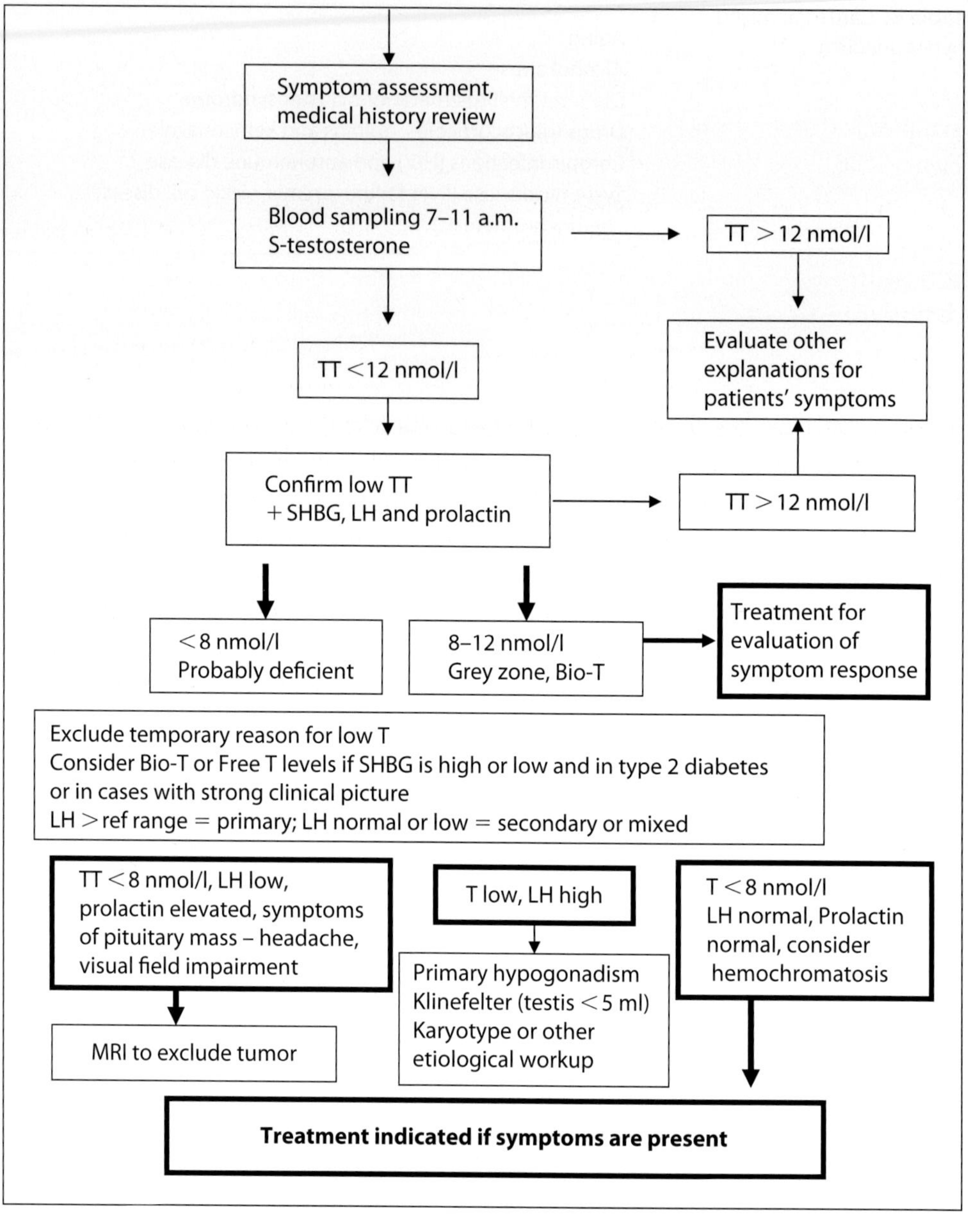

Fig. 4. Subjects with signs, symptoms or other reason for evaluation of eventual hypogonadism. T = Testosterone; TT = total testosterone.

mass expands laterally it can also affect the sinus cavernous and paralyze the occulomotor nerve without visual field defects. If the mass expands further laterally the fourth, fifth and sixth cranial nerve may be involved. It is therefore of importance that all patients with adenoma larger than 10 mm (macroadenomas) are carefully evaluated for visual impairment.

Conclusion

Hypogonadism is a clinical syndrome complex, which consists of the presence of symptoms with or without signs and biochemical confirmation of testosterone deficiency. Classical diagnosis of pituitary or testicular disease represents a minority of men with hypogonadism. The observed increase in hypogonadism with age seems to be more related to comorbidity and increments in BMI than age per se. Cohorts of men with various medical disorders, e.g. metabolic syndrome, type 2 diabetes, cardiovascular disease, COPD, chronic infections, and rheumatoid diseases, are all associated with a high prevalence of low testosterone levels and symptoms related to androgen deficiency. Diagnostic workup includes a review of symptoms, laboratory assessments, clarification of the etiological background and screening for potential absolute and relative contraindications. Symptom assessment questionnaires may be used to assist in symptom assessment and as a reference for the evaluation of therapeutic intervention. Laboratory analysis of serum testosterone is readily available but with some limitations. The lack of definitive levels defining testosterone deficiency and the difference in symptom-precipitating threshold levels for different testosterone-dependent pathways strongly underline the need for a careful clinical assessment of the patient. In general testosterone levels below 8 nmol/l probably signify a deficiency while levels above 12 nmol/l are most likely normal. Testosterone levels between 8 and 12 nmol/l may be further scrutinized with the determination of free or Bio-T. In the absence of contraindications patients may be given a limited trial period of adequate testosterone replacement therapy. Monitoring testosterone therapy includes prostate (PSA and digital examination) and hematological (hematocrit) safety assessment after the initial 3, 6, 9 and 12 months of therapy and on a yearly basis thereafter. Evaluation of efficacy endpoints may include subjective symptoms and signs and assessment of bone mineral density.

References

1 Nieschlag E, Swerdloff R, Behre HM, et al: Investigation, treatment, and monitoring of late-onset hypogonadism in males: ISA, ISSAM, and EAU recommendations. J Androl 2006;27:135–137.

2 Bhasin S, Woodhouse L, Casaburi R, et al: Older men are as responsive as young men to the anabolic effects of graded doses of testosterone on the skeletal muscle. J Clin Endocrinol Metab 2005;90:678–688.

3 Bhasin S, Cunningham GR, Hayes FJ, et al: Testosterone therapy in adult men with androgen deficiency syndromes: an endocrine society clinical practice guideline. J Clin Endocrinol Metab 2006;91: 1995–2010.

4 Zitzmann M, Faber S, Nieschlag E: Association of specific symptoms and metabolic risks with serum testosterone in older men. J Clin Endocrinol Metab 2006;91:4335–4343.

5 Corona G, Mannucci E, Petrone L, et al: ANDROTEST: a structured interview for the screening of hypogonadism in patients with sexual dysfunction. J Sex Med 2006;3:706–715.

6 Heinemann LAJ, Zimmerman T, Vermeulen A, Thiel C: A new 'aging male' symptoms' (AMS) rating scale. Aging Male 1999;2:105–114.

7 Morley JE, Charlton E, Patrick P, et al: Validation of a screening questionnaire for androgen deficiency in aging males. Metabolism 2000;49:1239–1242.

8 Smith KW, Feldman HA, McKinlay JB: Construction and field validation of a self-administered screener for testosterone deficiency (hypogonadism) in ageing men. Clin Endocrinol (Oxf) 2000;53:703–711.

9 Spratt DI, O'Dea LS, Schoenfeld D, et al: Neuroendocrine-gonadal axis in men: frequent sampling of LH, FSH, and testosterone. Am J Physiol 1988;254:E658–E666.

10 Tremblay RR, Dube JY: Plasma concentrations of free and non-TeBG bound testosterone in women on oral contraceptives. Contraception 1974;10:599–605.

11 Vermeulen A, Verdonck L, Kaufman JM: A critical evaluation of simple methods for the estimation of free testosterone in serum. J Clin Endocrinol Metab 1999;84:3666–3672.

12 Kapoor D, Aldred H, Clark S, et al: Clinical and biochemical assessment of hypogonadism in men with type 2 diabetes: correlations with bioavailable testosterone and visceral adiposity. Diabetes Care 2007;30: 911–917.

13 Zitzmann M: Mechanisms of disease: pharmacogenetics of testosterone therapy in hypogonadal men. Nat Clin Pract Urol 2007;4:161–166.

14 Citron JT, Ettinger B, Rubinoff H, et al: Prevalence of hypothalamic-pituitary imaging abnormalities in impotent men with secondary hypogonadism. J Urol 1996;155:529–533.

15 Buvat J, Lemaire A: Endocrine screening in 1,022 men with erectile dysfunction: clinical significance and cost-effective strategy. J Urol 1997;1585:1764–1767.

Prof. Stefan Arver
Centre for Andrology and Sexual Medicine
Karolinska University Hospital M52
SE–141 86 Stockholm (Sweden)
Tel. +46 8 5858 0446, Fax +46 8 5858 7076, E-Mail stefan.arver@ki.se

Jones TH (ed): Advances in the Management of Testosterone Deficiency.
Front Horm Res. Basel, Karger, 2009, vol 37, pp 21–31

Laboratory Measurement of Testosterone

Michael J. Diver

Department of Clinical Chemistry, Royal Liverpool University Hospital, Liverpool, UK

Abstract

Plasma testosterone concentrations in men, first quantified nearly half a century ago, are now measured routinely as a primary index of androgen status. Most clinical laboratories employ a multichannel, fully automated analyzer. Current evidence suggests that these analyzers are capable of satisfactorily quantifying the concentration of total plasma testosterone in men. Newer technology, in the form of tandem mass spectrometry, may, in the future, replace these automated platforms, providing a more specific estimate of testosterone concentration. When concentrations of plasma testosterone are found to be around the lower limit of normal (~9.0 nmol/l; μg/l = nmol/l × 0.288), some measure of bioactive testosterone should be sought. This may be a free (non-protein-bound) or bioavailable (free plus albumin-bound) testosterone and may be measured (laborious and time-consuming and therefore unsuited to routine clinical laboratories) or calculated using any one of a variety of mathematical expressions. Sampling for the estimation of plasma testosterone should be carried out in the morning, before 11:00 h, to obviate the effect of the marked diurnal variation in testosterone production. In samples found to have an equivocal concentration (7.0–12.5 nmol/l) at least one more estimate should be obtained to account for the possible significant intra-individual variability. Although it is generally accepted that the concentrations of total, free and bioavailable testosterone decline as men age, the majority of elderly men have testosterone levels in the young adult range (9.0–35 nmol/l) and some maintain a diurnal rhythm. Salivary testosterone offers a non-invasive estimate of free testosterone but there does not appear to be an immediate demand for a routine salivary testosterone service.

Although it is nigh on 50 years since testosterone concentration was first measured in human plasma the estimation still presents the laboratory with analytical problems. These are much more confounding in the analysis of female rather than male plasma, mainly because of the difference in circulating concentrations. As a rule of thumb, normal female concentrations of plasma total testosterone (~0.5–3.0 nmol/l) are around 10 times less than those in male plasma (~9.0–35 nmol/l). These problems were clearly manifest in a report [1] that identified a profound lack of confidence in the ability of modern-day multi-analyte automated platforms to reproducibly quantify testosterone at concentrations less than 1.7 nmol/l, indicating that current immunoassays for testosterone at such concentrations produce results that are little better than generating random numbers. Although this work dwelt mainly on measurement of female testosterone, the findings concluded that most methodologies currently in routine hospital laboratories were capable of quantifying testosterone concentration reasonably well in men. The Endocrine Society (Chevy Chase, Md., USA), concluding that most testosterone assays for men have adequate sensitivity and reasonable clinical utility, have supported this opinion in a recent position statement [2].

Testosterone circulates in the bloodstream in both protein-bound and non-protein-bound (free) moieties. In men approximately 20–30% is loosely bound to albumin, 50–70% is avidly bound to sex hormone-binding globulin (SHBG), 4% is bound to other proteins and 1–3% is free, non-protein-bound.

The estimated (measured) concentration of circulating testosterone is dependant on numerous variables. Factors that play an important role are:

- Method of measurement
- Intra-individual variation
- Time of the day
- Age

Most clinical laboratories estimate the circulating concentration of total testosterone (i.e. the free, non-protein-bound fraction, together with the albumin-bound and SHBG-bound components). In order to quantify all three components together, a method for displacing testosterone from protein needs to be incorporated in the methodology. This may involve disruption of the proteins, extraction of the steroid into an organic solvent or addition of a chemical agent that has a higher binding affinity than has testosterone for the binding proteins. Prior to assay, all the plasma testosterone to be measured should, therefore, be in the free, non-protein-bound state.

A number of biochemical indices are available to assess androgen status in men. These include total testosterone, free testosterone estimated by equilibrium dialysis, ultracentrifugation or direct immunoassay, bioavailable (free plus albumin-bound) testosterone, calculated free and bioavailable testosterone or the free androgen index (FAI), namely total testosterone × 100/SHBG.

Method of Measurement

Total Testosterone

Nowadays, measurement of total testosterone in man is a relatively simple laboratory procedure, carried out almost universally on multichannel, fully automated immunoassay analyzers. To this end the use of radioimmunoassay (RIA) for measuring testosterone is all but obsolete, as is, for reasons of health and safety, the use of organic solvent extraction prior to immunoassay. Few laboratories are registered with an appropriate licensing authority (in the UK: The Environment Agency) in order to use radioactivity as an endpoint in immunoassays.

Standard, well-authenticated immunoassay techniques are used on these automated platforms. Detailed methodologies are comprehensively described in previous reports [1, 3] with sample volumes ranging from 15 to 200 μl and incubation times varying from 15 min to 2 h. Most platforms incorporate solid phase separation of bound and free moieties using antibody-coated magnetic particles, beads or wells with chemiluminescent, enzyme-linked or immunofluometric endpoints to quantify the testosterone concentration.

Very few, 4 or 5 at the most, multichannel platforms provide around 95% of the total testosterone market with widespread use of limited technologies. Prominent among these multinational companies are Roche Diagnostics, Abbott Diagnostics, Siemens (incorporating Diagnostic Products Corporation and Bayer Diagnostics) and Beckman Corporation.

Very recently the advent into clinical laboratories of mass spectrometry (MS) has been seen either as isotope dilution-gas chromatography-mass spectrometry (IDGCMS) or as isotope dilution-liquid chromatography-tandem MS. At present this technology is used by very few centres, but may represent a major step forward in providing a more specific and more sensitive manner of measuring total plasma testosterone. Preliminary reports would tend to suggest that this technology may not be any more precise than currently available methodology for measuring total testosterone in the reference range for men [3, 4]. One report [5] indicates an interassay imprecision of 5.6% at critical male levels of 8.59 nmol/l, very close to the lower limit of their reference range (8.0 nmol/l). It is noteworthy that one of these reports [3] employs 2.0 ml of sample for analysis. In contrast other reports use much smaller volumes, e.g. 0.1 ml [6] but at the same time report that in healthy men results from immunoassays agreed with those from an MS-based method.

Individual laboratory reference ranges for total testosterone concentration will depend to a greater or lesser extent on the platform chosen and as can be seen from a recent comprehensive study, manufacturers' quoted values may not reflect those established in individual laboratories [7]. The same study suggested that the currently available commercial assays when compared to GC/MS assays are technically wanting and that their general performance is unable to confidently indicate androgen deficiency from eugonadism in men. Nevertheless a more recent study on a total of 122 samples [8] has indicated that although there were substantial differences in absolute levels of testosterone between RIA (in-house tritium-labelled tracer) and MS methods, both Pearson and Spearman correlation coefficients were near 1.0 and all were highly significant ($p < 0.001$). This lack of agreement between absolute results obtained on immunoassays and those obtained by IDGCMS may be due to a matrix effect (seen more often in direct assays), the effect of SHBG binding, methods used to displace protein-bound testosterone prior to immunoassay, or antibody recognition of steroids other than testosterone. These interferences are less likely to be detected in male plasma as most of any factitious increase in concentration is likely to be masked by producing a testosterone level still within the broader reference range.

Nevertheless, a reference range of approximately 9.0–35 nmol/l is in consensus with published data over the years [1, 7, 9–11]. It should, however, be emphasized that individual laboratories providing a clinical service for plasma testosterone should establish their own reference ranges on a well-constructed sample of the male population, ensuring that the selected cohort does not contain individuals with cryptic reproductive disorders. This advice is comprehensively discussed in a report by Sikaris et al. [7].

Following a study to evaluate up-to-date assays for total and free testosterone in the clinical setting, the Endocrine Society in the United States recently issued a position statement indicating that for diagnosis of hypogonadism in men, almost any total testosterone assay would suffice [2]. The exception to this recommendation lies in the detection of the subtle decrease in testosterone in the aging male when the testosterone is near the lower limit of the reference range. In these cases a calculated free testosterone may prove helpful. Most assays are capable of distinguishing differences in total testosterone concentrations between normal and hypogonadal men but should be measured before 11:00 h in the morning and on more than one occasion.

Free and/or Bioavailable Testosterone

A recent report testifies to total testosterone being the best marker of hypogonadism in men [12] but concedes that when total testosterone is borderline normal (between 7.0 and 12.0 nmol/l) the calculated indices of free or bioavailable testosterone may help to confirm the diagnosis. These conclusions were based on correlating measured or calculated bioavailable testosterone, using several derived equations, with total testosterone in order to predict hypogonadism in a series of 1,072 men. These findings are in accord with another opinion that suggests that unequivocally low levels of total testosterone, in all probability, indicate hypogonadism [13].

Nevertheless a very large body of opinion would now advocate the use of bioavailable testosterone as the best marker of androgen status [see 14 for references]. This index may be measured, usually by the ammonium sulphate precipitation method of Tremblay and Dube [15], or derived from measuring total testosterone and SHBG and applying an algorithm in a computer program. Numerous formulae, both simple and more complex, have been derived for calculation of either free or bioavailable testosterone. These are based on prior measurement of total testosterone and SHBG.

The original testosterone binding index which gives a measure of SHBG-bound testosterone was described by Vermeulen et al. [16] followed later by calculation of the 'apparent free testosterone concentration' [17].

A relatively simple expression for calculating % free testosterone was devised by Anderson et al. [18]: % free testosterone $= 2.28 - 1.38 \log \text{SHBG} \cdot 10^{-8}$.

While this equation was used mainly for calculating free testosterone in women, a not dissimilar equation was suggested for both male and female samples [19]: % free testosterone $= 6.11 - 2.38 \log \text{SHBG} \cdot 10^{-9}$.

Several groups have produced more complex computer-assisted algorithms to calculate both free and bioavailable testosterone [12, 20–22]. These calculations require input of concentrations of total testosterone, SHBG and albumin and the use of experimentally derived association constants for testosterone with both SHBG and albumin.

Recently, de Ronde et al. [23] used 5 different published algorithms [12, 21, 22, 24, 25] to estimate bioavailable and free testosterone concentrations in a group of 399 men and found that these algorithms showed large differences between the calculated results. They suggest that the algorithms should be revalidated in each local laboratory to avoid over- or underestimation of both free and bioavailable testosterone.

Use of these mathematical concepts to estimate concentrations of free and/or bioavailable testosterone are in all probability impractical for routine hospital laboratories and may be best applicable to experimental and research scenarios.

More recently, however, the WWW site of the International Society for the Study of the Aging Male (ISSAM) has provided a screen on the internet (www.isssam.ch) where both bioavailable and free testosterone concentrations are calculated automatically following insertion of concentrations of total testosterone, SHBG and albumin in pre-prepared calculator inserts. These calculations are based on the formula derived at the University of Ghent, Belgium [22]. Whether this method of calculating bioavailable testosterone in all men is the most appropriate has recently been questioned [26]. This report indicates an age-related discrepancy between measured and calculated bioavailable testosterone where the calculated concentration was found to be higher than the measured concentration, probably due to an age-related decrease in adrenal androgens.

The ammonium sulphate precipitation technique for measuring bioavailable testosterone, described by Tremblay and Dube [15], is universally recognized as a reliable estimate of the non-SHBG-bound fraction of testosterone. Several reports have testified to this measurement being a satisfactory index of androgen status in men, especially where total testosterone concentrations are borderline hypogonadal [12, 22–24, 26–29].

Many laboratories measure SHBG in conjunction with total testosterone and produce an FAI using a simple arithmetical formula:

$$\mathrm{FAI} = [\mathrm{testosterone}] \cdot 100/[\mathrm{SHBG}].$$

Although this index has found favour in discriminating hyperandrogenic females with normal total testosterone concentrations, its use as a reliable index of bioavailable testosterone in men has been questioned [22, 30]. The 'reference' method for estimating free testosterone is generally accepted as equilibrium dialysis [30] or centrifugal ultrafiltration [31], but these methods are time-consuming and labour-intensive and are unsuitable for a routine clinical service. Reports have suggested that the use of analogue RIA direct methods for measurement of free testosterone produces results at variance with those generally accepted as reflecting the free hormone concentrations

[30, 32–35]. A strongly worded statement has advised against the use of these methods for measuring free testosterone [36].

In summary, most automated immunoassays are capable of accurately measuring male levels of testosterone in serum. When the concentration is equivocally hypogonadal (7.0–12.0 nmol/l) some measure of bioactive testosterone (measured or calculated bioavailable or calculated free testosterone) may be required. Calculating these indices necessitates the measuring of SHBG and albumin concentrations in the same sample.

Salivary Testosterone

In all probability salivary testosterone reflects a measure of the concentration of free, non-protein-bound circulating testosterone with levels in the 200–400 pmol range.

To date it is unlikely that multichannel immunoassay analyzers can adapt plasma methodology to accommodate assays in saliva with such low concentrations and in a non-protein matrix. In light of the imprecision reported in plasma samples with concentrations <2.0 nmol/l [1] it would appear that a considerably more sensitive assay would be required. There may be scope for applying GC/MS techniques to salivary samples.

Although saliva sample collection would be less invasive and more convenient than collecting blood samples, introduction of this medium for routine assessment of gonadal status in men would necessitate all the rigorous procedures of methodology validation including quality control and quality assessment.

There may be, however, a role for salivary testosterone when multiple samples are required, e.g. for long-term studies or for more regular assessment of androgen status in men on testosterone replacement therapy. This, again, would require intensive studies in order to establish the level of salivary testosterone that represents adequate replacement and how to relate this salivary measurement to replacement dose.

As current opinion suggests that the quality of plasma assays is satisfactory enough to provide a more than adequate clinical service there does not appear to be a pressing requirement for establishing routine clinical services for salivary testosterone in men. A recent report, while conceding that salivary testosterone concentrations may adequately reflect androgen status in men, indicated that there was a strong correlation of salivary testosterone with total testosterone ($p < 0.002$), bioavailable testosterone ($p < 0.00001$) and calculated free testosterone ($p < 0.0001$) in plasma from a cohort of 1,454 men [37].

Intra-Individual Variation

Disagreement exists on the day-to-day constancy of testosterone concentration in normal males. Early work suggested marked day-to-day fluctuations in plasma testosterone levels even though samples were collected at the same time each day in different studies [38]. One report [39] concluded from a cohort of 169 men aged 40–80 years with plasma testosterone measured 8 times in 50 weeks that as the level in the initial sample correlated with the mean concentration a single estimate was adequate. This reflected earlier work recommending measuring testosterone on 3 occasions throughout the day in order to establish an overall daily concentration [40]. More recently, however, others have shown a marked week-to-week variability in both testosterone and bioavailable testosterone [28]. These findings are in accord with studies [14] where testosterone in normal males aged 25–60 years showed marked intra-individual variability in total testosterone in both morning and afternoon samples. In some individuals the values ranged from normal (14.0 nmol/l) to hypogonadal (8.0 nmol/l) (fig. 1). This evidence would suggest that unless the initial testosterone level is unequivocally normal (>12.5 nmol/l) or unequivocally abnormal (<7.0 nmol/l) more than one estimate of total testosterone should be obtained before classifying a result as indicating hypogonadism.

Diurnal Variation

Concentrations of plasma testosterone, total, free and bioavailable, display a circadian rhythm with the highest levels found in the morning and the lowest in the evening. This diurnal variation has been reported [41] to be blunted in elderly men, but a more recent study suggests that in fit healthy men this rhythm is maintained into the seventh decade [42]. This latter report describes a decrease of at least 43% in total testosterone from peak to nadir in all the men studied (fig. 2). It would, therefore, seem strongly advisable that when measuring testosterone in plasma in order to ascertain gonadal status that strict attention is paid to the time of sampling.

Effect of Age

It is generally accepted that, in men, advancing age is accompanied by a gradual diminution in circulating total testosterone. This decline is reported to be even more pronounced in both free and bioavailable testosterone, probably as a result of an increase in SHBG. Furthermore many reports testify to concentrations of total testosterone in old men well into the reference range for young adults [see 14 for list of references]. A more recent study has shown that as men age the lower limits of reference ranges decrease, but that up to 50% of the men in the study aged 70–79 years had a total testosterone >15 nmol/l [43]. In light of the conflicting evidence on the concentration of total testosterone found in elderly men it remains a moot point as to whether a separate reference range should be given for older men. More evidence would be required as to the cut-off age for defining 'elderly'.

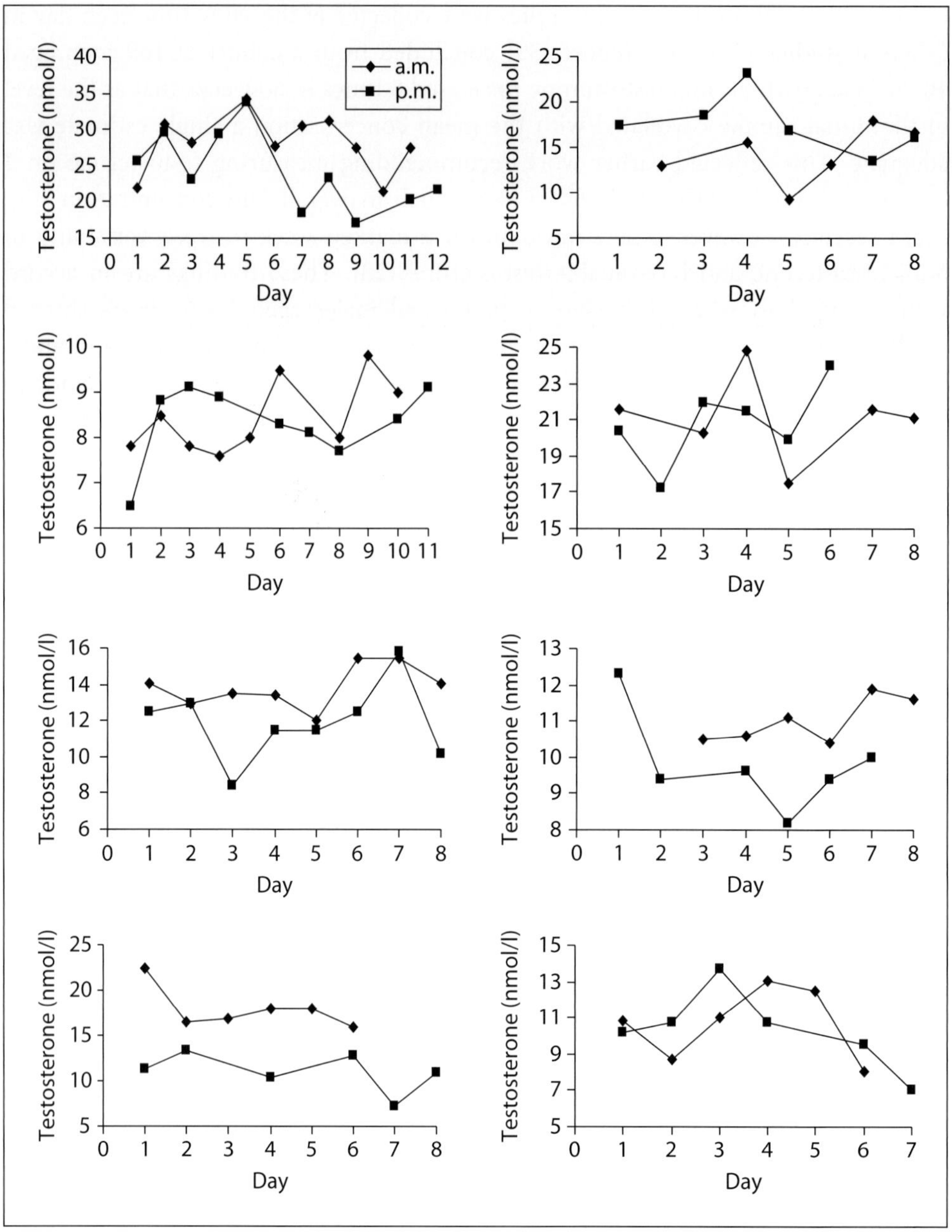

Fig. 1. Intra-individual variability in plasma testosterone in 8 normal men aged 25–60 years in samples taken between 09:00 and 10:00 h and between 16:00 and 17:00 h on at least 6 separate days over a 1-month period [reproduced from 14].

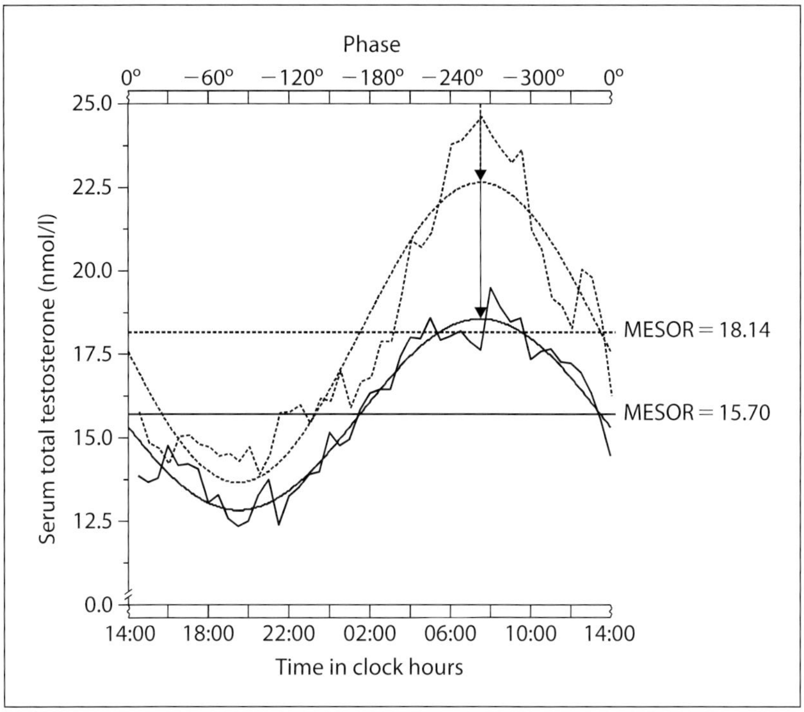

Fig. 2. Cosinor-derived circadian rhythmometry (Chronolab) for plasma total testosterone concentration in 10 young men (----) and in 8 middle-aged men (—) showing the diurnal rhythm maintained in both groups of men [from 42, reproduced by permission of *Clinical Endocrinology*].

Conclusions

(1) Unless equivocal (7.0–12.5 nmol/l), total plasma testosterone measured on an automated analyzer will provide a true reflection of androgen status in men. Newer technology (tandem MS) may offer more specific assessment of testosterone levels.

(2) Where equivocal levels of total testosterone are revealed more than one estimate should be obtained.

(3) The laboratory should offer some measure of assessment of free or bioavailable testosterone concentration.

(4) Samples for estimation of plasma testosterone concentration should be obtained in the early morning (before 11:00 h).

(5) The majority of elderly men have total testosterone concentrations in the reference range for young men.

(6) It is unlikely that salivary testosterone offers any benefit at present to the routine assessment of androgen status.

References

1 Taieb J, Mathian B, Millot F, Patricot M-C, Mathieu E, Queyrel N, Lacroix I, Somma-Delperro C, Boudou P: Testosterone measured by 10 immunoassays and by isotope-dilution gas chromatography-mass spectrometry in sera from 1116 men, women and children. Clin Chem 2003;49:1381–1395.

2 Rosner W, Auchus RJ, Azziz R, Sluss PM, Raff H: Utility, limitations and pitfalls in measuring testosterone: an Endocrine Society Position Statement. J Clin Endocrinol Metab 2007;92:405–413.

3 Wang C, Catlin DH, Demers LM, Starcevic B, Swerdloff RS: Measurement of total serum testosterone in adult men: comparison of current laboratory methods versus liquid chromatography-tandem mass spectrometry. J Clin Endocrinol Metab 2004; 89:534–543.

4 Matsumoto AM, Bremner WJ: Editorial: serum testosterone assays – accuracy matters. J Clin Endocrinol Metab 2004;89:520–524.

5 Cawood ML, Field HP, Ford CG, Gillingwater S, Kicman A, Cowan D, Barth JH: Testosterone measurement by isotope-dilution liquid chromatography-tandem mass spectrometry: validation of a method for routine clinical practice. Clin Chem 2005;51:1472–1479.

6 Kushmir MM, Rockwood AL, Roberts WL, Pattison EG, Bunker AM, Fitzgerald RL, Meikle AW: Performance characteristics of a novel tandem mass spectrometry assay for serum testosterone. Clin Chem 2006;52:120–128.

7 Sikaris K, McLachlan RI, Kazlauskas R, de Krester D, Holden CA, Handelsman DJ: Reproductive hormone reference intervals for healthy fertile young men: evaluation of automated platform assays. J Clin Endocrinol Metab 2005;90:5928–5936.

8 Hsing AW, Stanczyk FZ, Belanger A, Schroeder P, Chang L, Falk RT, Fears TR: Reproducibility of serum sex steroid assays in men by RIA and mass spectrometry. Cancer Epidemiol Biomarkers Prev 2007;16:1004–1008.

9 Harman SM, Metter JE, Tobin JD, Pearson J, Blackman MR: Longitudinal effects of aging on serum total and free testosterone levels in healthy men. J Clin Endocrinol Metab 2001;86:724–731.

10 Kaufman JM, Vermeulen A: Declining gonadal function in elderly men. Clin Endocrinol Metab 1997;11:289–309.

11 Ismail AAA, Astley P, Burr WA, Cawood M, Short F, Wakelin K, Wheeler M: The role of testosterone measurement in the investigation of androgen disorders. Ann Clin Biochem 1986;23:113–134.

12 Morris PD, Malkin CJ, Channer KS, Jones TH: A mathematical comparison of techniques to predict biologically available testosterone in a cohort of 1072 men. Eur J Endocrinol 2004;151:241–249.

13 Snyder PJ: Hypogonadism in elderly men – what to do until the evidence comes. N Engl J Med 2004; 350:440–442.

14 Diver MJ: Analytical and physiological factors affecting the interpretation of serum testosterone concentration in men. Ann Clin Biochem 2006;43:3–12.

15 Tremblay RR, Dube JY: Plasma concentration of free and non-TEBG bound testosterone of women on oral contraceptives. Contraception 1974;10:599–605.

16 Vermeulen A, Verdonck L, van der Straeten M, Orie N: Capacity of the testosterone-binding globulin in human plasma and influence of specific binding of testosterone on its metabolic clearance rate. J Clin Endocrinol Metab 1969;29:1470–1480.

17 Vermeulen A, Stoica T, Verdonck L: The apparent free testosterone concentration, an index of androgenicity. J Clin Endocrinol Metab 1971;33:759–767.

18 Anderson DC, Thorner MO, Fisher RA: Effects of hormonal treatment on plasma unbound androgen levels in hirsute women. Acta Endocrinol 1985;224 (suppl 199):224.

19 Nanjee MN, Wheeler MJ: Plasma free testosterone – is an index sufficient? Ann Clin Biochem 1985;22: 387–390.

20 Pearlman WH, Crepy O: Steroid-protein interaction with particular reference to testosterone binding by human serum. J Biol Chem 1967;2:182–189.

21 Sodergard R, Backstrom T, Shanbag V, Cartensen H: Calculation of free and bound fractions of testosterone and estradiol 17β to human plasma protein at body temperature. J Steroid Biochem 1982;26:801–810.

22 Vermeulen A, Verdonck L, Kaufman JM: A critical evaluation of simple methods for the estimation of free testosterone in serum. J Clin Endocrinol Metab 1999;84:3666–3672.

23 de Ronde W, van der Schouw YT, Pols HAP, Gooren LJG, Muller M, Grobbee DE, de Jong FH: Calculation of bioavailable and free testosterone in men: a comparison of 5 published algorithms. Clin Chem 2006; 52:1777–1784.

24 Emadi-Konjin P, Bain J, Bromberg IL: Evaluation of an algorithm for calculation of serum 'bioavailable' testosterone. Clin Biochem 2003;36:591–596.

25 Ly P, Handelsman DJ: Empirical estimation of free testosterone from testosterone and sex hormone binding globulin immunoassays. Eur J Endocrinol 2005;152:471–478.

26 Dechaud H, Denuziere D, Rinaldi S, Bocquet J, Lejeune H, Pugeat M: Age-associated discrepancy between measured and calculated bioavailable testosterone in men. Clin Chem 2007;53:723–728.
27 Dechaud H, Lejeune H, Garoscio-Cholet M, Mallien R, Pugeat M: Radioimmunoassay of testosterone not bound to sex-steroid binding protein in plasma. Clin Chem 1989;35:1609–1614.
28 Morley JE, Patrick P, Perry HM 3rd: Evaluation of assays to measure free testosterone. Metabolism 2002; 51:554–559.
29 Giton F, Fiet J, Guechot J, Ibrahim F, Bronsard F, Chopin D, Raynaud J-P: Serum bioavailable testosterone: assayed or calculated? Clin Chem 2006;52: 474–481.
30 Kapoor P, Luttrell BM, Williams D: The free androgen index is not valid for adult males. J Steroid Biochem Mol Biol 1993;45:325–326.
31 Hammond GL, Nisker JA, Jones LA, Siiteri PK: Estimation of the percentage of free steroid in undiluted serum by centrifugal ultrafiltration-dialysis. J Biol Chem 1980;255:5023–5026.
32 Rosner W: Errors in the measurement of plasma free testosterone. J Clin Endocrinol Metab 1997;82: 2014–2015.
33 Winders SJ, Kelley DE, Goodpaster B: The analog free testosterone assay: are the results in men clinically useful? Clin Chem 1986;44:2178–2182.
34 Cheng RW, Reed MJ, James VHT: Plasma free testosterone: equilibrium dialysis vs. direct radioimmunoassay. Clin Chem 1986;32:1411.
35 Wilke TJ, Utley DJ: Total testosterone, free-androgen index, calculated free testosterone and free testosterone by analog RIA compared in hirsute women and in otherwise-normal women with altered binding of sex-hormone-binding globulin. Clin Chem 1987;33:1372–1375.
36 Rosner W: An extraordinarily inaccurate assay for free testosterone is still with us. J Clin Endocrinol Metab 2001;86:2903.
37 Morley JE, Perry HM 3rd, Patrick P, Dollbaum CM, Kells JM: Validation of salivary testosterone as a screening test for male hypogonadism. Aging Male 2006;9:165–169.
38 Fox CA, Ismail AAA, Love DN, Kirkham KE, Loraine JA: Studies on the relationship between plasma testosterone levels and human sexual activity. J Endocrinol 1972;52:51–58.
39 Vermeulen A, Verdonck G: Representative of a single point plasma testosterone level for long term hormonal milieu. J Clin Endocrinol Metab 1992;74: 939–942.
40 Neischlag E, Ismail AAA: Diurnal variations of plasma testosterone in normal and pathological conditions as measured by the technique of competitive protein binding. J Endocrinol 1970;46:ii–iv.
41 Bremner WJ, Vitiello MV, Prinz PN: Loss of circadian rhythmicity in blood testosterone levels in normal men. J Clin Endocrin Metab 1983;56:1278–1281.
42 Diver MJ, Imtiaz KE, Ahmad AM, Vora JP, Fraser WD: Diurnal rhythms of serum total, free and bioavailable testosterone and of SHBG in middle-aged men compared with those in young men. Clin Endocrinol 2003;58:710–717.
43 Mohr BA, Guay AT, O'Donnell AB, McKinlay JB: Normal, bound and nonbound testosterone levels in normally ageing men: results from the Massachusetts Male Ageing Study. Clin Endocrinol 2005;62:64–73.

Dr. Michael J. Diver
Department of Clinical Chemistry
Royal Liverpool University Hospital, Prescot Street
Liverpool L7 8XP (UK)
Tel. +44 151 706 4305, Fax +44 151 706 5813, E-Mail mjdiver@liv.ac.uk

Jones TH (ed): Advances in the Management of Testosterone Deficiency.
Front Horm Res. Basel, Karger, 2009, vol 37, pp 32–51

Advances in Testosterone Replacement Therapy

Louis J.G. Gooren

Department of Endocrinology, VU University Medical Centre,
Amsterdam, The Netherlands

Abstract

The major goal of androgen substitution is to replace testosterone at levels as close to physiological concentrations as is possible. The mainstay of testosterone susbstitution are parenteral testosterone esters (enanthate and cypionate) to be administered every 2–3 weeks. A major disadvantage is the strongly fluctuating levels of plasma testosterone which are at least 50% of the time not in the physiological range. A significant improvement is parenteral testosterone undecanoate producing normal plasma testosterone for 12 weeks. Subcutaneous testosterone implants provide the patient, depending on the dose of implants, with normal plasma testosterone for 3–6 months. Its use is, however, not widespread. Oral testosterone undecanoate dissolved in oil bypasses the liver via its lymphatic absorption, but resulting plasma levels are erratic. Transdermal testosterone preparations have already been available for two decades. Transdermal testosterone gel produces attractive pharmocokinetic serum testosterone profiles and offers greater flexibility in dosing. Transdermal gel has been recommended in elderly males. In case of complications its use can be discontinued immediately. Oromucosal testosterone preparations are being developed. Testosterone replacement is usually of long duration, and patient compliance is of utmost importance. Therefore, the patient must be involved in the selection of the type of testosterone preparation.

The Various Testosterone Preparations for Treatment of Hypogonadal Men

Soon after its chemical identification more than 70 years ago, the male hormone testosterone became available pharmaceutically. But it has taken considerable time before convenient and safe preparations were developed. Three approaches have been used to make testosterone therapeutically effective: (1) routes of administration, (2) esterification in the 17β-position and (3) chemical modification of the molecule, or a combination of these approaches. In clinical practice, particularly in the perception of the patient, the route of administration is most relevant, and is used to categorize the preparations described here. Recent reviews of treatment modalities may be recommended [1, 2].

Free unesterified testosterone is absorbed well from the gut but is effectively metabolized and inactivated in the liver before it reaches the target organs. Pharmacological changes of the testosterone molecule in the 17α position render the molecule orally effective. Alkylated derivatives of testosterone including methyltestosterone and fluoxymesterone are administered orally or sublingually. They are metabolized by the liver, like natural testosterone, but more slowly, and, like testosterone, interact directly with androgen receptors. Clinical responses are variable and plasma levels cannot be determined accurately, because alkylated androgens are not recognized by most testosterone assays. The prolonged use (especially the 17α-alkylated androgens) has been associated with hepatotoxicity including hepatocellular adenoma, cholestatic jaundice and hemorrhagic liver cysts [1, 3].

Oral Testosterone Undecanoate

Testosterone undecanoate (TU) is testosterone esterified in the 17β position with a long aliphatic side chain, undecanoic acid, dissolved in oil and encapsulated in soft gelatin. Of the 40-mg capsules 63% (25 mg) is testosterone. After ingestion, for a portion (around 5%) of the administered dose, the route of absorption from the gastrointestinal tract is shifted from the portal vein to the thoracic duct. Due to its aliphatic chain it travels with lipids in the lymph and reaches the general circulation via the subclavian vein thus avoiding a first pass through the liver and subsequent metabolism of testosterone [4]. The dosing is as a rule 2 times 80 mg/day.

For its adequate absorption from the gastrointestinal tract it is essential that oral TU is taken with a meal that contains dietary fat. Maximum serum levels are reached 2–6 h after ingestion, and result in fluctuating serum testosterone levels [for a review, see 4]. To increase shelf life, the preparation was recently reformulated and the oil in the capsule is now castor oil. Recent studies show that there is dose proportionality between serum testosterone levels and the dose range of 20–80 mg. With a dose of 120–240 mg/day over 80% of hypogonadal men showed plasma testosterone levels in the normal range over 24 h [5].

Transbuccal Testosterone Administration

Transbuccal administration of testosterone provides a means of oral administration. It is marketed as a biopellet to be pressed on the gum above the incisor tooth; then, the buccal film which develops is put between the lower gum and the cheek. The resorption of testosterone through the oral mucosa avoids intestinal absorption and subsequent hepatic inactivation of testosterone. In a 7-day study transbuccal testosterone efficiently elevated serum testosterone and 5α-dihydrotestosterone (DHT) levels in hypogonadal men within the first day of application,

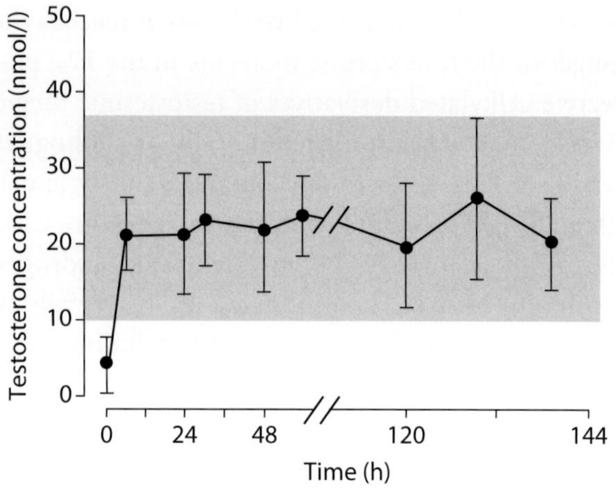

Fig. 1. Serum testosterone levels on repeat dosing with buccal testosterone 30 mg b.d. over 6 days. Reproduced with permission from Ross et al. [6].

achieved a steady state within 24 h and maintained serum testosterone in the normal range with a twice-daily treatment [6] (fig. 1). In an informative study, Dobs et al. [7] compared treatment with the testosterone buccal system (Striant®) 30 mg twice daily to a transdermal gel delivery system, 5 g containing 1% (50 mg) testosterone daily for 14 days in androgen-deficient men. 92.3% of testosterone buccal system and 83.3% of testosterone gel patients had C(ave(0–24)) within the normal range of 10.4–36.4 nmol/l (3.0–10.5 ng/ml). Mean total testosterone values were not different in the testosterone buccal system group [C(ave (0–24)) 16.7 ± 4.7 nmol/l; 4.8 ± 1.4 ng/ml] compared to the testosterone gel group [C(ave (0–24)) 15.9 ± 4.8 nmol/l; 4.6 ± 1.4 ng/ml]. The effects of buccal testosterone on sexual functioning were comparable to those of parenteral testosterone enanthate (TE) [8].

Sublingual Testosterone Administration

Sublingual application of testosterone has been tested with the inclusion of the hydrophobic testosterone molecule with 2-hydroxypropyl-β-cyclodextrin (HPBCD). HPBCD enhances testosterone solubility and absorption but HPBCD itself is not absorbed [9]. The integrated DHT/testosterone ratio was normal. Serum E_2 remained in the normal range. There were no accumulations of steroid hormones over the 7-day test period [9, 10]. Effects on sexual behavior were comparable to those of parenteral administration of 200 mg TE every 20 days.

Transdermal Delivery

Testosterone can be delivered to the circulation through intact skin, both genital and nongenital [1, 2]. Transdermal administration delivers testosterone at a controlled rate into the systemic circulation avoiding hepatic first pass and reproducing the diurnal rhythm of testosterone secretion, without the peak and through levels observed in long-acting testosterone injections.

Scrotal Testosterone Patch

Scrotal patches were first designed to deliver testosterone through the scrotal skin, where the permeability is 5 times greater than for other skin sites [4]. Clinical results were satisfactory. Transdermal scrotal testosterone administration is associated with high levels of DHT as a result of high concentrations of 5α-reductase in the scrotal skin [4]. The patch may be irritating and its use is not feasible if there is not sufficient scrotal surface. The scrotal patches sometimes fell off the scrotum leaving the patient undersubstituted. To overcome these limitations, nonscrotal skin patches have been developed.

Nonscrotal Testosterone Patch

These patches have a reservoir containing testosterone with a permeation-enhancing vehicle and gelling agents [11]. Clinical efficacy was as good as with conventional testosterone ester injections. Though satisfactory pharmacokinetically and clinically, there are adverse effects such as local skin reactions. Fifty percent of men participating in a clinical trial reported transient, mild-to-moderate erythema at some time during the therapy [11].

Testosterone Gel

When testosterone patches appeared less attractive to patients (skin irritations, visibility), we investigated whether the application of a gel would be a treatment option. When testosterone is applied to the skin surface as a hydroalcoholic gel, the gel dries rapidly and the steroid is absorbed into the stratum corneum, which serves as a reservoir. The reservoir in the skin releases testosterone slowly into the circulation over a period of several hours, resulting in steady-state serum levels of the hormones. Testosterone gel has become a prominent option for replacement therapy. Testosterone gel is hydroalcoholic, 1% (10 mg testosterone/g gel) and between 5 and 10 g gel/day is administered, amounting to 50 and 100 mg testosterone per application. The gel

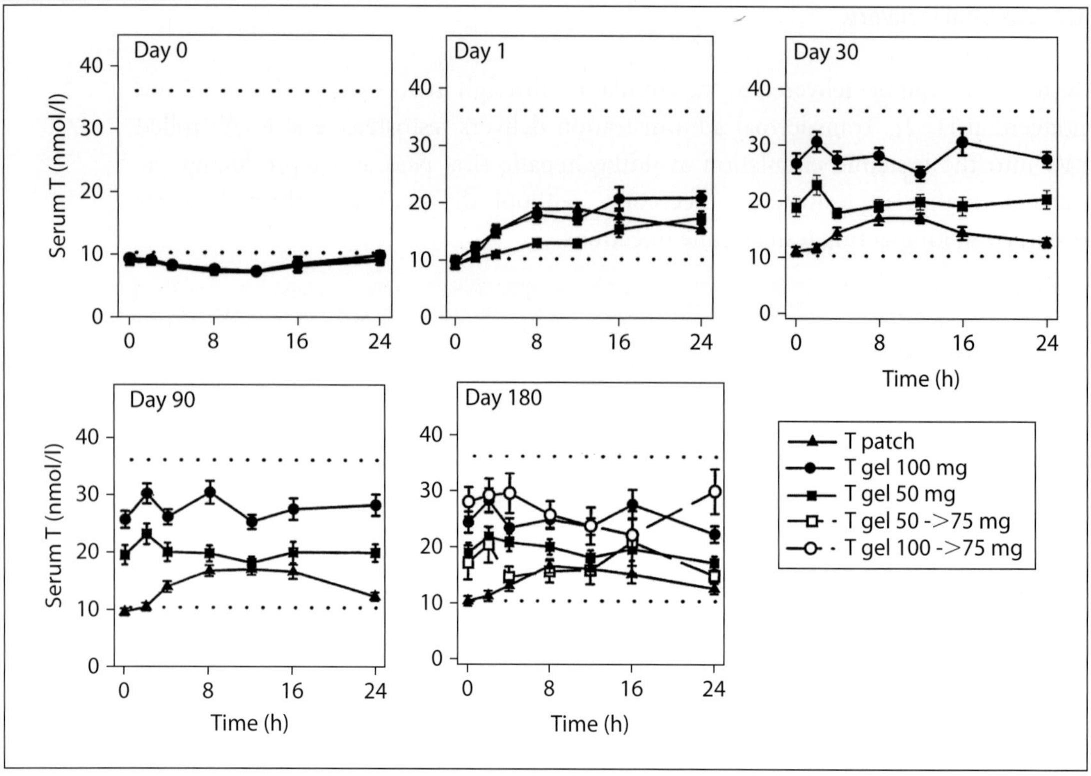

Fig. 2. Long-term pharmacokinetics of testosterone (T) gel in hypogonadal men (n = 227). Reproduced with permission from Swerdloff et al. [16].

should be applied to the abdomen, shoulders or upper arms daily. It has been available in the USA and Europe for several years and its use has been well studied [12–14]. It is marketed as Testogel® (Schering AG, Germany; AndroGel®, Solvay Pharmaceuticals). More recently developed gels are Tostrex® (ProStrakan) and Testocur®.

Pharmacokinetics

The pharmacokinetics of testosterone gel have been extensively studied [15], both in short- and long-term pharmacokinetic studies of Testogel 50, 75 and 100 mg [16–18]. In short-term (7–14 days) pharmacokinetic studies of testosterone transdermal hydroalcoholic gels peak levels of testosterone were measured 18–24 h after initial application. Serum testosterone levels rose 2- to 3-fold 2 h after application and rose further to 4- to 5-fold 24 h after application. Steady-state testosterone levels were achieved 48–72 h after the first application [12] (fig. 2). Thereafter, serum testosterone remained steadily in the upper range of normal and returned to baseline within 4 days after termination of the application of testosterone gel [15]. Later studies showed that 9–14% of the testosterone administered is bioavailable. The remaining

85–90% of the applied testosterone may be metabolized in the skin to products not measured by the assays used. Part of it is probably reduced to DHT. Studies demonstrated that application of the testosterone gel at a single site versus four separate sites resulted in a similar delivery rate of testosterone, indicating that the site of application and its related properties of the skin do not represent a barrier to testosterone absorption [17]. The formulation of the testosterone gel allows easy dose adjustments (50-, 75- and 100-mg testosterone gel) [19], though in most countries only the 50-mg gel is available commercially. Fluctuations in testosterone absorption from the skin have been noted and may be ascribed to its clearance rate and to fluctuations in skin blood flow, skin temperature, perspiration or other local environmental factors [14].

Long-term pharmacokinetics, with hormone levels measured after 30, 90 and 180 days of treatment, revealed remarkably constant and steady serum levels of testosterone (fig. 2), DHT and estradiol, with only small and variable peaks of serum testosterone after each daily application. When application of testosterone was suspended, serum testosterone levels gradually declined over 48–96 h, indicating that some accumulation of testosterone had occurred, and that this treatment mode generates a reservoir of testosterone which protects the patient from a strong decline of serum testosterone when an application of the gel has been forgotten [16]. This contrasts with the testosterone levels attained with the testosterone patch where no evidence of accumulation of testosterone with repeated application was encountered.

With continued application of testosterone gel, there were no further increases of accumulation of testosterone adding further support to the favorable properties of this treatment mode and probably rendering this system of delivery more safe [14].

The dose of testosterone recommended by manufacturers is 50 mg (5 g of gel) per day, and in most countries this is the only marketed dose. With this dose approximately 20% of patients may not attain a stable serum testosterone concentration in the young adult reference range. There are some unresolved questions with regard to testosterone replacement with the gels. In the studies by Swerdloff et al. [12, 16], it was not rare that in patients who were changed from a dose of testosterone gel of 50 to 75 mg/day, serum testosterone levels remained similar or even lower than those receiving the 50-mg testosterone gel in spite of an increase of the administered dose by 50% [19]. The authors could not ascertain whether the men who did not attain eugonadal values of testosterone upon application of the 50-mg testosterone gel were less compliant or were biologically different. It cannot be ruled out that some patients have a lower than average absorption and/or a high clearance rate of testosterone either in the basal state or after following a stimulus induced by exogenous testosterone. By contrast, patients who had supranormal serum testosterone levels upon application of the 100-mg dose of the gel and who were shifted to 50 mg showed promptly normal testosterone levels. Overall, the findings of pharmacokinetic studies show that the average patient is well served with a 50-mg dose of testosterone gel and in those men who will not have a normalization of their serum testosterone will not necessarily respond favorably to an increase of the dose. In some recent studies on the testosterone gel, the testosterone levels achieved during treatment were somewhat lower than previously reported [20, 21], confirming that absorption cannot be assumed to be equal for every subject. In the most recently developed gels (Tostrex and Testocur), the testosterone concentration in the gel has been increased from 1 to 2 and 2.5%, respectively. It may be the case that in a minority of patients the available transdermal preparations will not generate reference values of testosterone levels and that they are better off with injectable esters [22].

Pharmacokinetic studies have shown that DHT and estradiol levels increase steadily after the first application. Following application of testosterone gel the mean serum level of DHT tripled after the application of 50-mg testosterone gel and increased nearly 5-fold with the application of 100-mg testosterone gel, which is considerably higher than observed with patches. It is not clear whether this must be ascribed to a higher delivery of bioavailable testosterone, a higher conversion of testosterone to DHT in the skin which expresses 5α-reductase activity, or is a result of the application of the gel to a larger area of skin surface compared with the very small area of skin exposed to the nonscrotal testosterone patch, although DHT is lower than observed with scrotal patches. It has been confirmed in other studies that the testosterone gels generate higher DHT levels compared with patches [20, 23]. Increases in DHT after testosterone gel application constitute a risk which remains to be established but which is unlikely. Administration of DHT as a gel appears to have a favorable safety profile [24]. Serum estradiol levels showed small and proportionate increases following transdermal testosterone application. The biological relevance of estrogens for serum lipid levels, vascular endothelium reactivity, sexual function, body composition and bone mass have been documented over the last decade [25].

Clinical Efficacy

The clinical efficacy of testosterone replacement with transdermal testosterone gel on various androgen-dependent target organ systems is now well documented. The efficacy of various testosterone treatment options on the symptoms of hypogonadism has been reviewed in two recently published meta-analyses of randomized controlled trials. Two large-scale, open-label, well-performed studies documented the benefits of the application of the 1% testosterone gel for sexual function, mood, muscle strength, body composition and bone mineral density in men with hypogonadism of various etiologies. More importantly, improvements in these features persisted when treatment was extended ≤3 years [12, 16, 19]. The increases in bone mineral density observed after 6 months of treatment were 1% in the hip and 2% in the spine, and appeared to be dependent on the testosterone level achieved. A randomized, placebo-controlled study with 22 patients established that 1% testosterone gel, when added to patients' existing antidepressant regimens, is significantly superior to placebo in reducing scores on the Hamilton Depression Rating and Clinical Global Impression Scale, in patients with treatment-resistant depression [21]. Other studies showed that testosterone gel treatment significantly improved depressive symptoms, but a statistical difference between testosterone and placebo treatment could not be demonstrated. These data suggest that responses in depressed subjects have been variable [26, 27].

Safety

Safety data are available for the 1% testosterone gel [16]. After 3 years of treatment, levels of total cholesterol, low-density lipoprotein cholesterol, high-density lipoprotein cholesterol and triglycerides remained unchanged. Levels of prostate-specific antigen (PSA) rose in proportion to the increase of testosterone levels but did not exceed normal values. These data collected in prospective well-designed large-scale studies are relatively rare in the area of testosterone treatment of male hypogonadism. Consequently, the testosterone gel may be considered an appropriate therapy for patients with classical hypogonadism, but also for elderly men with LOH. It offers the opportunity of flexibility and of instant discontinuation in the event of safety problems. Skin irritation was noted in 5.5% of patients in the study [19].

Patients need to minimize the amount used as a precaution for transfer of testosterone to partners by skin contact. However, the likelihood of gel transfer has been found to be low, and it is reduced by washing the application site after it has dried [28]. After intense skin-to-skin contact between volunteers, one of whom had applied testosterone gel to his forearm, no increase in serum testosterone levels could be found in the other volunteer, in whom endogenous testosterone production had been suppressed using norethisterone enanthate. So, transfer from one person to another is likely to be insignificant [28]. However, three cases of transfer from fathers to their children have recently been reported [29].

Place of the Testosterone Gel in Testosterone Substitution Treatment

The testosterone gel appears to be a major improvement in the treatment of hypogonadism thanks to its favorable pharmacokinetic profile, its safety and its convenience. Patients are instructed not to apply the gel to the genital area. The gel dries within 5 min, and having a shower or swimming 4–6 h later does not affect the blood levels [30]. Very little testosterone is washed off the skin after evaporation of the alcoholic vehicle, and bathing or swimming after the gel has dried is unlikely to negatively affect serum testosterone levels [16]. Patient compliance with gel administration appears markedly better than that with patch administration, and considerably fewer cases of skin reactions occurred with the gel. As application of the gel is simple, convenient and almost free of local reactions, and does not require assistance of medical personnel as is the case with injections, a large number of patients prefer this application mode over intramuscular injections. Timing of application of the gel is not crucial as gels reach a steady-state level after the first few days. Most patients prefer to apply the gel in the morning. Then it will result in physiological serum levels almost mimicking the normal diurnal rhythm. The biological significance of the circadian rhythm has, however, not been established. Most men feel that with an application in the morning the risk of transfer to others will be less than with an application in the evening.

Androgen Replacement with DHT

The effects of testosterone are mediated directly as testosterone or after conversion to either DHT or estradiol locally in target tissues. The reduction of testosterone to DHT is an amplification mechanism of the androgenizing effects of testosterone. DHT binds to the same receptor as testosterone but its receptor binding is stronger resulting in a considerably higher biopotency than testosterone itself. DHT, as opposed to testosterone, cannot be aromatized to estradiol and acts, therefore, as a pure androgen. In certain clinical conditions a pure androgen might have advantages over aromatizable testosterone, such as in cases of a microphallus, hypogonadal men with a susceptibility to gynecomastia or constitutionally delayed puberty in boys. Estrogens are pivotal in the closure of the epiphyses at puberty, and a nonaromatizable androgen might allow some extra gain in height by slowing the closure of the pubertal epiphyses. Estrogen effects on the prostate might be deleterious [31] and in this regard DHT might be the preferred androgen for the androgen-deficient aging male. Studies of DHT administration to hypogonadal men show that DHT maintains sex characteristics, increases muscle mass and improves sexual functions without significant increases in prostate size [32, 33].

Subcutaneous/Intramuscular Administration

Testosterone Implants

Subdermal pellet implantation was among the earliest effective treatment modalities for clinical use of testosterone and became an established form of androgen replacement by 1940 [for a review, see 34]. Several reports have outlined its desirable pharmacological properties but its use and merits and its complications (such as infection and extrusion) have been best documented by the group of Handelsman [34].

Testosterone Esters

The most commonly used forms of androgen replacement therapy include 17β-hydroxyl esters of testosterone administered with slow release, oil-based vehicles. Commonly used intramuscular injectable testosterone esters are TE and cypionate [1, 2, 4].

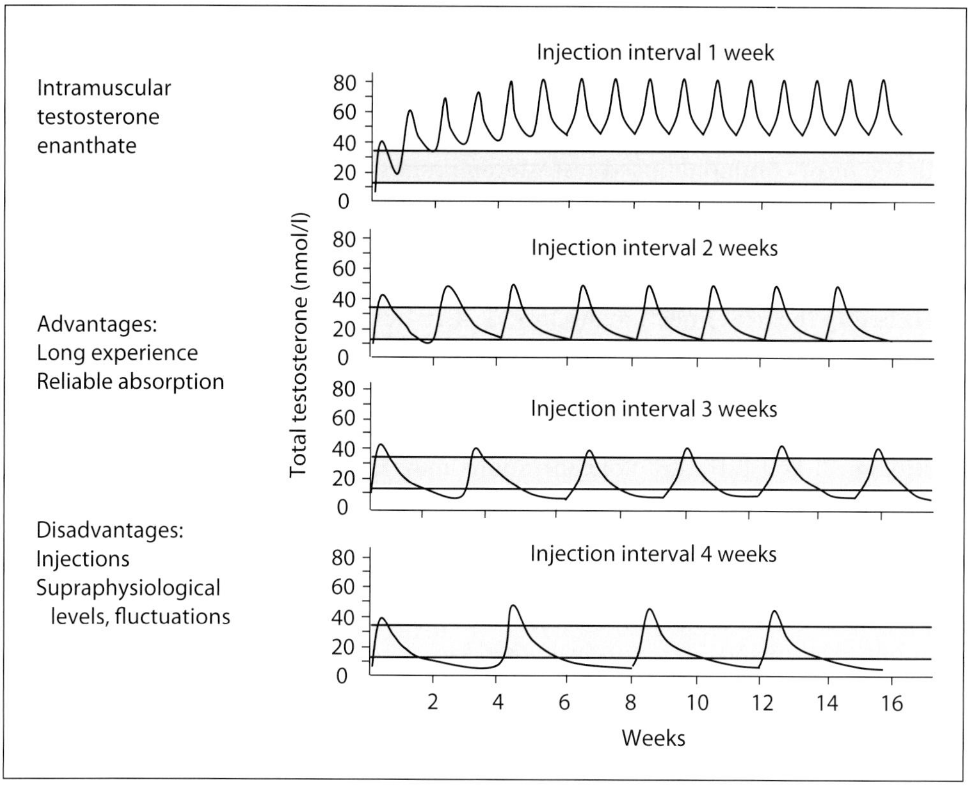

Fig. 3. Pharmacokinetics of intramuscular TE demonstrating wide fluctuations in serum testosterone levels. Reproduced with permission from Nieschlag et al. [60].

TE is one of the most widely used intramuscular testosterone esters. At a dose of 200–250 mg the optimal injection interval is 2–3 weeks but peak and through values are clearly above and below the normal range (fig. 3).

Testosterone propionate has a terminal half-life of only 19 h. After a single injection of 50 mg the maximum concentration is reached after approximately 14 h [4]. On the basis of this profile, injection intervals are only 2–3 days with peak and through values above and below the normal range and therefore not suitable for monotherapy of testosterone deficiency. Alternatively, 100 mg weekly may be given. Other testosterone esters are testosterone cypionate and testosterone cyclohexanocarboxylate. The pharmacokinetics of these testosterone esters are very similar to those of TE [4]. Administration of 200 mg every 2 weeks provides an acceptable form of testosterone replacement.

Several commercially available testosterone preparations contain a number of short and longer acting testosterone esters aiming to deliver more even serum testosterone levels. Pharmacokinetic studies of these preparations show that this goal has not been achieved. The peak values are higher than in single testosterone ester preparations and resulting plasma testosterone levels show even larger fluctuations [4]. So, most intramuscular presentations of testosterone are not ideal. With the most commonly used testosterone esters a maximum concentration follows approximately 72 h after injection. Testosterone levels slowly diminish during the following 10–14 days showing an exponential decline of serum testosterone levels reaching baseline approximately at day 21 [4]. As a result the testosterone levels before the next injection are low [1, 4]. The normal pattern of the circadian rhythm of testosterone is not achieved, though it is questionable whether the circadian rhythm has much therapeutic relevance. The injections are painful [1]. Although levels of DHT are normal, androgen metabolites are frequently not physiological and estradiol concentrations may become excessive in some men. The profile of testosterone levels may be accompanied by disturbed fluctuations in sexual function, energy level, and mood [1, 2]. High postinjection levels of testosterone predispose the patient to acne and polycythemia, and elevated estradiol predisposes to gynecomastia. In some patients, injections may be associated with bleeding or bruising [2]. However, these long-acting testosterone preparations have for a long time been the mainstay of testosterone treatment and they are the most cost-effective methods, with the administration of 200–400 mg every 2–4 weeks. The 200-mg injection will maintain normal testosterone for approximately 2 weeks while 300-mg doses are required for eugonadal ranges for approximately 3 weeks [4].

New Developments in Parenteral Testosterone Esters

In search of better intramuscular long-acting testosterone preparations for male contraception, it appeared that testosterone esterified with undecanoic acid (TU) showed more favorable long-term kinetics than the traditional testosterone esters [4, 35]. In contrast to the conventional fatty acid esters, the kinetics for side chain cleavage of the saturated aliphatic fatty acid undecanoic acid with 11 carbon atoms turned out to be considerably longer permitting much longer injection intervals, at the same time preventing supra- or subphysiological serum testosterone levels.

Like in the traditional testosterone esters, the active pharmacological principle of TU is testosterone itself [36]. Therefore, in principle, the toxicology of TU is the same as for other cleavable testosterone fatty acid esters such testosterone propionate, testosterone enanthate or testosterone cypionate. TU as an oral preparation has been available for more than 30 years. It is well-tolerated, but the bioavailability of testosterone leaves much to be desired. It requires careful dosing at least 2 times a day and it must be taken with fatty meals in order to achieve acceptable plasma testosterone levels [5].

Pharmacokinetics in Men

There is now long-term experience with TU of more than 8 years [37, 38]. Individual dosing intervals ranged from 10 to 14 weeks. Serum trough levels of testosterone were generally within the low normal range, indicating sufficient substitution. In contrast to short-acting testosterone esters, sensations of fluctuations in androgen serum concentrations were rarely observed. If this was the case, it occurred during the last 2 weeks before the next injection indicating a loss of androgenic psychotropic effects. Summarizing a key study [39] the following administration regimen is recommended for TU therapy in hypogonadal men. After the 1st injection of 1,000 mg TU, the 2nd injection of 1,000 mg TU is to be administered 6 weeks after the 1st injection (loading dose) followed by injections every 12 weeks. While this schedule will generally be adequate, an individualization of TU therapy may be desirable [37, 38]. If the testosterone serum concentration before the 4th injection lies between 10 and 15 nmol/l then the injection interval should be every 12 weeks. Should the testosterone serum concentration at this time be lower than10 nmol/l, then the injection interval is shortened to every 10 weeks. If the testosterone level is greater than 15 nmol/l, then the injection interval should be extended to every 14 weeks. Additionally, clinical symptoms should be considered for the individualization of injection intervals with TU therapy. The loading dose of TU achieved by the first 2 injections with an interval of 8 weeks is also recommended for patients who are transferred from short-acting testosterone injections (e.g. TE 250 mg) to treatment with TU.

Efficacy Studies Including Any Comparative Studies

The efficacy of TU has been compared to the previous gold standard of 250 mg TE i.m. per 3 weeks in a 30-week controlled, prospective, randomized, parallel-group study [39]. During the first 30 weeks of the comparative phase, 40 hypogonadal men with testosterone levels below 5 nmol/l were randomly assigned to either 250 mg TE i.m. every 3 weeks (n = 20) or TU 3 times in 6-week intervals followed by a 9-week interval. Following the first 30 weeks of the comparative part of the study, all patients received TU every 12 weeks in the one-arm follow-up study over an additional 30 months. In the first 30 weeks there were no differences in sexual parameters (spontaneous morning erections, total erections, ejaculations) between the two groups. After 30 weeks, serum PSA levels in both treatment groups had risen slightly, but remained stable during long-term TU administration and stayed within the normal range over the entire observation period. Prostate volume increased during the first 30 weeks to a similar degree with both testosterone preparations but then remained stable until the end of the follow-up study [40].

It is now clear that TU is at least as effective and safe as the standard injectable formulation and requires only 4 injections per year in long-term treatment while

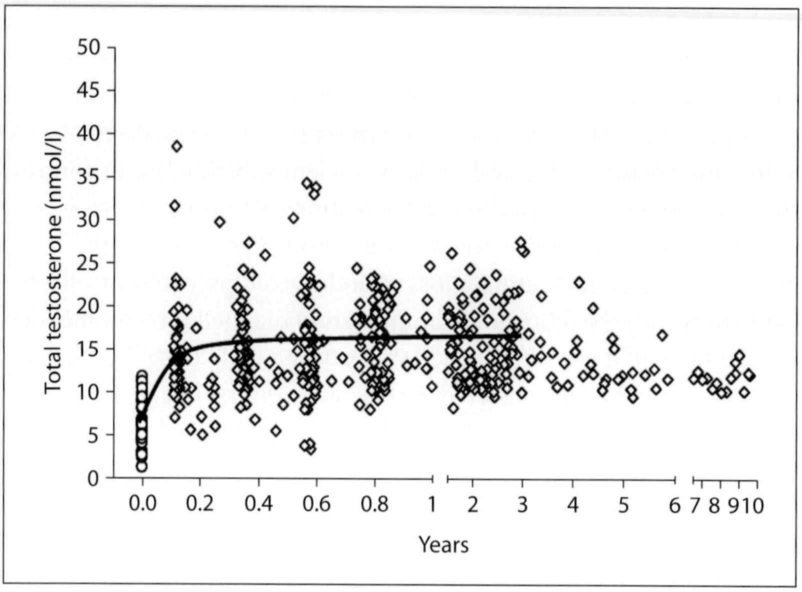

Fig. 4. Total serum testosterone concentrations displaying 515 data points of 66 hypogonadal men before (○) and during substitution therapy with TU i.m. (◇; nadir levels). Reproduced with permission from Zitzmann et al. [41].

maintaining serum testosterone levels within the physiological range [39, 41] (fig. 4). There are data to confirm the safety and efficacy of long-term TU therapy of hypogonadal patients treated over a period of more than 8 years [37, 40]. The study included 22 patients who received TU for up to 8.5 years at injection intervals of approximately 12 weeks. Patients reported restoration of sexual functions and positive changes in mood patterns. In contrast to short-acting TE preparations, patients rarely reported perceptions of fluctuations in androgen concentrations. Over the whole treatment period, PSA concentrations did not exceed the normal range and prostate size remained below 30 ml in all patients (fig. 3). Hemoglobin and hematocrit increased initially during treatment but remained within the normal range over the entire treatment period. Computer tomography of the lumbar spine showed that bone density improved in all patients during the first 2 years and remained stable thereafter. Body mass index decreased during the first 2 years of treatment. Serum total cholesterol levels did not change over the treatment period and serum LDL levels decreased slightly, concurring with the decrease of body mass index, and serum HDL levels increased slightly over time. There were no relevant changes in blood pressure or heart rate. Overall, treatment with intramuscular TU appeared to have beneficial effects on body composition and lipid profile [42, 43].

Treatment of Erectile Dysfunction with TU

There is a new interest in the treatment of erectile dysfunction with testosterone. Apart from its well-known effects on libido, testosterone appears to have significant direct effects on anatomical and physiological properties of erectile tissue [44, 45], and there are some interesting new observations. In support of a direct effect of testosterone on penile tissues, treatment with TU appeared to improve venoocclusive dysfunction evidenced by cavernosographic changes in hypogonadal patients with severe erectile dysfunction, diabetes mellitus, obesity and/or metabolic syndrome who had earlier not responded to PDE-5 inhibitors and intracavernosal alprostadil injections [46, 47]. One patient having venous leakage upon testosterone administration received treatment with TU at 12- to 14-week intervals following a loading dose of 6 weeks. The patient showed improved sexual function after 9 weeks of treatment and repeated cavernosography after 12 weeks revealed that the venous leakage had receded [46]. This finding was replicated in 5 out of 12 hypogonadal patients [47] and could have suggested the correction of a venous leak; this could be at least in part a metabolic lesion rather than a mechanical one, such as in venous anatomic abnormality or venous valve dysfunction, and could perhaps clarify the higher recurrence rate in penile venous surgery. These results confirm data obtained from animal studies showing that androgen insufficiency leads to venoocclusive dysfunction which cannot be restored with PDE-5 inhibitor treatment alone [48].

Safety and Tolerability

TU is generally well tolerated. Local irritation at the site of injection is moderate, does not last longer than 3 days and can be minimized by administering TU slowly over a period of at least 1 min. Very few patients reported irritation or pain at the sight of injection despite the large volume of the injection of 4 ml. No patient discontinued treatment due to problems of local discomfort. TU should be injected deeply into the gluteal muscle. The patient should be in a prone position. During the first year of TU treatment, for safety reasons, erythropoiesis parameters and prostate size and serum PSA as well as International Prostate Symptoms Score (IPSS) should be monitored in men above the age of 45 years at quarterly intervals and then yearly thereafter [49].

The conventional injectable testosterone esters, such as TE with injection intervals of 2–3 weeks, are associated with supraphysiological peak values shortly after the injection and with subphysiological levels in the days before the new injection. This often leads to mood swings or emotional instability. Another important consequence of the supraphysiological testosterone levels under treatment with TE is the induction of elevations of hematocrit. Of 70 older men with low serum testosterone receiving 200 mg of TE every other week, 30% developed a hematocrit greater than 52% [50, 51]. In another study of 32 hypogonadal men receiving 200 mg TE every other week,

14 patients (43.8%) had at least one occurrence of an elevated hematocrit value [52]. The evidence that elevated hematocrit values may lead to thromboembolic events is not very well documented. It is clear now that TU is at least as effective and safe as the standard injectable formulation and eventually requires only 4 injections per year while maintaining serum testosterone levels within the physiological range. There are data to confirm the safety and efficacy of long-term TU therapy in hypogonadal patients treated over a period of more than 8 years.

No major adverse effects were encountered in the clinical trials of TU. This is not surprising since the pharmaceutically active component is testosterone itself. Common side effects of testosterone administration, such as gynecomastia, breast tenderness and acne, were reported in only a minority of patients. This absence of side effects is probably to be ascribed to the largely normal physiological levels of T, and its derivatives DHT and estradiol, achieved with TU. Adverse effects were observed in the initial studies when the dosing schedule had not yet been well established and the higher frequency of administration of TU led to higher than normal levels of testosterone. Significant increases in PSA and prostate size were noted in some of these trials; however, this is due to the fact that hypogonadal men have subnormal PSA values and small prostate sizes at baseline and it is observed with every treatment modality of testosterone administration upon normalization of plasma testosterone levels [53, 54]. In a systematic review of the effect of testosterone administration on the prostate in hypogonadal men, the average PSA increase after initiation of testosterone therapy was 0.3 ng/ml in young hypogonadal men and 0.44 ng/ml in older men [55].

In the further course of treatment with TU, PSA levels and prostate size remained stable and within the normal range. Similarly, increases of parameters of erythropoiesis to eugonadal values were observed, but there was no occurrence of polycythemia as observed in studies with the more traditional testosterone esters [50, 52]. Only one study showed a transient decline in serum HDL cholesterol; however, its value remained within the normal range [for a review, see 56]. So, TU appears to be a safe modality of testosterone treatment, which can be ascribed to the fact that with the dosage regimen established at present plasma testosterone levels remain in the physiological range.

Several of the recommendations of testosterone administration to elderly men with late onset hypogonadism argue in favor of short-acting testosterone preparations [49]. The reasoning is that in case an intercurrent disease develops, such as prostate malignancy, the impact of the extra androgens provided by the administration of testosterone will be short-lived. It is questionable whether this recommendation is rational (1) in view of the fact that there is an early diagnosis in this group of men who supposedly are monitored, following the guidelines, with an absolute minimum of digital rectal examination + PSA determination once a year. (2) In view of the fact that delays between diagnostic biopsies and treatment of several months up to 1 year did not affect the recurrence rate as measured by PSA levels. Modern testosterone preparations generate physiological testosterone levels for a maximum duration of 10–14 weeks. So, it would seem that the choice of longer-acting testosterone preparation is not of great pathophysiological relevance [57–59]. (3) With the modern testosterone preparations, plasma testosterone remains in the normal range, so that there is no overexposure of the prostate to testosterone. (4) Even with the traditional testosterone esters, with supraphysiological levels shortly after administration, no cause and effect of prostate cancer related to treatment with testosterone has been found. (5) Men diagnosed with prostate cancer do not routinely undergo androgen ablation treatment. Therefore, it would seem that there is no serious objection to treating elderly men with a long-acting testosterone preparation.

Patients' Perspectives

Most medical conditions requiring androgen therapy are irreversible. As a consequence, androgen replacement therapy often extends over many decades. Therefore, patient compliance is of utmost importance.

After a recommended loading dose of 2 injections with a 6-week interval, TU is the first intramuscular agent that can be administered every 12 weeks thus maintaining physiological plasma testosterone levels. Depending on the trough plasma testosterone level immediately before the next injection and clinical symptoms of the patient, adjustment of the injection interval is desirable, rarely by shortening (every 10–11 weeks) but more often by prolonging (every 13–14 weeks) the interval between 2 injections. TU produces fewer peaks and troughs in serum testosterone levels in comparison to the traditional testosterone esters. Hypogonadal men treated with TU report a general sense of well-being and normal sexual function during treatment. These parameters were not different when evaluated in the middle of an injection interval versus at the end of an injection interval. This suggests that normal physiological testosterone values were maintained throughout the 12-week period without major fluctuations. As a result, patients did not report mood swings or emotional instability, which is a common complaint with other testosterone preparations.

A major advantage of TU is that it only requires 4 injections/year compared with 26 injections/year of TE (if taken at a dose of 200 or 250 mg every 2 weeks which is necessary if the plasma testosterone levels are to be kept in the physiological range; though, with this frequency, plasma testosterone levels will exceed to the supraphysiological range in the days following an injection). The physician sees the patient every 12 weeks for safety and efficacy monitoring. With a 2- to 3-weekly injection of TE, the frequency is so high that efficacy and safety of testosterone administration will not be assessed at every visit. The clinical experience with TU meets the requirements spelled out in the consensus on testosterone as well as other recommendations regarding safety and efficacy monitoring of testosterone administration. Therefore, TU is also very suitable for elderly men because these patients will be examined 4 times/year and prostate malignancy and other reasons for the discontinuation of the therapy can be diagnosed in good time. There was no impairment of uroflow.

Conclusions

Treatment with unmodified testosterone molecules is preferred by opinion leaders, with a treatment modality and in a dose which maintain serum testosterone in the physiological range for the full 24 h of the day. Studies so far have shown that both the testosterone gel and parenteral TU fulfill these requirements and represent effective, safe and well-tolerated means of androgen treatment in hypogonadal men. At present, clinical experience is available with testosterone gels over 15 years and with TU treatment over 9 years. In view of their favorable pharmacokinetic profiles, both the testosterone gels and TU have been well received. The advantages of TU over the more conventional injectable testosterone preparations are obvious. The injection frequency is as little as 4 per year. The large fluctuations of plasma testosterone with the conventional testosterone esters are subjectively experienced as unpleasant by many patients. TU, with its more favorable pharmacokinetic profile, did not have these side effects in clinical trials. So the merits of TU are manifest.

From a pharmacotherapeutic perspective, both testosterone gels and TU are equivalent and physicians may not have a strong preference for one over the other. It appears, however, that patients have preferences for certain treatment modalities; so for the sake of compliance it is important to present them with the options available. Changing from one treatment modality presents no great problem. Both the testosterone gels and TU are more expensive than the conventional parenteral testosterone esters which were developed some 50–60 years ago. Health economics may delay a wide introduction of testosterone gels and TU in the short term in spite of the obvious advantages over the traditional testosterone esters.

The open questions are related to testosterone therapy in general and apply to all testosterone preparations and to prostate cancer. There is no evidence that testosterone causes prostate cancer. But larger, longer-term clinical studies with more patients (ideally comprising 6,000 men followed up for 6–8 years) are required to find definitive answers regarding the interrelationships between testosterone serum levels following testosterone administration and the pathophysiology of prostate cancer. However, experts agree that it is responsible clinical practice to treat elderly hypogonadal men with testosterone provided the existing guidelines for monitoring are followed.

References

1 Gooren LJ, Bunck MC: Androgen replacement therapy: present and future. Drugs 2004;64:1861–1891.

2 Nieschlag E: Testosterone treatment comes of age: new options for hypogonadal men. Clin Endocrinol (Oxf) 2006;65:275–281.

3 Bagatell CJ, Bremner WJ: Androgen and progestagen effects on plasma lipids. Prog Cardiovasc Dis 1995;38:255–271.

4 Behre HM, Wang C, Handelsman DJ, Nieschlag E: Pharmacology of testosterone preparations; in Nieschlag E, Behre HM (eds): Testosterone: Action, Deficiency, Substitution. Cambridge, Cambridge University Press, 2004, pp 405–444.

5 Bagchus WM, Hust R, et al: Important effect of food on the bioavailability of oral testosterone undecanoate. Pharmacotherapy 2003;23:319–325.

6 Ross RJ, Jabbar A, et al: Pharmacokinetics and tolerability of a bioadheive testosterone tablet in hypogonadal men. Eur J Endocrinol 2004;150:57–63.

7 Dobs AS, Matsumoto AM, et al: Short-term pharmacokinetic comparison of a novel testosterone buccal system and a testosterone gel in testosterone deficient men. Curr Med Res Opin 2004;20:729–738.

8 Wang C, Swerdloff R, et al: New testosterone buccal system (Striant) delivers physiological testosterone levels: pharmacokinetics study in hypogonadal men. J Clin Endocrinol Metab 2004;89:3821–3829.

9 Stuenkel CA, Dudley RE, et al: Sublingual administration of testosterone-hydroxypropyl-beta-cyclodextrin inclusion complex simulates episodic androgen release in hypogonadal men. J Clin Endocrinol Metab 1991;72:1054–1059.

10 Wang C, Eyre DR, et al: Sublingual testosterone replacement improves muscle mass and strength, decreases bone resorption, and increases bone formation markers in hypogonadal men – a clinical research center study. J Clin Endocrinol Metab 1996; 81:3654–3662.

11 Meikle AW, Arver S, et al: Pharmacokinetics and metabolism of a permeation-enhanced testosterone transdermal system in hypogonadal men: influence of application site – a clinical research center study. J Clin Endocrinol Metab 1996;81:1832–1840.

12 Wang C, Swerdloff RS, et al: Transdermal testosterone gel improves sexual function, mood, muscle strength, and body composition parameters in hypogonadal men. J Clin Endocrinol Metab 2000;85: 2839–2853.

13 Kuhnert B, Byrne M, et al: Testosterone substitution with a new transdermal, hydroalcoholic gel applied to scrotal or non-scrotal skin: a multicentre trial. Eur J Endocrinol 2005;153:317–326.

14 Mazer N, Bell D, et al: Comparison of the steady-state pharmacokinetics, metabolism, and variability of a transdermal testosterone patch versus a transdermal testosterone gel in hypogonadal men. J Sex Med 2005;2:213–226.

15 Meikle AW, Matthias D, et al: Transdermal testosterone gel: pharmacokinetics, efficacy of dosing and application site in hypogonadal men. BJU Int 2004; 93:789–795.

16 Swerdloff RS, Wang C, et al: Long-term pharmacokinetics of transdermal testosterone gel in hypogonadal men. J Clin Endocrinol Metab 2000;85:4500–4510.

17 Wang C, Berman N, et al: Pharmacokinetics of transdermal testosterone gel in hypogonadal men: application of gel at one site versus four sites: a General Clinical Research Center Study. J Clin Endocrinol Metab 2000;85:964–969.

18 Wang C, Iranmanesh A, et al: Comparative pharmacokinetics of three doses of percutaneous dihydrotestosterone gel in healthy elderly men – a clinical research center study. J Clin Endocrinol Metab 1998; 83:2749–2757.

19 Wang C, Cunningham G, et al: Long-term testosterone gel (AndroGel) treatment maintains beneficial effects on sexual function and mood, lean and fat mass, and bone mineral density in hypogonadal men. J Clin Endocrinol Metab 2004;89:2085–2098.

20 Mazer N, Fisher D, et al: Transfer of transdermally applied testosterone to clothing: a comparison of a testosterone patch versus a testosterone gel. J Sex Med 2005;2:227–234.

21 Pope HG Jr, Cohane GH, et al: Testosterone gel supplementation for men with refractory depression: a randomized, placebo-controlled trial. Am J Psychiatry 2003;160:105–111.

22 Jockenhovel F: Testosterone supplementation: what and how to give. Aging Male 2003;6:200–206.

23 Dean JD, Carnegie C, et al: Long-term effects of testim(r) 1% testosterone gel in hypogonadal men. Rev Urol 2004;6(suppl 6):S22–S29.

24 Sakhri S, Gooren LJ: Safety aspects of androgen treatment with 5alpha-dihydrotestosterone. Andrologia 2007;39:216–222.

25 Steidle C, Schwatrz S, et al: North American AA2500 T Gel Study Group: AA2500 testosterone gel normalizes androgen levels in ageing males with improvements in body composition and sexual function. J Clin Endocrinol Metab 2003;88:2673–2681.

26 Orengo CA, Fulleton L, et al: Safety and efficacy of testosterone gel 1% augmentation in depressed men with partial response to antidepressant therapy. J Geriatr Psychiatry Neurol 2005;18:20–24.

27 Carnahan RM, Perry PJ: Depression in ageing men: the role of testosterone. Drugs Aging 2004;21: 361–376.

28 Rolf C, Knie U, et al: Interpersonal testosterone transfer after topical application of a newly developed testosterone gel preparation. Clin Endocrinol (Oxf) 2002;56:637–641.

29 Brachet C, Vermeulen J, et al: Children's virilization and the use of a testosterone gel by their fathers. Eur J Pediatr 2005;164:646–647.

30 Margo K, Winn R: Testosterone treatments: why, when, and how? Am Fam Physician 2006;73: 1591–1598.

31 Carruba G: Estrogens and mechanisms of prostate cancer progression. Ann NY Acad Sci 2006;1089: 201–217.

32 Ly LP, Jimenez M, et al: A double-blind, placebo-controlled, randomized clinical trial of transdermal dihydrotestosterone gel on muscular strength, mobility, and quality of life in older men with partial androgen deficiency. J Clin Endocrinol Metab 2001;86:4078–4088.
33 Wang C, Swerdloff RS: Should the nonaromatizable androgen dihydrotestosterone be considered as an alternative to testosterone in the treatment of the andropause? J Clin Endocrinol Metab 2002;87:1462–1466.
34 Kelleher S, Howe C, et al: Testosterone release rate and duration of action of testosterone pellet implants. Clin Endocrinol (Oxf) 2004;60:420–428.
35 Herz JE, Torres JV, et al: Potential long-acting contraceptive agents: esters and ethers of testosterone with alpha- and/or beta-chain branching. Steroids 1985;46:947–953.
36 Horst HJ, Holtje WJ, et al: Lymphatic absorption and metabolism of orally administered testosterone undecanoate in man. Klin Wochenschr 1976;54:875–879.
37 Zitzmann M, Nieschlag E: Long-term experience of more than 8 years with a novel formulation of testosterone undecanoate (Nebido) in substitution therapy of hypogonadal men. Aging Male 2006;5:5.
38 Saad F, Kamischke A, et al: More than eight years' hands-on experience with the novel long-acting parenteral testosterone undecanoate. Asian J Androl 2007;9:291–297.
39 Schubert M, Minnemann T, et al: Intramuscular testosterone undecanoate: pharmacokinetic aspects of a novel testosterone formulation during long-term treatment of men with hypogonadism. J Clin Endocrinol Metab 2004;89:5429–5434.
40 Minnemann T, Schubert M, et al: A four-year efficacy and safety study of the long-acting parenteral testosterone undecanoate. Aging Male 2007;10:155–158.
41 Zitzmann M, Nieschlag E: Androgen receptor gene CAG repeat length and body mass index modulate the safety of long-term intramuscular therapy in hypogonadal men. J Clin Endocrinol Metab 2007;92:3844–3853.
42 Saad FG, Haider LJ, Yassin A: An exploratory study of the effects of 12 month administration of the novel long-acting testosterone undecanoate on measures of sexual function and the metabolic syndrome. Arch Androl 2007;53:353–357.
43 Saad F, Gooren LJ, et al: A dose-response study of testosterone on sexual dysfunction and features of the metabolic syndrome using testosterone gel and parenteral testosterone undecanoate. J Androl 2008;29:102–105.
44 Gooren LJ, Saad F: Recent insights into androgen action on the anatomical and physiological substrate of penile erection. Asian J Androl 2006;8:3–9.
45 Traish AM, Guay AT: Are androgens critical for penile erections in humans? Examining the clinical and preclinical evidence. J Sex Med 2006;3:382–407.
46 Yassin AA, Saad F: Dramatic improvement of penile venous leakage upon testosterone administration. A case report and review of literature. Andrologia 2006;38:34–37.
47 Yassin AA, Saad F, et al: Testosterone undecanoate restores erectile function in a subset of patients with venous leakage: a series of case reports. J Sex Med 2006;3:727–735.
48 Traish AM, Toselli P, et al: Adipocyte accumulation in penile corpus cavernosum of the orchiectomized rabbit: a potential mechanism for veno-occlusive dysfunction in androgen deficiency. J Androl 2005;26:242–248.
49 Nieschlag E, Swerdloff R, et al: Investigation, treatment and monitoring of late-onset hypogonadism in males: ISA, ISSAM, and EAU recommendations. Int J Androl 2005;28:125–127.
50 Dobs AS, Meikle AW, et al: Pharmacokinetics, efficacy, and safety of a permeation-enhanced testosterone transdermal system in comparison with bi-weekly injections of testosterone enanthate for the treatment of hypogonadal men. J Clin Endocrinol Metab 1999;84:3469–3478.
51 Gui YL, He CH, et al: Male hormonal contraception: suppression of spermatogenesis by injectable testosterone undecanoate alone or with levonorgestrel implants in Chinese men. J Androl 2004;25:720–727.
52 Jockenhovel F, Vogel E, et al: Effects of various modes of androgen substitution therapy on erythropoiesis. Eur J Med Res 1997;2:293–298.
53 Behre HM, Bohmeyer J, et al: Prostate volume in testosterone-treated and untreated hypogonadal men in comparison to age-matched normal controls. Clin Endocrinol (Oxf) 1994;40:341–349.
54 Bhasin S, Cunningham GR, et al: Testosterone therapy in adult men with androgen deficiency syndromes: an endocrine society clinical practice guideline. J Clin Endocrinol Metab 2006;91: 1995–2010.
55 Bhasin S, Singh AB, et al: Managing the risks of prostate disease during testosterone replacement therapy in older men: recommendations for a standardized monitoring plan. J Androl 2003;24:299–311.

56 Harle L, Basaria S, et al: Nebido: a long-acting injectable testosterone for the treatment of male hypogonadism. Expert Opin Pharmacother 2005;6: 1751–1759.

57 Boorjian SA, Bianco FJ Jr, et al: Does the time from biopsy to surgery affect biochemical recurrence after radical prostatectomy? BJU Int 2005;96: 773–776.

58 Graefen M, Walz J, et al: Reasonable delay of surgical treatment in men with localized prostate cancer – impact on prognosis? Eur Urol 2005;47:756–760.

59 Morgentaler A, Rhoden EL: Prevalence of prostate cancer among hypogonadal men with prostate-specific antigen levels of 4.0 ng/mL or less. Urology 2006;68:1263–1267.

60 Behre HM, Wang C, Handelsman DJ, Nieschlag E: Pharmacology of testosterone preparations; in Nieschlag E, Behre HM, Nieschlag S (eds): Testosterone, Action, Deficiency, Substitution, 3rd edition. Cambridge, Cambridge University Press, 2004.

Prof. Louis J.G. Gooren
Department of Endocrinology
VU University Medical Center, PO Box 7057
NL–1007 MB Amsterdam (The Netherlands)
Tel. +662 653 8066, Fax +31 20 4440502, E-Mail louisjgooren@gmail.com

Jones TH (ed): Advances in the Management of Testosterone Deficiency.
Front Horm Res. Basel, Karger, 2009, vol 37, pp 52–61

The Role of the CAG Repeat Androgen Receptor Polymorphism in Andrology

Michael Zitzmann

Institute of Reproductive Medicine, Universitätsklinikum Münster, Münster, Germany

Abstract

A dysfunctional androgen receptor is able to cause variable phenotypes of androgen insensitivity or androgenicity in humans. In addition, also a polymorphism, the CAG repeat polymorphism in exon 1 of the androgen receptor gene (CAG)n, modulates androgen effects: androgen-induced target activities are attenuated corresponding to the length of triplet residues. Clinically, the (CAG)n polymorphism causes marked modulations of androgenicity in eugonadal men in various tissues and psychological traits and may cause the clinical picture of hypogonadism in the presence of normal testosterone concentrations. Also pharmacogenetic implications might exist in this regard: there appears to be a significant role of testosterone treatment of hypogonadal men as treatment effects have been demonstrated to be modulated by the number of (CAG)n in retrospective approaches.

After binding of testosterone or dihydrotestosterone (DHT) to the androgen receptor (AR) and its consequent dimerization, the following steps in the cellular cascade of normal male sexual differentiation are initiated by activation of androgen-responsive target tissues via transcription of target genes. As complete insensitivity to androgens leads to a female phenotype [e.g. 1], maleness in general can be described as the sublimate of gender difference. Testosterone and its 5α-reductase metabolite DHT exert their effects on gene expression via the AR. A vast range of clinical conditions starting with complete androgen insensitivity have been correlated with mutations in the AR [1, 2].

More subtle modulations of the transcriptional activity induced by the AR have been observed as well and can frequently be assigned to a polyglutamine stretch of variable length within the n-terminal domain of the receptor protein. This stretch is encoded by a variable number of (CAG)n in exon 1 of the AR gene being located on the X-chromosome (fig. 1). First observations of pathologically elongated (CAG)n repeats in patients with X-linked spinobulbar muscular atrophy (X-SBMA) showing marked hypoandrogenic traits [3] were supplemented by findings of clinical significance also within the normal range of (CAG)n length.

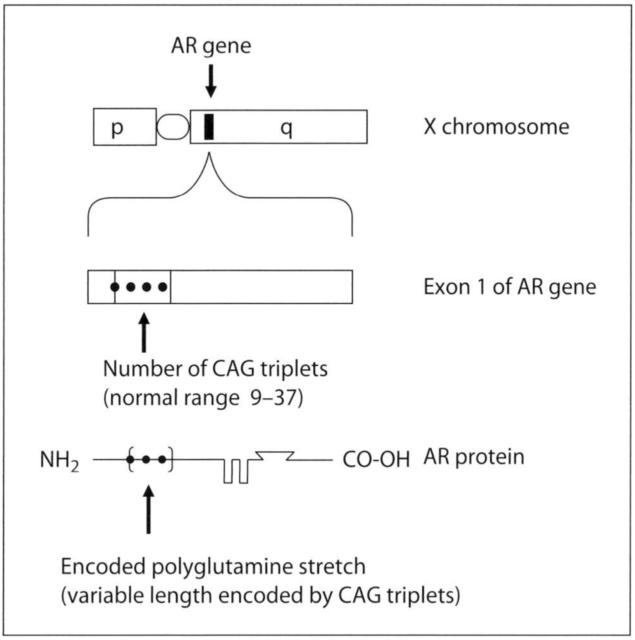

Fig. 1. X chromosome with the AR gene is shown. Exon 1 contains a variable number of (CAG)n encoding a polyglutamine stretch of variable length in the receptor protein. The number of (CAG)n or length of polyglutamine residues is inversely associated with the transcriptional activity of androgen- dependent genes, hence androgen effects in target tissues.

The modulatory effect on androgen-dependent gene transcription is most likely to be linear and mediated by causing a differential affinity of coactivator proteins to the encoded polyglutamine stretch. ARA24 and p160 are, for example, such proteins [4, 5]. As these proteins are ubiquitously but, notwithstanding, nonuniformly expressed, the modulatory effect of the (CAG)n polymorphism on AR target genes is most likely not only dependent on androgenic saturation and AR expression, but also varies between tissues. To date, an involvement of multiple human tissues has been demonstrated in this regard.

General Aspects of AR Functionality and Androgen Insensitivity in Humans

The AR is a ligand-activated transcription factor of androgen-regulated target genes. It is commonly assumed – although not precisely and experimentally proven – that a controlled temporal and spatial expression of androgen-regulated genes during early embryogenesis provokes a spectrum of functional and structural alterations of the internal and external genitalia ultimately resulting in the irreversible formation of the male phenotype [6].

The AR belongs to the intracellular group of structurally closely related steroid hormone receptors. Transcriptional regulation mediated by the AR is a complex and multistep process involving androgen binding, conformational changes of the protein (dimerization), receptor phosphorylation, nuclear trafficking, DNA binding, cofactor interaction and finally transcription activation. The human AR gene had been cloned and mapped to the short arm of the X chromosome (Xq11–12) [7–12]. It spans approximately 90 kb and comprises 8 exons. Transcription of the AR gene and subsequent splicing usually results in specific AR mRNA populations in various target tissues.

The AR shares its particular composition of three modular functional domains with the other steroid hormone receptors. A large n-terminal domain precedes the DNA-binding domain, followed by the c-terminal ligand-binding domain. Additionally, functional subdomains could be identified by in vitro investigation of artificially truncated and post-hoc deleted ARs [1]. Upon entering target cells, androgens interact specifically with the ligand-binding pocket of the AR, initiating a cascade of conformational changes and the consequent nuclear translocation of the AR. Prior to receptor binding to target DNA, homodimerization of two AR proteins occurs. This is mediated by sequences within the second zinc finger of the DNA-binding domain as well as through specific structural N-C-terminal interactions. The AR homodimer binds to hormone-responsive elements which usually consist of two palindromic sequences within the promoter regions of androgen-regulated genes. Through chromatin remodeling, an interaction with other transcription factors and specific coactivators and corepressors, a steroid receptor-specific modulation of the assembly of the preinitiation complex is achieved, which ultimately results in specific activation or repression of target gene transcription.

A multitude ($n > 350$) of mutations have been identified in androgen insensitivity syndroms (http://ww2.mcgill.ca/androgendb/). Extensive structural alterations of the AR can result from complete or partial deletions of the AR gene while smaller deletions introduce a frame shift into the open reading frame leading to a premature stop codon downstream of the mutation. Likewise, molecular consequences arise from the direct introduction of a premature stop codon due to point mutations. Such alterations usually lead to severe functional defects of the AR and are associated with androgen insensitivity syndromes. Extensive disruption of the AR protein structure can also be due to mutations leading to aberrant splicing of the AR mRNA [13, 14]. However, as aberrant splicing can be partial and thus enable expression of the wild-type AR, the phenotype is not necessarily complete but may also present partial androgen insensitivity [14]. However, the most common molecular defects of the AR gene are missense mutations [2].

The Role of CAG Repeat Polymorphisms of the AR in Various Target Organs: Subtle Modulation of Androgen Effects

A Mouse Model of the AR (CAG)n Polymorphism

To directly assess the functional significance of the AR (CAG)n polymorphism, the mouse AR, normally containing only one CAG repeat, was converted to the human sequence by germline gene targeting, introducing alleles with 12, 21 or 48 (CAG)n. The resulting three humanized AR mouse lines exhibited markedly different seminal vesicle weights as classic indicator of androgen effects in the presence of equivalent serum testosterone levels. Molecular analysis of AR-dependent target gene expression demonstrated in the prostate probasin, Nkx3.1 and clusterin mRNAs as being influenced by the number of (CAG)n. When crossed with transgenic adenocarcinoma of mouse prostate mice, genotype-dependent differences in prostate cancer prevalence were observed [15]. This confirms findings of AR (CAG)n-modulated gene expression in human prostate cancer cells [16].

Kennedy Syndrome: X-SBMA

X-SBMA or Kennedy syndrome is a rare inherited neurodegenerative disease which is characterized by progressive neuromuscular weakness due to a loss of motor neurons mainly in the spinal cord. Onset of the disease usually starts in the 3rd to 5th decade of life and is likely to be preceded by muscular cramps on exertion, tremor of the hands and elevated muscle creatine kinase. The initial description of individuals affected with Kennedy syndrome also includes gynecomastia, a symptom of hypoandrogenicity [17]. Reports that followed emphasized the presence of symptoms indicating the development of androgen insensitivity in men with X-SBMA exhibiting various degrees of gynecomastia, testicular atrophy, disorders of spermatogenesis, elevated serum gonadotropins and also diabetes mellitus [e.g. 18]. Hence, the AR was regarded as candidate gene for X-SBMA and the expansion of the polyglutamine repeat within the n-terminal region was later recognized as the cause [3]. The longer the CAG repeat tract in the AR gene, the earlier is the onset of the disease; furthermore, (CAG)n length correlates with electrophysiological motor and sensory dysfunctionality in SBMA as well as severity of symptoms of hypogonadism [19, 20]. The absence of any neuromuscular deficit or degeneration in patients with complete androgen insensitivity [1] suggests that neurological deficits in X-SBMA are not caused by a lack of androgen influence but rather by a neurotoxic effect associated with the pathologically elongated number of (CAG)n, which causes irregular processing of the AR protein and accumulation of end products [21].

Prostate Development and Malignancy

The prostate is an androgen-sensitive organ. Henceforth, it can be assumed that a polymorphism of the AR with the capacity to modulate androgen effects has an influence on the fate of malignant cells in the prostate. Epidemiological findings in humans concerning the incidence of prostate cancer suggest an influence by (CAG)n polymorphism: a review of numerous studies described an odds ratio of 1.19 for prostate cancer with decreasing (CAG)n [22], corroborating the findings in mouse models (see A Mouse Model of the AR (CAG)n Polymorphism above). Epidemiological findings in humans concerning the incidence of prostate cancer suggest an influence by this AR polymorphism in different human races [23].

The putative relation between benign hyperplasia of the prostate (BPH) and the (CAG)n polymorphism of the AR gene is another aspect. BPH consists of the overgrowth of tissue within the transition zone and periurethral area of the prostate. This is histologically defined as epithelial and fibromuscular hyperplasia. The putative relation between BPH and the (CAG)n polymorphism of the AR gene has been investigated. The two largest studies comparing matched healthy controls and BPH patients describe the odds ratio for BPH surgery or an enlarged prostate gland to be 1.92 when comparing (CAG)n <20 to >24 or more. For a six-repeat decrement in CAG repeat length, the odds ratio for moderate or severe urinary obstructive symptoms from an enlarged prostate gland was 3.62 [24, 25]. Similarly, adenoma or organ size was found to be inversely associated with (CAG)n length in various approaches [26, 27].

Reproductive Functions

The stimulation of Sertoli cells by FSH is a prerequisite in primate spermatogenesis and, thus, intratesticular androgen activity represents an important cofactor that has a positive effect on the support function of Sertoli cells. Hence, it can be assumed that the (CAG)n polymorphism might have an influence on spermatogenesis. Such an effect can be observed as severely impaired spermatogenesis in X-SBMA patients [18]. The investigation of the possible influence of a polyglutamine stretch within the normal length on sperm production requires a sample of carefully selected patients in whom significant confounders such as obstructive symptoms due to infections, congenital aplasia of the vas deferens, impaired spermatogenesis due to chromosome or hormone disorders or deletions in one of the azoospermia-associated regions of the Y chromosome have been ruled out. A recent meta-analysis summarizing the results of such approaches reports a negative association of (CAG)n length with the efficacy of spermatogenesis [28].

Bone Tissue

Androgen activity influences bone metabolism and respective observations apply to the (CAG)n polymorphism of the AR gene: in 110 healthy younger males, a high number of (CAG)n was significantly associated with lower bone density [29]. This result is corroborated by a negative association between (CAG)n length and bone density at the femoral neck in a group of 508 Caucasian men aged over 65 years [30]. The same workgroup also observed an increased vertebral fracture risk among older men with longer (CAG)n [31]. In a group of 140 Finnish men aged 50–60 years, lumbar and femoral bone mineral density values were higher in those men with shorter (CAG)n in comparison to those with longer (CAG)n [32]. The differences reached statistical significance when the groups with (CAG)n of 15–17 and (CAG)n of 22–26 were compared directly. A higher risk for osteoporotic fractures was also observed in a large cohort of postmenopausal women with longer (CAG)n [33].

Psychological Implications

Testosterone supplementation in hypogonadal men attenuates melancholic or depressive aspects [34]. Accordingly, treatment with testosterone gel improves symptoms in men with refractory depression [35]. In addition, it has been demonstrated in 1,000 older men that this mood dependency on androgen levels is modified by the (CAG)n polymorphism. Depression scores were significantly and inversely associated with testosterone levels in subjects with shorter (CAG)n, while this was not observed in men with moderate and longer polyglutamine stretches in the AR protein. Low versus high testosterone in such men was associated with a 5-fold increased likelihood of depressive mood [36].

In a sample of 172 Finnish men aged 41–70 years, there was a significant association independent of testosterone levels of the length of (CAG)n with symptom scores concerning depression, as expressed by the wish to be dead, depressed mood, anxiety and deterioration of general well-being [37]. This is corroborated by a recent interracial approach to depression [38].

Male Patients with Abnormal Karyotype (Klinefelter 47,XXY and 46,XX Males)

In Klinefelter patients, who have two AR alleles due to their 47,XXY karyotype, the shorter CAG repeat allele is preferentially inactive. In this group of patients, CAG repeat length is positively associated with body height, while bone density and the relation of arm span to body height are inversely related to CAG repeat length. The presence of long CAG repeats was seen as predictive for gynecomastia, while shorter CAG repeats were associated with a stable partnership and professions requiring higher standards of education [39]. Also aspects of puberty and masculinization of younger Klinefelter patients seem to be influenced by this polymorphism, with those boys with longer CAG repeats exhibiting mitigated androgen effects [40, 41].

In addition, in men with the abnormal karyotype of 46,XX, the so-called XX males, associations of (CAG)n length with hormone constellations and hematocrit as a marker of androgenization can be observed [42].

Pharmacogenetic Aspects of Testosterone Therapy

Considering the observations in eugonadal men, it can be assumed that testosterone therapy in hypogonadal men should have a differential impact on androgen target tissue, depending on (CAG)n length. A longitudinal pharmacogenetic study in 131 hypogonadal men demonstrated that prostate volume is influenced before and under androgen substitution. The length of (CAG)n, sex hormone levels and anthropometric measures were investigated. Initial prostate size of hypogonadal men was dependent on age and baseline testosterone levels, but not the (CAG)n polymorphism. However, when prostate size increased significantly during therapy, prostate growth per year and absolute prostate size under substituted androgen levels were strongly dependent on the polymorphism, with lower treatment effects in longer repeats. Other modulators of prostate growth were age and testosterone level being treated. This first pharmacogenetic study on androgen substitution in hypogonadal men demonstrates a marked influence of the CAG repeat polymorphism on prostate growth [43]. In subsequent evaluations of men receiving long-acting preparations of the intramuscular testosterone undecanoate, it was demonstrated that the increment of hematocrit, which is usually observed upon replenishment of androgen resources in hypogonadal men, is strongly modulated by the (CAG)n polymorphism [44].

A retrospective approach concerning pharmacogenetic influences in hormonal male contraception demonstrated that, as spermatogenesis is partially dependent on intratesticular androgen activity, sperm counts are more easily suppressed by various pharmacological regimens in men with longer (CAG)n in the subgroup with remnant gonadotropin activity [45].

Another aspect of the pharmacogenetic influence of the CAG repeat polymorphism is the susceptibility of male pattern baldness to the treatment with finasteride. Men with shorter CAG repeat tracts respond significantly better to this treatment than men with longer CAG repeats. However, the effect may not be pharmacogenetic, but rather a selection phenomenon: the men with shorter repeat tracts are probably those with androgenically induced baldness and are thus more susceptible to a reduction of DHT [46]. Also the increase in bone mineral density in postmenopausal women receiving hormone replacement therapy is more significant in those women with shorter (CAG)n [47].

Outlook

Further decoding of the molecular and biochemical pathways is necessary for a comprehensive understanding of normal and abnormal sexual determination and differentiation, especially in regard to AR coactivators and corepressors. Based on molecular defects of impaired human sexual development, achievements in the field of genomics and proteomics offer unique opportunities to identify the genetic programs downstream of known androgen pathways which are ultimately responsible for structure and function of a normal or abnormal genital phenotype.

The highly polymorphic nature of glutamine residues within the AR protein, which is encoded by the (CAG)n polymorphism of the AR gene, causes a subtle gradation of androgenicity among individuals. As the pharmacogenetic implication of this polymorphism seems to play an important role as modulator of treatment effects in hypogonadal men, it has become evident that these insights are important enough to become part of individually useful laboratory assessments.

References

1 Quigley CA, De Bellis A, Marschke KB, el-Awady MK, Wilson EM, French FS: Androgen receptor defects: historical, clinical, and molecular perspectives. Endocr Rev 1995;16:271–321.

2 Hiort O, Sinnecker GHG, Holterhus PM, Nitsche EM, Kruse K: The clinical and molecular spectrum of androgen insensitivity. Am J Med Genet 1996; 63:218–222.

3 La Spada AR, Wilson EM, Lubahn DB, Harding AE, Fischbeck KH: Androgen receptor gene mutations in X-linked spinal and bulbar muscular atrophy. Nature 1991;352:77–79.

4 Hsiao PW, Thin TH, Lin DL, Chang C: Differential regulation of testosterone vs. 5alpha-dihydrotestosterone by selective androgen response elements. Mol Cell Biochem 2000;206:169–175.

5 Irvine RA, Ma H, Yu MC, Ross RK, Stallcup MR, Coetzee GA: Inhibition of p160-mediated coactivation with increasing androgen receptor polyglutamine length. Hum Mol Genet 2002;9:267–274.

6 Holterhus PM, Hiort O, Demeter J, Brown PO, Brooks JD: Differential gene-expression patterns in genital fibroblasts of normal males and 46,XY females with androgen insensitivity syndrome: evidence for early programming involving the androgen receptor. Genome Biol 2003;4:R37.

7 Chang C, Kokontis J, Liao S: Structural analysis of complementary DNA and amino acid sequences of human and rat androgen receptors. Proc Natl Acad Sci USA 1988;85:7211–7215.

8 Chang C, Kokontis J, Liao S: Molecular cloning of human and rat complementary DNA encoding androgen receptors. Science 1988;240:324–326.

9 Lubahn DB, Joseph DR, Sar M, Tan J-A, Higgs HN, Larson RE, French FS, Wilson EM: The human androgen receptor: complementary deoxyribonucleic acid cloning, sequence analysis and gene expression in prostate. Mol Endocrinol 1988;2:1265–1275.

10 Lubahn DB, Joseph DR, Sullivan PM, Willard HF, French FS, Wilson EM: Cloning of human androgen receptor complementary DNA and localization to the X chromosome. Science 1988;240:327–330.

11 Tilley WD, Marcelli M, Wilson JD, McPhaul MJ: Characterization and expression of a cDNA encoding the human androgen receptor. Proc Natl Acad Sci USA 1989;86:327–331.

12 Trapman J, Klaassen P, Kuiper GGJM, van der Korput JAGM, Faber PW, van Rooij HCJ, Geurts van Kessel A, Voorhorst MM, Mulder E, Brinkmann AO: Cloning, structure and expression of a cDNA encoding the human androgen receptor. Biochem Biophys Res Commun 1988;153:241–248.

13 Hellwinkel OJ, Bull K, Holterhus PM, Homburg N, Struve D, Hiort O: Complete androgen insensitivity caused by a splice donor site mutation in intron 2 of the human androgen receptor gene resulting in an exon 2-lacking transcript with premature stop-codon and reduced expression. J Steroid Biochem Mol Biol 1999;68:1–9.

14 Hellwinkel OJC, Holterhus PM, Struve D, Homburg N, Hiort O: A unique exonic splicing mutation in the human androgen receptor gene demonstrates the physiologic relevance of regular androgen receptor transcript variants. J Clin Endocrinol Metab 2001; 86:2569–2575.

15 Albertelli MA, Scheller A, Brogley M, Robins DM: Replacing the mouse androgen receptor with human alleles demonstrates glutamine tract length-dependent effects on physiology and tumorigenesis in mice. Mol Endocrinol 2006;20:1248–1260.

16 Coutinho-Camillo CM, Miracca EC, dos Santos ML, Salaorni S, Sarkis AS, Nagai MA: Identification of differentially expressed genes in prostatic epithelium in relation to androgen receptor CAG repeat length. Int J Biol Markers 2006;21:96–105.

17 Kennedy WR, Alter M, Sung JH: Progressive proximal spinal and bulbar muscular atrophy of late onset. Neurology 1968;18:671–680.

18 Arbizu T, Santamaria J, Gomez JM, Quilez A, Serra JP: A family with adult onset spinal and bulbar muscular atrophy X-linked inheritance and associated testicular failure. J Neurol Sci 1983;59:371–382.

19 Dejager S, Bry-Gauillard H, Bruckert E, Eymard B, Salachas F, LeGuern E, Tardieu S, Chadarevian R, Giral P, Turpin G: A comprehensive endocrine description of Kennedy's disease revealing androgen insensitivity linked to CAG repeat length. J Clin Endocrinol Metab 2002;87:3893–3901.

20 Suzuki K, Katsuno M, Banno H, Takeuchi Y, Atsuta N, Ito M, Watanabe H, Yamashita F, Hori N, Nakamura T, Hirayama M, Tanaka F, Sobue G: CAG repeat size correlates to electrophysiological motor and sensory phenotypes in SBMA. Brain 2008;131: 229–239.

21 Abdullah A, Trifiro MA, Panet-Raymond V, Alvarado C, de Tourreil S, Frankel D, Schipper HM, Pinsky L: Spinobulbar muscular atrophy: polyglutamine-expanded androgen receptor is proteolytically resistant in vitro and processed abnormally in transfected cells. Hum Mol Genet 1998;7:379–384.

22 Zeegers MP, Kiemeney LA, Nieder AM, Ostrer H: How strong is the association between CAG and GGN repeat length polymorphisms in the androgen receptor gene and prostate cancer risk? Cancer Epidemiol Biomarkers Prev 2004;13:1765–1771.

23 Giwercman C, Giwercman A, Pedersen HS, Toft G, Lundin K, Bonde JP, Lundberg GY: Polymorphisms in genes regulating androgen activity among prostate cancer low-risk Inuit men and high-risk Scandinavians. Int J Androl 2008;31:25–30.
24 Giovannucci E, Stampfer MJ, Chan A, Krithivas K, Gann PH, Hennekens CH, Kantoff PW: CAG repeat within the androgen receptor gene and incidence of surgery for benign prostatic hyperplasia in U.S. physicians. Prostate 1999;39:130–134.
25 Giovannucci E, Platz EA, Stampfer MJ, Chan A, Krithivas K, Kawachi I, Willett WC, Kantoff PW: The CAG repeat within the androgen receptor gene and benign prostatic hyperplasia. Urology 1999;53: 121–125.
26 Mitsumori K, Terai A, Oka H, Segawa T, Ogura K, Yoshida O, Ogawa O: Androgen receptor CAG repeat length polymorphism in benign prostatic hyperplasia (BPH): correlation with adenoma growth. Prostate 1999;41:253–257.
27 Larré S, Hamadeh H, Azzouzi AR, Vallancien G, Cochand-Priollet B, Cancel-Tassin G, Cussenot O: Genetic impact on prostate anatomical variability during ageing: role of CYP17, SRD5A2 and androgen receptor genes polymorphisms. BJU Int 2007; 100:679–684.
28 Davis-Dao CA, Tuazon ED, Sokol RZ, Cortessis VK: Male infertility and variation in CAG repeat length in the androgen receptor gene: a meta-analysis. J Clin Endocrinol Metab 2007;92:4319–4326.
29 Zitzmann M, Brune M, Kornmann B, Gromoll J, Junker R, Nieschlag E: The CAG repeat polymorphism in the androgen receptor gene affects bone density and bone metabolism in healthy males. Clin Endocrinol 2001;55:649–657.
30 Zmuda JM, Cauley JA, Kuller LH, Newman AB, Robbins J, Harris T, Ferrell RE: Androgen receptor CAG repeat polymorphism: a novel marker of osteoporotic risk in men. Osteoporosis Int 2000;11:S151.
31 Zmuda JM, Cauley JA, Kuller LH, Zhang X, Palermo L, Nevitt MC, Ferrell RE: Androgen receptor CAG repeat length is associated with increased hip bone loss and vertebral fracture risk among older men. J Bone Miner Res 2000;15:S491, M141.
32 Remes T, Vaisanen SB, Mahonen A, Huuskonen J, Kroger H, Jurvelin JS, Penttila IM, Rauramaa R: Aerobic exercise and bone mineral density in middle-aged Finnish men: a controlled randomized trial with reference to androgen receptor aromatase and estrogen receptor alpha gene polymorphisms. Bone 2003;32:412–420.
33 Langdahl BL, Stenkjaer L, Carstens M, Tofteng CL, Eriksen EF: A CAG repeat polymorphism in the androgen receptor gene is associated with reduced bone mass and increased risk of osteoporotic fractures. Calcif Tissue Int 2003;73:237–243.
34 Burris AS, Banks SM, Carter CS, Davidson JM, Sherins RJ: A long-term prospective study of the physiologic and behavioural effects of hormone replacement in untreated hypogonadal men. J Androl 1992;13:297–304.
35 Pope HG, Cohane GH, Kanayama G, Siegel AJ, Hudson JI: Testosterone Gel supplementation for men with refractory depression: a randomized placebo-controlled trial. Am J Psychiatry 2003;160: 105–111.
36 Seidman SN, Araujo AB, Roose SP, McKinlay JB: Testosterone level androgen receptor polymorphism and depressive symptoms in middle-aged men. Biol Psychol 2001;50:371–376.
37 Harkonen K, Huhtaniemi I, Makinen J, Hübler D, Irjala K, Koskenvuo M, Oettel M, Raitakari O, Saad F, Pollanen P: The polymorphic androgen receptor gene CAG repeat pituitary-testicular function and andropausal symptoms in ageing men. Int J Androl 2003;26:187–194.
38 Colangelo LA, Sharp L, Kopp P, Scholtens D, Chiu BC, Liu K, Gapstur SM: Total testosterone, androgen receptor polymorphism, and depressive symptoms in young black and white men: the CARDIA Male Hormone Study. Psychoneuroendocrinology 2007;32:951–958.
39 Zitzmann M, Depenbusch M, Gromoll J, Nieschlag E: X-chromosome inactivation patterns and androgen receptor functionality influence phenotype and social characteristics as well as pharmacogenetics of testosterone therapy in Klinefelter patients. J Clin Endocrinol Metab 2004;89:6208–6217.
40 Zinn AR, Ramos P, Elder FF, Kowal K, Samango-Sprouse C, Ross JL: Androgen receptor CAGn repeat length influences phenotype of 47,XXY (Klinefelter) syndrome. J Clin Endocrinol Metab 2005;90:5041–5046.
41 Wikstrom AM, Painter JN, Raivio T, Aittomaki K, Dunkel L: Genetic features of the X chromosome affect pubertal development and testicular degeneration in adolescent boys with Klinefelter syndrome. Clin Endocrinol (Oxf) 2006;65:92–97.
42 Vorona E, Zitzmann M, Gromoll J, Schüring AN, Nieschlag E: Clinical, endocrinological, and epigenetic features of the 46,XX male syndrome, compared with 47,XXY Klinefelter patients. J Clin Endocrinol Metab 2007;92:3458–3465.
43 Zitzmann M, Depenbusch M, Gromoll J, Nieschlag E: Prostate volume and growth in testosterone-substituted hypogonadal men are dependent on the CAG repeat polymorphism of the androgen receptor gene: a longitudinal pharmacogenetic study. J Clin Endocrinol Metab 2003;88:2049–2054.

44 Zitzmann M, Nieschlag E: Androgen receptor gene CAG repeat length and body mass index modulate the safety of long-term intramuscular testosterone undecanoate therapy in hypogonadal men. J Clin Endocrinol Metab 2007;92:3844–3853.
45 Von Eckardstein S, Schmidt A, Kamischke A, Simoni M, Gromoll J, Nieschlag E: CAG repeat length in the androgen receptor gene and gonadotrophin suppression influence the effectiveness of hormonal male contraception. Clin Endocrinol 2002;57: 647–655.
46 Wakisaka N, Taira Y, Ishikawa M, Nakamizo Y, Kobayashi K, Uwabu M, Fukuda Y, Taguchi Y, Hama T, Kawakami M: Effectiveness of finasteride on patients with male pattern baldness who have different androgen receptor gene polymorphism. J Investig Dermatol Symp Proc 2005;10:293–294.
47 Retornaz F, Paris F, Lumbroso S, Audran F, Tigoulet F, Michelon C, Jeandel C, Sultan C, Blain H: Association between androgen receptor gene polymorphism and bone density in older women using hormone replacement therapy. Maturitas 2006;55: 325–333.

Prof. Dr. Michael Zitzmann, MD, PhD
Institute of Reproductive Medicine
Universitätsklinikum Münster, Domagkstrasse 11
DE–48149 Münster (Germany)
Tel. +49 251 83 56 104, Fax +49 251 83 56 093, E-Mail Michael.Zitzmann@ukmuenster.de

Jones TH (ed): Advances in the Management of Testosterone Deficiency.
Front Horm Res. Basel, Karger, 2009, vol 37, pp 62–73

Late-Onset Hypogonadism

Louis J.G. Gooren

Department of Endocrinology, VU University Medical Center, Amsterdam, The Netherlands

Abstract

With aging, a significant percentage of men over the age of 60 years have serum testosterone levels below the lower limits of young adult men. Testosterone is not only pivotal for male reproductive/sexual functioning but plays also a significant role in the maintenance of bone and muscle mass and is a determinant of glucose homeostasis and lipid metabolism. The metabolic syndrome, erectile dysfunction and patterns of testosterone in aging men are intertwined. Testosterone is a factor in libido but also exerts essential effects on the anatomical and physiological substrate of penile erection. With these recent insights, the health problems of elderly men must be placed in a context that allows an integral approach. Treatment of testosterone deficiency is to become part of this approach. Recently, professional organizations have published guidelines in an attempt to define the condition and provide treatment. Despite this, much confusion still exists regarding the appropriate approach to diagnosing late-onset hypogonadism. Side effects concern mainly the prostate and erythropoeisis, but the currently available literature indicates that there is no increased risk of developing prostate cancer in men receiving testosterone treatment. Administration of testosterone to elderly men with testosterone deficiency is an acceptably safe practice.

Aging can be viewed as a time-related functional decline of health into the frailty of old age, with an ever-increasing vulnerability to disease and eventually to death. Age changes will occur in every human being given sufficient time to live. Probably, all we can do about aging is to: '*prevent the preventable and delay the inevitable*' [1].

Among the many processes of aging, endocrine changes are relatively easy to identify and quantify with the presently available methods for determining hormone levels, which are reliable and sensitive. The question has been raised whether a counterpart to menopause exists in the male. It has become clear that levels of testosterone do, indeed, show an age-related decline but the characteristics of this age-related decline of testosterone are so fundamentally different from the menopause that drawing parallels generates more confusion than clarity. In men, testosterone production is affected in a slowly progressive way as part of the normal aging process. It will rarely be manifest in men under the age of 50 years and usually becomes only quantitatively significant in men over 60 years of age (for review, see Kaufman and

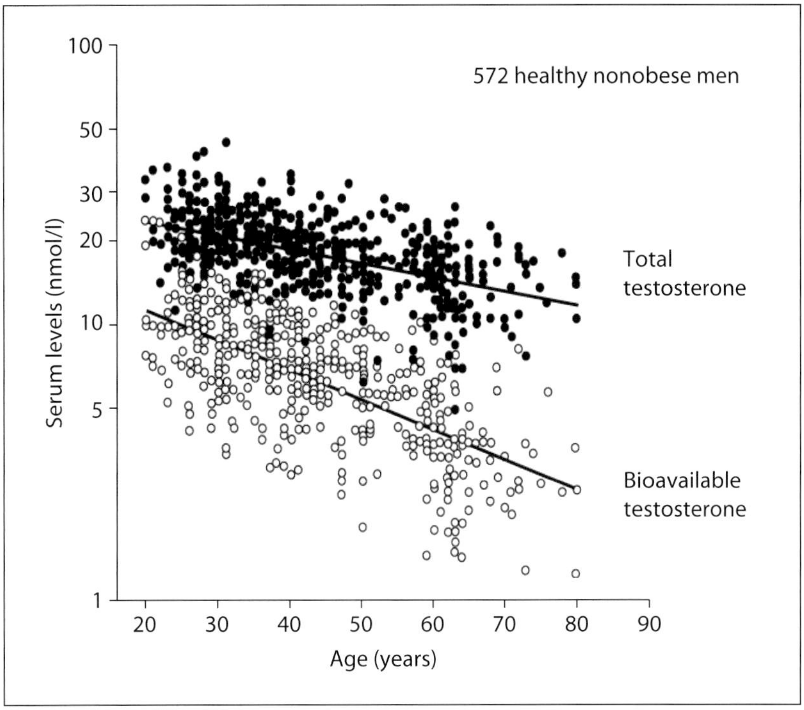

Fig. 1. Age-related changes of testosterone in healthy men [3].

Vermeulen [2]). This age-related decline of testosterone shows considerable interindividual variation. Some men in their 80s will still have fairly normal testosterone levels [3] (fig. 1). Disease is a strong predictor of the age-related decline of plasma testosterone [4–6]. It has been argued that lifestyle changes (reduction/prevention of obesity) may decelerate the age-related decline of plasma testosterone [7].

Unlike the menopause, the age-associated decline of testosterone does not present itself in an 'all or none' fashion. The vast majority of women are able to retrospectively identify their age of menopause. Men are unable to pinpoint the start of their decline of testosterone. So, the age-related decline of testosterone calls for terminology not reminiscent of the female menopause.

Adequate Terminology

The discourse of a certain condition may go through profound changes in the light of certain developments, outcomes of studies, and, more importantly, how these findings are subsequently interpreted and construed by the community of experts, the media and patient interest groups. This applies to the conceptualization of the hormonal changes of the aging male. Much of the conceptualization of the pathophysiological relevance of these hormonal changes and of the potential risks/benefits of androgen replacement in old age has been profoundly influenced by the scientific discourse of the menopause. First and foremost its conceptualization and designation as 'male menopause' or 'climacterium virile'. The first reports by Werner [8] in 1939, Heller and Myers [9] in 1944, and about 10 years later McGavack [10] drew a close parallel with the female menopause. The male climacteric 'strikes at the core of what it is to be a man [...] his youthful sexual drive and performance' and includes such symptoms as hot flushes, depression, insomnia, mood swings, irritability, impotence, decreased libido, weakness, lethargy and loss of bone mass. Because of the inadequacy of the terms male menopause and male climacterium, the term 'andropause' has been proposed which is still widely used and the term generates a large amount of articles when used as a search term in databases, even though it is an inappropriate term to describe the events of hormonal changes in aging men. For the reasons given above, they should not be used. (Partial) androgen decline in the aging male (ADAM or PADAM) is a better description, but is also ambiguous. The term late-onset hypogonadism (LOH) is probably now the preferred term [11, 12]. While being an acceptable term, it is of note that the testosterone deficiency in LOH is usually less profound and less manifest than in other hypogonadal states, but may nevertheless be clinically significant and deserves the attention of the medical profession.

In a recent paper, some authorities in the field of health issues of the aging male have eloquently argued for more accurate terminology of the age-related decline in testosterone levels [13]. Firstly, the authors point out that the decline makes a start in mid-life [4], not in old age, arguing that it is more fitting not to include age or late onset (as in 'late-onset hypogonadism') in the terminology. It may be counter-argued that admittedly plasma testosterone starts to decline in midlife, but at that stage plasma testosterone does not fall below levels which qualify as hypogonadal, levels that as yet have not been established in clinical trials. Secondly, an even more important point was in their view that decline of testosterone levels is not a universal or inevitable effect of aging [13]. Thirdly, they argue not to use the term androgens but testosterone: for the diagnosis of testosterone deficiency plasma levels of testosterone are determined, and in cases of severe enough deficiency, treatment with testosterone is supplied. They advise against the use of the term hypogonadism in this context arguing that hypogonadism is synonymous with pathological testosterone deficiency arising from specific diseases or dysfunctions of the hypothalamic-pituitary-testicular axis which generally require specialized investigations, in their view quite different from the age-related decline in testosterone in terms of both etiology and severity. Their recommendation is to adopt the term 'testosterone deficiency syndrome' (TDS) and where necessary to compliment TDS by 'in the elderly' or 'in diabetes', etc. [13]. Though there is statistically, a decline of plasma testosterone levels with aging, the authors have a valid point in stressing that aging per se, is not the main determinant of the statistical decline of plasma testosterone but age-associated conditions such as the metabolic syndrome or ailments common in aging men. They advise against use of the term hypogonadism (as, in for instance, 'late onset hypogonadism') but use of the term hypogonadism makes clear that only those men with a testosterone deficiency of such a severity that qualifies as hypogonadism are of concern, and not those men, at least with the present insight into the matter, whose testosterone have been declining with aging and of whom it is less than certain that they as a category will benefit from testosterone treatment. For the latter category, it remains to be demonstrated whether they constitute a clinically relevant entity. Further, the value of inclusion of the 'aging', 'age-related' or 'late onset' in the terminology draws attention to the possibility that a limited number of elderly men, suffering from ailments, have such low plasma testosterone levels that they might qualify for testosterone treatment. If 'aging' or 'late onset' is not included in the terminology these men will be overlooked in medical practice, as has been the case until recently when an awareness of the potentiality of a clinically significant decline of testosterone levels with aging has emerged. So, while debunking that aging as such is an indication for androgen treatment, the authors should not forget that ailments of which aging is the most powerful predictor, might lead to a state of testosterone deficiency qualifying for testosterone treatment. It is difficult to coin adequate terminology as long as only the contours of the problem are clear but the details remain uncharted. If there is a clinically relevant problem with the decline of plasma testosterone in elderly men, it is predominantly found in elderly men who are not healthy [2, 4, 5]. Elderly men in good health statistically have plasma testosterone levels within the reference range.

The notion of an andropause or male menopause, or as it is termed now LOH, is not rarely viewed with some skepticism by the medical profession [14]. This is a concept that all too readily lends itself to opportunistic exploitation by anti-aging entrepreneurs, usually working outside the public health sector, who tout 'rejuvenation cures'. The history of this field, which includes names like Voronoff and Lespinasse and, surprisingly, even such reputable scientists as Brown-Sequard and Steinach, is not a proud one [15]. It is feared that those who peddle the indiscriminate use of androgens, growth hormone, melatonin and adrenal androgens will perpetuate this quackery in the present time [14]. Only well-designed studies into the endocrinology of aging, with clear clinical objectives and proper terminology, can ensure that history does not repeat itself and that the baby is not thrown out with the bathwater. Questions as to who will benefit from testosterone treatment, and how safe testosterone treatment of elderly males is, are therefore timely and important.

Neuroendocrine Mechanisms Explaining the Decline of Testosterone with Aging

Most of the hormone deficiencies associated with aging are based on neuroendocrine mechanisms [16]. One of the best known examples of an age-related decline of hormones is the menopause. Originally believed to result from 'exhaustion of the ovary', it is becoming clear that neuroendocrine mechanisms orchestrate the loss of reproductive capacity in women. Its sequels can be alleviated by the administration of estrogens, the end products of ovarian hormone production, though this clinical practice is now hotly debated [17, 18]. The basis of the decline of testosterone is also to a large extent, but not exclusively, explained by neuroendocrine mechanisms, all leading to a diminished stimulation of the pituitary to produce the stimulatory hormone of the peripheral endocrine gland. Healthy elderly men maintain high-frequency but low-amplitude LH secretion patterns. Further, there is evidence that, with the same circulating levels of testicular steroids, the feedback signal to the hypothalamus is stronger than in younger men, thus diminishing the output of LH when testosterone levels decline [2, 19]. The patterns of LH release are significantly more disorderly. These observations indicate that age reduces hypothalamic LHRH outflow (release and delivery) to the gonadotrope cells in the pituitary [20]. Most studies agree that the capacity of the pituitary to secrete LH and FSH is not seriously affected with aging. It has also been found in obese men that that there is an attenuated pulse amplitude of luteinizing hormone (LH) while the LH pulse frequency is unaffected, thus producing a less strong stimulation of testicular testosterone production [21, 22].

It is not only the reproductive hormones that decline with aging. The production of the sleep-related pineal hormone melatonin declines with aging. Adrenal androgens levels start to decline in both sexes from the age of 30 years (adrenopause), becoming very low at and beyond age 80 years. The levels of the main adrenal hormone cortisol do not fall with aging. The question has arisen whether the imbalance between the catabolic cortisol and anabolic testosterone contributes to the sarcopenia of old age [23]. Growth hormone secretion also undergoes an age-related decline (somatopause). While insulin levels generally do not fall with aging, sensitivity to the biological action of insulin decreases considerably with aging. Changes in calcium, water and electrolyte metabolism and thyroid function all characterize aging. These changes often have clinical relevance. Hypothyroidism or hyperthyroidism may be associated with forms of senile dementia, a diagnosis that can often be overlooked. Asthenia and muscle weakness may find their cause in disturbances of the electrolytes or androgen and growth hormone physiology. Therefore, the relationship between aging and hormonal changes is a two-way street: aging affects the endocrine system but age-related endocrine dysfunction also produces symptoms of the aging process.

Obviously, it would be simple-minded to interpret all age-related changes of hormones as deficiencies awaiting correction [24]. There is still substantial research to be done to ascertain whether the replacement of age-related reductions in hormone production is meaningful and, even more so, whether it is safe. Hormones such as estrogens, androgens and growth hormone are potential factors in the development and growth of tumors that occur in old age.

Factors Acting at the Level of the Leydig Cell Accounting for the Decline of Testosterone with Aging

There are primary testicular changes leading a diminished testicular secretory capacity; Stimulation with human chorionic gonadotropin (hCG) [25], with pulsatile administration of GnRH [26], or with biosynthetic LH after downregulation of endogenous LH secretion with leuprolide [26] has consistently revealed a diminished secretory capacity of the Leydig cells in the elderly compared with young men. This decrease in testicular secretory reserve appears to involve a reduction of the number of Leydig cells [27]. In old rats at least, all enzymes involved in the synthesis of testosterone are decreased with aging, as is the steroidogenic acute regulatory protein, which is involved in the transport of cholesterol into mitochondria [28]. There is also evidence for a shift in testicular androgen biosynthesis favoring the Δ 4 over the Δ 5 steroids, analogous to the situation for the adrenals [29]. In healthy, community-dwelling men over age 75 years, mean testicular volume is reduced by about 30% relative to that in young men [30].

Aging is very commonly associated with an increase in body weight and adiposity appears to contribute to a less-efficacious steroidogenesis of the Leydig cell. The adipocyte functions as an endocrine cell and produces molecules with regulatory potential, the so-called adipocytokines/adipokines of which leptin is a prominent member. Leptin may be a factor in the association between adiposity and decreased testosterone levels. In men there is a correlation between body mass index and fat mass on the one hand and leptin levels on the other. Leptin receptors are present on the Leydig cell and inhibit the testosterone generated by administration of human chorionic gonadotropin [31, 32]. These findings were supported by studies that found a negative correlation between adiposity, insulin and leptin on the one hand and testosterone levels on the other [33, 34]. Insulin is an important determinant of leptin levels. Feeding and overfeeding increase insulin levels which leads, in turn, to an increase in leptin, and vice versa [35].

Hyperinsulinemia as encountered in insulin resistance might impair testosterone secretion by the Leydig cell, maybe directly since there are insulin receptors on the Leydig cell [36]. Insulin and IGF-1 promotes T responsiveness to hCG, so hyperinsulinemia as a reflection of insulin resistance may lead to an impairment of testosterone secretion. In large epidemiological studies obesity appears indeed to be a factor in a larger age-related decline of plasma testosterone [4–7].

Correlation studies cannot unravel the cause and effect relationships between the correlates whether low testosterone/low SHBG induces visceral fat deposition or whether a large visceral fat depot leads to low testosterone levels but a combination is likely. Therefore, the effects of weight changes are illuminating. Weight gain in men leads to a preferential accumulation of fat in the visceral depot. It is associated with a decrease in plasma SHBG and usually with a decrease in plasma testosterone but at least there is a significant negative correlation between changes of visceral fat and of plasma testosterone. A further positive correlation that appeared was between fasting insulin and changes in abdominal fat and in testosterone [37]. Plasma levels of insulin are negatively correlated with SHBG and testosterone [38]. Conversely, weight loss, either produced an increase of testosterone itself [39] and/or an increase in SHBG. The rise in testosterone levels correlated inversely with loss of abdominal fat and with plasma insulin. Collectively, these studies suggest that a high degree of visceral adiposity is associated with high insulin levels and low SHBG levels and low total plasma testosterone and with an increase of metabolites of testosterone, and vice versa. The above observations were in healthy young men, but similar observations have been made in men with the metabolic syndrome [40, 41]. Therefore, the conclusion seems warranted that increases/decreases in body weight are associated with higher/lower insulin levels and with lower/higher SHBG levels and with lower/higher plasma testosterone.

Role of Sex Hormone-Binding Globulin

With aging, in general an Increase of plasma levels of sex hormone-binding globulin (SHBG) is observed. This provides an explanation why the plasma levels total testosterone fall less then levels of bioavailable and free testosterone in aging men. In young men an increase of binding capacity will be compensated for through the testosterone feedback regulation and total serum testosterone will increase and free testosterone levels will be maintained, as is the case, for instance, in young adult men with thyrotoxicosis [42]. In the healthy elderly, however, the increase in plasma testosterone-binding capacity is accompanied by a decrease of the nonspecifically bound fractions of testosterone, because it occurs against the background of the aforementioned testicular and neuroendocrine changes operating in aging. The substantial age-related increase of SHBG (about 1.2%/year) is somewhat paradoxical. Most aging show a degree of obesity and an increase of fat mass and insulin levels are strong negative determinants of SHBG levels [43]. It seems unlikely that the decreased plasma testosterone or the associated decrease of the plasma testosterone/estradiol ratio would be the explanation, because the increase of SHBG seems to begin at a younger age [37]. The mechanisms accounting for the age-associated increase of serum SHBG are yet to be determined. An attractive hypothesis is the age-related decline in the activity of the somatotropic axis, but this hypothesis presently supported only by indirect evidence, such as the existence of a negative association between serum levels of SHBG and IGF-I [43] and the normalization of elevated serum SHBG levels in adults with GH deficiency who receive substitution with adequate doses of GH or IGF-I, respectively [43].

There is a wide variety of plasma SHBG levels in elderly men but one study in healthy elderly men with rather normal plasma total testosterone found that with increasing levels of SHBG there was an increase of plasma total T but the levels of testosterone not bound to SHBG were stable across the spectrum of SHBG concentrations [44]. These were healthy men with rather normal plasma testosterone levels.

I would like to add some published data showing that free or biovaialable testosterone are a better indicator of androgenicity than total testosterone, in other words that the increase of SHBG with aging is clinically significant.

Can the Age-Related Decline of Testosterone Be Prevented or Reversed?

As indicated above, the age-related changes in neuroendocrine functioning leading to a diminished efficacy of LH stimulation of the Leydig cell and impairments of the steroidogenic process of testosterone synthesis are probably inherent factors in the age-related decline of circulating testosterone levels. One of the early studies concluded that aging is the main factor in this process [45]. But increasingly there is insight that disease [4, 46] significantly contributes to the age-related decline of testosterone [47]. Numerous studies have found associations between features of the metabolic syndrome and plasma testosterone [48–51], and changes in lifestyle (diet/exercise) might partially prevent or redress the decline of androgen levels with aging [6, 7, 52].

Guidelines for Administration of Androgens to Elderly Men

Professional organizations recognize that androgen deficiency in the aging male should receive due interest and debate, not least because the demographics clearly demonstrate the increasing percentage of the population that is in the older age groups. The progressive decline of testosterone is now supported by scientific evidence. With age, a significant percentage of men over the age of 60 years have serum testosterone levels that are below the lower limits of young adult (aged 20–30 years) men. Whether older hypogonadal men will benefit from testosterone treatment and what will be the risks associated with such intervention can only be resolved by sufficiently powered studies. In the views of the above professional bodies, these studies are timely since studies in the past decade have produced evidence of the benefit of androgen treatment on multiple target organs of hypogonadal men, and recent studies show short-term beneficial effects of testosterone in older men that are similar to those in younger men. Long-term data on the effects of testosterone treatment in the older population are limited, and specifically data on the risks of prostate and cardiovascular disease are needed. Answers to key questions regarding the functional benefits of testosterone administration to retard frailty of the elderly are not yet available but are urgently needed. A diagnosis of androgen deficiency should be based on consistent symptoms and signs and unequivocally low serum testosterone levels. It is recommended to measure morning total testosterone level by a reliable assay as the initial diagnostic test. In case there is no clear-cut outcome, confirmation of the diagnosis by repeating the measurement of morning total testosterone is recommended, in some patients complemented by measurement of the free or bioavailable testosterone level. The use of accurate assays is pivotal for a proper diagnosis. Testosterone therapy is given with the aim to induce and maintain secondary sex characteristics and to improve sexual function, sense of well-being, muscle mass and strength, and bone mineral density. It should be reserved for symptomatic men with androgen deficiency, who have low testosterone levels. Professional organizations have formulated guidelines/recommendations for the administration of testosterone to elderly men. One set of guidelines has been adopted by the International Society of Andrology, the International Society for the Study of the Aging Male and the European Association of Urology [11, 12]. The other one has been proposed by a task force of the Endocrine Society [53].

One set of guidelines defines the reference values of testosterone as follows: normal = total testosterone >12 nmol/l (346 ng/dl) and free testosterone >250 pmol/l (72 pg/ml). Treatment may be considered if there are symptoms and the value of total testosterone 8–12 nmol/l (231–346 ng/dl). A value of total testosterone <8 nmol/l (231 ng/dl) and free T <180 pmol/l (52 pg/ml) is an indication for treatment [11, 12]. The guidelines of the Endocrine Society specify that there is as yet no consensus on what constitutes low testosterone values but values of total testosterone <6.9–10.4 nmol/l (200–300 ng/dl) and free testosterone <0.17 nmol/l (50 pg/ml) are regarded as low [53]. According to the above guidelines, when testosterone therapy is instituted, achieved testosterone levels during treatment should be in the mid-normal range [53–55]. The formulation of testosterone should be chosen on the basis of the patient's preference, consideration of pharmacokinetics, treatment burden, and cost [53]. Men receiving testosterone therapy should be monitored using a standardized plan, as detailed in the above guidelines.

Conclusion

There is now solid evidence that statistically a decline of (free) testosterone levels occurs in aging men. A number of men continue to have normal testosterone levels well into high age, but a proportion are androgen deficient and their quality of life might be improved with androgen supplementation. The identification of aging men with androgen deficiency remains a difficult problem in routine clinical practice. Aging men often show clinical signs of hypogonadism (loss of muscle mass/strength, reduction in bone mass and an increase in visceral fat). These manifestations might indicate androgen deficiency but often near-normal plasma testosterone levels are found. But there is increasing insight that symptoms accumulate gradually with decreasing testosterone levels, with the levels of testosterone differing between individuals, and, within a subject, not all symptoms of testosterone deficiency will manifest themselves at the same blood testosterone levels. In order to let aging testosterone-deficient men benefit from androgen supplementation, their identification should be guided by clinical signs of androgen deficiency: loss of lean body mass and bone mass, increase in (visceral) fat mass, and decline in psychological and sexual functioning and biochemical evidence of testosterone deficiency. The first studies of androgen supplement administration in aging men have been encouraging.

References

1 Lunenfeld B: The Aging Male. Aging Male 2002;5:73.
2 Kaufman JM, Vermeulen A: The decline of androgen levels in elderly men and its clinical and therapeutic implications. Endocr Rev 2005;26:833–876.
3 Leifke E, Gorenoi V, et al: Age-related changes of serum sex hormones, insulin-like growth factor-1 and sex-hormone binding globulin levels in men: cross-sectional data. Clin Endocrinol 2000;53:689–695.
4 Gray A, Feldman HA, et al: Age, disease, and changing sex hormone levels in middle-aged men: results of the Massachusetts Male Aging Study.' J Clin Endocrinol Metab 1991;73:1016–1025.
5 Feldman HA, Longcope C, et al: Age trends in the level of serum testosterone and other hormones in middle-aged men: longitudinal results from the Massachusetts male aging study. J Clin Endocrinol Metab 2002;87:589–598.
6 Svartberg J, Midtby M, et al: The associations of age, lifestyle factors and chronic disease with testosterone in men: the Tromso Study. Eur J Endocrinol 2003;149:145–152.
7 Travison TG, Shabsigh R, et al: The natural progression and remission of erectile dysfunction: results from the Massachusetts Male Aging Study. J Urol 2007;177:241–246; discussion 246.
8 Werner A: The male climacteric. JAMA 1939;112: 1441–1443.
9 Heller C, Myers GB: The male climacteric, its symptomatology, diagnosis and treatment. JAMA 1944; 126:472–477.
10 McGavack T: The male climacterium. J Am Geriatric Soc 1955;3:639–655.
11 Nieschlag E, Swerdloff R, et al: Investigation, treatment and monitoring of late-onset hypogonadism in males. Aging Male 2005;8:56–58.
12 Nieschlag E, Swerdloff R, et al: Investigation, treatment and monitoring of late-onset hypogonadism in males. ISA, ISSAM, and EAU recommendations. Eur Urol 2005;48:1–4.
13 Morales A, Schulman CC, et al: Testosterone deficiency syndrome (TDS) needs to be named appropriately: the importance of accurate terminology. Eur Urol 2006;50:407–409.
14 Handelsman DJ, Liu PY: Andropause: invention, prevention, rejuvenation. Trends Endocrinol Metab 2005;16:39–45.
15 Schultheiss D, Jonas U, et al: Some historical reflections on the ageing male. World J Urol 2002;20: 40–44.
16 Smith RG, Betancourt L, et al: Molecular endocrinology and physiology of the aging central nervous system. Endocr Rev 2005;26:203–250.
17 NIH State-of-the-Science Conference Statement on Management of Menopause-Related Symptoms. NIH Consens State Sci Statements 2005;22:1–38.
18 Harman SM, Naftolin F, et al: Is the estrogen controversy over? Deconstructing the Women's Health Initiative Study: a critical evaluation of the evidence. Ann NY Acad Sci 2005;1052:43–56.
19 Veldhuis JD, Iranmanesh A: Short-term aromatase-enzyme blockade unmasks impaired feedback adaptations in luteinizing hormone and testosterone secretion in older men. J Clin Endocrinol Metab 2005;90:211–218.
20 Veldhuis JD, Iranmanesh A, et al: Age and testosterone feedback jointly control the dose-dependent actions of gonadotropin-releasing hormone in healthy men. J Clin Endocrinol Metab 2005;90: 302–309.
21 Vermeulen A, Kaufman JM, et al: Attenuated luteinizing hormone (LH) pulse amplitude but normal LH pulse frequency, and its relation to plasma androgens in hypogonadism of obese men. J Clin Endocrinol Metab 1993;76:1140–1146.
22 Lima N, Cavaliere H, et al: Decreased androgen levels in massively obese men may be associated with impaired function of the gonadostat. Int J Obes Relat Metab Disord 2000;24:1433–1437.
23 Crawford BA, Liu PY, et al: Randomized placebo-controlled trial of androgen effects on muscle and bone in men requiring long-term systemic glucocorticoid treatment. J Clin Endocrinol Metab 2003; 88:3167–3176.
24 Lamberts SW, Romijn JA, et al: The future endocrine patient. Reflections on the future of clinical endocrinology. Eur J Endocrinol 2003;149:169–175.

25 Harman SM, Tsitouras PD: Reproductive hormones in aging men. I. Measurement of sex steroids, basal luteinizing hormone, and Leydig cell response to human chorionic gonadotropin. J Clin Endocrinol Metab 1980;51:35–40.
26 Mulligan T, Iranmanesh A, et al: Pulsatile iv infusion of recombinant human LH in leuprolide-suppressed men unmasks impoverished Leydig-cell secretory responsiveness to midphysiological LH drive in the aging male. J Clin Endocrinol Metab 2001; 86:5547–5553.
27 Neaves WB, Johnson L, et al: Age-related change in numbers of other interstitial cells in testes of adult men: evidence bearing on the fate of Leydig cells lost with increasing age. Biol Reprod 1985;33: 259–269.
28 Culty M, Luo L, et al: Cholesterol transport, peripheral benzodiazepine receptor, and steroidogenesis in aging Leydig cells. J Androl 2002;23:439–447.
29 Vermeulen A, Deslypere JP: Intratesticular unconjugated steroids in elderly men. J Steroid Biochem 1986;24:1079–1083.
30 Mahmoud AM, Goemaere S, et al: Testicular volume in relation to hormonal indices of gonadal function in community-dwelling elderly men. J Clin Endocrinol Metab 2003;88:179–184.
31 Caprio M, Isidori AM, et al: Expression of functional leptin receptors in rodent Leydig cells. Endocrinology 1999;140:4939–4947.
32 Isidori AM, Caprio M, et al: Leptin and androgens in male obesity: evidence for leptin contribution to reduced androgen levels. J Clin Endocrinol Metab 1999;84:3673–3680.
33 Soderberg S, Olsson T, et al: A strong association between biologically active testosterone and leptin in non-obese men and women is lost with increasing (central) adiposity. Int J Obes Relat Metab Disord 2001;25:98–105.
34 Van Den Saffele JK, Goemaere S, et al: Serum leptin levels in healthy ageing men: are decreased serum testosterone and increased adiposity in elderly men the consequence of leptin deficiency? Clin Endocrinol (Oxf) 1999;51:81–88.
35 Doucet E, St-Pierre S, et al: Fasting insulin levels influence plasma leptin levels independently from the contribution of adiposity: evidence from both a cross-sectional and an intervention study. J Clin Endocrinol Metab 2000;85:4231–4237.
36 Pitteloud N, Hardin M, et al: Increasing insulin resistance is associated with a decrease in Leydig cell testosterone secretion in men. J Clin Endocrinol Metab 2005;90:2636–2641.
37 Pritchard J, Despres JP, et al: Plasma adrenal, gonadal, and conjugated steroids before and after long-term overfeeding in identical twins. J Clin Endocrinol Metab 1998;83:3277–3284.
38 Vermeulen A, Kaufman JM, et al: Influence of some biological indexes on sex hormone-binding globulin and androgen levels in aging or obese males. J Clin Endocrinol Metab 1996;81:1821–1826.
39 Pritchard J, Despres JP, et al: Plasma adrenal, gonadal, and conjugated steroids following long-term exercise-induced negative energy balance in identical twins. Metabolism 1999;48:1120–1127.
40 Strain G, Zumoff B, et al: The relationship between serum levels of insulin and sex hormone-binding globulin in men: the effect of weight loss. J Clin Endocrinol Metab 1994;79:1173–1176.
41 Niskanen L, Laaksonen DE, et al: Changes in sex hormone-binding globulin and testosterone during weight loss and weight maintenance in abdominally obese men with the metabolic syndrome. Diabetes Obes Metab 2004;6:208–215.
42 Vermeulen A, Stoica T, et al: The apparent free testosterone concentration, an index of androgenicity. J Clin Endocrinol Metab 1971;33:759–767.
43 Gomez JM, Maravall FJ, et al: Determinants of sex hormone-binding globulin concentrations in a cross-sectional study of healthy men randomly selected. J Nutr Health Aging 2007;11:60–64.
44 de Ronde W, van der Schouw YT, et al: Serum levels of sex hormone-binding globulin (SHBG) are not associated with lower levels of non-SHBG-bound testosterone in male newborns and healthy adult men. Clin Endocrinol (Oxf) 2005;62:498–503.
45 Vermeulen A, Deslypere JP: Testicular endocrine function in the ageing male. Maturitas 1985;7: 273–279.
46 Handelsman DJ: Testicular dysfunction in systemic disease. Endocrinol Metab Clin N Am 1994;23: 839–856.
47 Travison TG, Araujo AB, et al: The relative contributions of aging, health, and lifestyle factors to serum testosterone decline in men. J Clin Endocrinol Metab 2007;92:549–555.
48 Mohr BA, Bhasin S, et al: The effect of changes in adiposity on testosterone levels in older men: longitudinal results from the Massachusetts Male Aging Study. Eur J Endocrinol 2006;155:443–452.
49 Rodriguez A, Muller DC, et al: Aging, androgens, and the metabolic syndrome in a longitudinal study of aging. J Clin Endocrinol Metab 2007.
50 Allan CA, Strauss BJ, et al: The association between obesity and the diagnosis of androgen deficiency in symptomatic ageing men. Med J Aust 2006;185: 424–427.
51 Kaplan SA, Meehan AG, et al: The age related decrease in testosterone is significantly exacerbated in obese men with the metabolic syndrome: what are the implications for the relatively high incidence of erectile dysfunction observed in these men? J Urol 2006;176:1524–1527; discussion 1527–1528.

52 Isidori AM, Lenzi A: Risk factors for androgen decline in older males: lifestyle, chronic diseases and drugs. J Endocrinol Invest 2005;28(3 suppl):14–22.
53 Bhasin S, Cunningham GR, et al: Testosterone therapy in adult men with androgen deficiency syndromes: an endocrine society clinical practice guideline. J Clin Endocrinol Metab 2006;91: 1995–2010.
54 Jacobeit JW, Gooren LJ, et al: Long-acting intramuscular testosterone undecanoate for treatment of female-to-male transgender individuals. J Sex Med 2007;4:1479–1484.
55 Saad F, Gooren LJ, et al: A dose response study of testosterone on sexual dysfunction and on features of the metabolic syndrome using testosterone gel and parenteral testosterone undecanoate. J Androl 2008;29:102–105.

Prof. Louis J.G. Gooren
Department of Endocrinology
VU University Medical Center, PO Box 7057
NL–1007 MB Amsterdam (The Netherlands)
Tel. +662 653 8066, Fax +31 20 4440502, E-Mail louisjgooren@gmail.com

Jones TH (ed): Advances in the Management of Testosterone Deficiency.
Front Horm Res. Basel, Karger, 2009, vol 37, pp 74–90

Testosterone in Obesity, Metabolic Syndrome and Type 2 Diabetes

Roger D. Stanworth · T. Hugh Jones

Centre for Diabetes and Endocrinology, Barnsley Hospital NHS Foundation Trust, Barnsley, and Academic Unit of Diabetes, Endocrinology and Metabolism, University of Sheffield Medical School, Sheffield, UK

Abstract

Testosterone levels are reduced in obesity, the metabolic syndrome and type 2 diabetes. Low testosterone levels are now being recognised as an independent risk factors for these conditions. Findings from men undergoing androgen suppression as treatment for prostate cancer confirm that the hypogonadal state increases body fat mass and serum insulin and there is a high rate of developing new diabetes in this population. Clinical trial data are consistent in showing reductions in body fat mass during testosterone replacement therapy. There are also trials showing improvements in insulin resistance and glycaemic control with testosterone. Most of the trials in this area to date have been of small size and the promising results require confirmation in larger trials, which are underway. In the longer term, large trials should be conducted to assess the potentially beneficial effects of testosterone on cardiovascular risk in this and other patient groups. In the meantime physicians involved in the care of men with diabetes should remain vigilant for the symptoms and signs of hypogonadism. Testosterone replacement therapy should be considered for those men with subsequently confirmed hypogonadism.

The prevalence of obesity, metabolic syndrome and type 2 diabetes continues to rise sharply which poses an international health challenge of grave proportions. The main causes of this worsening situation are thought to be changes in lifestyle including greater consumption of energy-rich foods and increased sedentary behaviour.

Insulin resistance caused primarily by visceral adiposity is recognised as the central pathological abnormality in the development of the metabolic syndrome and diabetes. Adipose tissue is highly metabolically active and produces numerous substances which mediate the links between obesity, insulin resistance, diabetes and vascular disease as well as other conditions. These adipocyte-derived hormones are collectively known as adipocytokines and have redefined the adipose tissue as an important component of the endocrine system. The most abundant adipocytokines in humans are leptin which is high in obesity and adiponectin which is low in the condition.

There is now convincing evidence that low testosterone is an independent risk factor for the development of obesity, metabolic syndrome and diabetes in men. There is also evidence that normalisation of these low testosterone levels improves obesity and has beneficial effects on other components of the metabolic syndrome as well as important parameters such as insulin resistance and glycaemic control in type 2 diabetes.

Obesity Link to Insulin Resistance and the Metabolic Syndrome

Body mass index is the most widely used measurement of overall obesity but central obesity, as clinically determined by waist circumference or waist-to-hip ratio, is a stronger predictor of insulin resistance and diabetes as well as cardiovascular disease. This is because central obesity is strongly linked to visceral adiposity. There are a number of specific characteristics which account for the observation that visceral but not subcutaneous fat is proportional to insulin resistance. Visceral adipocytes are metabolically more active than subcutaneous fat cells. Venous drainage from the abdominal viscera occurs via the portal vein directly to the liver. Visceral fat is responsible for delivering free fatty acids and adipocytokines to the liver leading to inhibition of hepatic insulin binding and gluconeogenesis.

The metabolic syndrome is a constellation of cardiovascular risk factors which has been shown to strongly predict the future development of cardiovascular disease or type 2 diabetes. The syndrome is formed around the core features of central obesity and insulin resistance but has been variously defined to incorporate a number of cardiovascular risk factors, mainly low serum HDL cholesterol, raised triglycerides and hypertension (table 1). The IDF and the NCEP ATP definitions are the main ones in clinical use. It remains controversial whether the concept of the metabolic syndrome is useful in clinical practice. A key argument within the controversy centres on whether the presence of the syndrome predicts cardiovascular risk better than its component parts. Difficulties also centre on the different definitions which can be used to describe the syndrome. Nevertheless, the idea of the metabolic syndrome does seem useful in reminding practitioners that cardiovascular risk factors tend to cluster together and that interventions to improve cardiovascular risk factors must do so within the context of the whole patient rather than an individual risk factor.

Clinical measurements of central obesity do not fully correlate with visceral obesity as they are also affected by the presence of fat in the subcutaneous tissues around the abdomen and back. Radiological methods such as CT, MRI and DEXA scanning are able to make this distinction but are not appropriate for routine clinical use. Total body fat mass can be derived by similar methods or by bioelectrical impedance measurements.

Table 1. Definition of the metabolic syndrome

	WHO	IDF	NCEP III
Essential feature	diabetes, impaired glucose tolerance or insulin resistance[a]	central obesity (men >94 cm waist, women >80 cm waist)	no essential feature
Diagnosis requires	essential feature plus 2 from: hypertension (>140/90) hypertriglyceridaemia (>1.7 mmol/l) low HDL cholesterol[b] central obesity[c] microalbuminuria[d]	essential feature plus 2 from; hypertension (>130/85) hypertriglyceridaemia (>1.7 mmol/l) low HDL cholesterol (<1.03 mmol/l) raised fasting glucose (>5.6 mmol/l)	diagnosis requires three factors from; hypertension (>130/85) hypertriglyceridaemia (>1.7 mmol/l) low HDL cholesterol (<1.03 mmol/l) raised fasting glucose (>5.6 mmol/l) central obesity[e]

WHO = World Health Organisation definition of the metabolic syndrome; IDF = International Diabetes Federation definition of the metabolic syndrome; NCEP = National Cholesterol Education Program Expert Panel III definition of the metabolic syndrome.

[a]Impaired glucose tolerance = glucose >7.8 mmol on 2-hour glucose tolerance test. Insulin resistance = in highest quartile of relevant population.

[b]HDL cholesterol <0.9 mmol/l in men, <1.0 mmol/l in women.

[c]Waist-to-hip ratio >0.9 in men, >0.85 in women or BMI greater than 30.

[d]Albumin-creatinine ratio >30.

[e]Waist circumference >102 cm in men, >88 cm in women.

Epidemiological Studies

Testosterone and Obesity

Studies consistently show significant relationships between serum testosterone and body fat in healthy or obese individuals [1]. Free testosterone levels have been shown to be inversely related to obesity in a number of studies with the link most often being seen with central obesity. Most of these studies report correlations with waist-to-hip ratios but one study of 23 men confirmed that visceral fat level assessed by CT scan, was negatively correlated with free and total testosterone [2]. The link between obesity and total testosterone levels is even stronger. Obesity is associated with low SHBG levels which results in lower total testosterone levels for a given level of free testosterone in obese men. In a subgroup of 217 healthy men from the HERITAGE family study low total testosterone and SHBG were levels were predictors of greater obesity and visceral fat levels on CT scan [3]. Another approach is to compare hypogonadal men with control cases. One study compared CT-derived fat distribution in 26 hypogonadal men with 17 controls matched for age and BMI [4]. Hypogonadal men had an increase in subcutaneous fat mass versus controls but there was no difference in visceral fat levels.

Low testosterone levels are also linked to abnormalities in glucose metabolism. In a study of 1,292 healthy non-diabetic men, there was an inverse correlation of total testosterone with insulin levels which remained significant after adjustment for age and obesity [5]. Results from a group of 178 men from the San Antonio Heart study confirmed the inverse relationship of total testosterone with insulin levels and also demonstrated that free testosterone levels were inversely related to insulin and glucose levels [6]. Total and free testosterone were also found to be inversely associated with insulin resistance in a group of 87 men from a Finnish population study [7].

Testosterone and Diabetes

Studies dating back nearly 30 years have described low total testosterone in men with type 2 diabetes. A meta-analysis of 21 studies including data from 3,825 men confirmed this and suggested that levels were on average 2.66 nmol/l lower in men with diabetes compared with controls [8].

Until recently, the situation with regard to free and bioavailable testosterone fractions was less clear. The known association of insulin resistance with low SHBG levels led to suggestions that reductions of total testosterone in diabetes merely reflected changes in SHBG and that bioavailable testosterone was not affected. Contrary to this hypothesis meta-analysis of data from 2,500 men found no significant reductions in SHBG levels of men with diabetes compared to controls although levels were non-significantly lower in diabetic men (−5.07 nmol/l, $p = 0.15$). This is in contrast to details from diabetic women showing significant average reductions of 16.2 nmol/l in SHBG. Furthermore, free testosterone levels as assessed by the 'gold standard' method of equilibrium dialysis were found to be low in 33% of diabetic men in one study [9] and recently published data from a UK diabetic population of 355 men showed that 50% had low bioavailable or free testosterone levels [10]. Recent data from 1,413 men in the Third National Health and Nutrition survey (NHANES III) showed that men in the lower tertile of free or bioavailable testosterone were approximately four times more likely to have diabetes than those in the upper tertile after adjustment for age, obesity and ethnicity [11]. Low total testosterone levels also increased the likelihood of diabetes but this was not independent of other factors in this group.

Few studies have assessed the relationship between testosterone levels in men with diabetes and symptoms of hypogonadism. Assessment is confounded by the fact that many symptoms of hypogonadism are prevalent in the male diabetic population as a whole regardless of hypogonadism: particularly erectile dysfunction which is contributed to by vascular disease, neuropathy, medications commonly used in diabetes such as antihypertensives and psychosocial factors. Recent data has confirmed a high

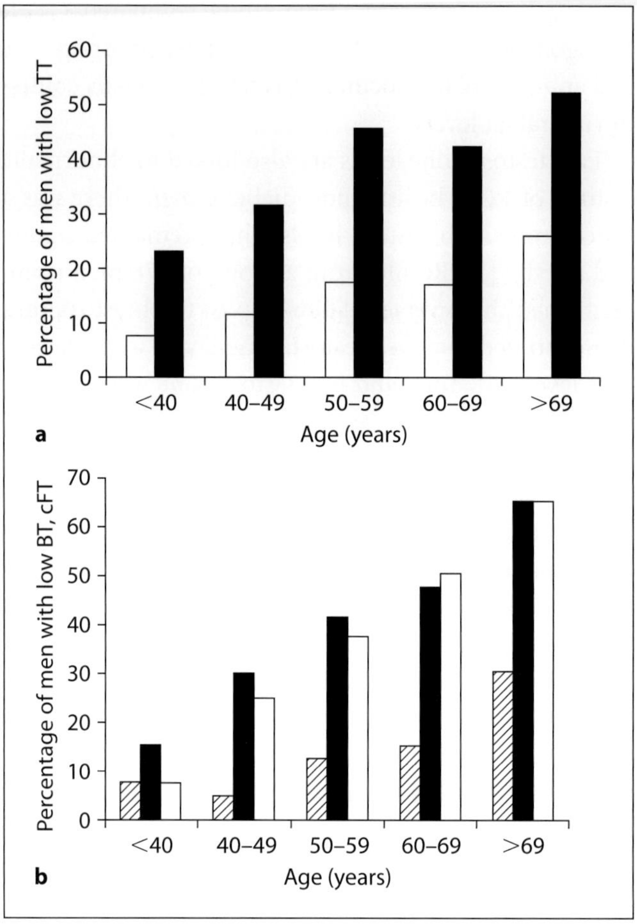

Fig. 1. Data from the Barnsley Study of the prevalence of hypogonadism in men with type 2 diabetes. The figures show the percentage of men with a positive symptom score and biochemical evidence of low total testosterone (**a** black TT <12 nmol/l, white TT <8 nmol/l) or bioactive testosterone (**b** black BT <4 nmol/l, hatched BT <2.5 nmol/l, white cFT < 0.255 nmol/l). TT = Total testosterone, BT = bioavailable testosterone, cFT = free testosterone. ©American Diabetes Association from Diabetes Care 2007, vol. 33, pp. 911–917.

prevalence of hypogonadism defined clinically by positive ADAM questionnaire and biochemically by reduced serum testosterone levels although there was no control group without diabetes in this study [10] (fig. 1).

The mechanisms linking testosterone with insulin resistance and type 2 diabetes have also been considered. A study assessed insulin resistance by the gold-standard method of hyperinsulinaemic-euglycaemic clamps in 60 men with a range of glucose tolerance from normal to diabetic [12]. Correlations were sought between testosterone and other parameters. The findings confirmed an inverse association of total testosterone with insulin resistance and also demonstrated positive correlations of testosterone with maximal aerobic capacity on exercise testing and ubiquinol cytochrome c reductase-binding protein (UQCRB) gene expression in muscle biopsies. Expression of UQCRB is known to be reduced in muscle from diabetic men and is an important indicator of mitochondrial function in this context. Maximal aerobic capacity is also known to be reduced in type 2 diabetes and insulin resistance and it is postulated by the authors that impairment of mitochondrial function may be a mechanism whereby low testosterone levels result in insulin resistance and type 2 diabetes. Many of the associations in this study were not independent of obesity and it may be that obesity may instead be the common link between low testosterone levels and insulin resistance and diabetes.

In vitro data also suggest that testosterone has a role in modulating insulin secretion. Investigators found that physiological testosterone concentrations acted to induce insulin secretion from isolated pancreatic β-cells [13]. The effect occurred rapidly suggesting that testosterone was acting via a membrane bound receptor rather than the classical nuclear androgen receptor.

As described above study findings vary as to whether the association of testosterone with diabetes occurs independently of obesity but meta-analysis of nine studies which matched their control groups for body mass index and/or waist-to-hip ratio show that testosterone were reduced in diabetic men of equivalent anthropomorphics [8].

Testosterone and Metabolic Syndrome

Low testosterone is associated with the presence of the metabolic syndrome in men. In a cohort study of 1,896 non-diabetic Finnish men free and total testosterone levels were significantly lower in those men with the metabolic syndrome, defined by WHO criteria [14] (table 1). They found that men with free testosterone levels in the lowest tertile were over 2.5 times more likely to have the metabolic syndrome. These findings are consistent with data from the Quebec Family study where higher levels of bioavailable and total testosterone were associated with increased insulin sensitivity and a reduced risk of the metabolic syndrome in a group of 130 men [15].

A study of 803 men including 236 with the metabolic syndrome showed that hypogonadism was more common in those with metabolic syndrome [16]. Data were also considered after splitting men into groups according to the number of metabolic syndrome features they demonstrated. Testosterone levels were sequentially lower with increasing numbers of components.

Low testosterone levels are associated with all main constituents of the metabolic syndrome as well as the overall syndrome. Associations with obesity and insulin resistance have already been discussed. HDL-cholesterol (HDL-C) has been shown to correlate positively with testosterone in a number of well-sized epidemiological studies so that higher testosterone levels are associated with beneficially higher levels of HDL-C. In one of these studies free testosterone was a more powerful predictor of HDL-C than either SHBG or oestradiol in regression analysis [17]. Testosterone levels correlate inversely with triglyceride levels across a number of published studies. Amongst the largest studies is a recently reported group of 1,274 men from the Tromso study which found a significant relationship despite using non-fasting samples [18]. Data from the Tromso group has also confirmed previous data linking low testosterone levels with hypertension. This study found an inverse association between testosterone and left ventricular mass [19].

Associations of low testosterone with cardiovascular risk are potentially of greater importance in men from groups with a high risk of cardiovascular disease such as type 2 diabetes where 80% of patients die of cardiovascular disease.

Low Testosterone as a Risk Factor for Obesity, the Metabolic Syndrome and Diabetes

Evidence from several longitudinal population studies suggests that low testosterone is an independent risk factor for the future development of obesity, the metabolic syndrome and type 2 diabetes. The data implicate low testosterone levels with the future accumulation of visceral adiposity. Baseline testosterone levels correlated inversely with the accumulation of visceral fat but not other fat depots on CT scan after 7.5 years follow-up in a group of 110 men [20] and there was a similar relationship of baseline testosterone with waist-to-hip ratio after 12 years of follow-up in a separate cohort of 511 men [21].

A cohort study from The Massachusetts Male Aging Study (MMAS) [22] and a case control study from the Multiple Risk Factor Intervention Trial (MRFIT) [23] have demonstrated that low baseline total testosterone and SHBG are both independent risk factors for the future development of diabetes in middle-aged men. Low total testosterone was also a risk factor for diabetes during 8 years of follow-up in The Rancho-Bernado Study [24]. The study also demonstrated significant inverse correlations of baseline total testosterone with glucose and insulin levels from fasting and 2-hour samples on the Oral Glucose Tolerance Test. The prospective data linking total testosterone to incident diabetes has been the subject of meta-analysis which showed that men developing diabetes during follow-up had total testosterone levels 2.48 nmol/l lower than those who did not [8]. Furthermore, after splitting the data into upper and lower dichotomies it was found that men with higher testosterone levels had a 42% reduction in the risk of developing diabetes during follow-up.

Data from a group of healthy Finnish men showed that low baseline total and free testosterone and SHBG levels predicted the development of the Metabolic Syndrome (according to NCEP definition) as well as diabetes during 11 years of follow-up [25]. Development of the metabolic syndrome after 15 years of follow up (NCEP definition) was also linked to baseline low testosterone and SHBG in 950 men from the MMAS [26]. The effect was most marked in non-obese men so that in these individuals, changes in testosterone predated obesity as well the metabolic syndrome. This supports the idea that low testosterone levels are linked to diabetes and the metabolic syndrome independently as well as through their common link with obesity.

Interestingly, further prospective data from the Finnish group show that men with the metabolic syndrome at baseline have an increased risk of developing hypogonadism during 11 years of follow-up [27]. This data is consistent with a synergistic relationship between obesity, the metabolic syndrome, diabetes and hypogonadism.

Effects of Androgen Suppression on Obesity and Diabetes

Study of individuals undergoing artificial induction of a hypogonadal state as part of treatment for prostate cancer can give information about the metabolic consequences of hypogonadism. Observational and retrospective studies suggest that there are clinically significant effects of this induced hypogonadism on glucose metabolism. In a study of 73,196 men with prostate cancer, treatment with androgen deprivation was associated with a significant hazard ratio of 1.44 of incident diabetes compared to other treatments [28]. A study involving 396 men with prostate cancer and known diabetes showed a high incidence of worsening glycaemic control following androgen deprivation [29]. These large data sets are supported by findings of smaller studies in men being commenced on androgen deprivation therapy. Initiation of either GnRH agonist or anti-androgen therapy in 22 men with prostate cancer led to increases in serum insulin after 3 months. Arterial stiffness and body fat mass also increased and there was a 1.9-kg increase in fat mass over the full 6 months' duration of the trial [30]. Increases in glucose, insulin and insulin resistance were also found in a longer-term study with a follow up of one year [31] and diabetic men treated with androgen ablation therapy for prostate cancer were found to have deteriorating glycaemic control and cardiovascular risk factors with a need for a significant increase in their diabetic medication during treatment [32].

A related approach has been to induce androgen deprivation with GnRH agonists during short-term studies in healthy men and then replace with testosterone at different doses with the aim of producing a range of serum testosterone levels. Groups can then be compared with the aim of determining the effect of different testosterone levels on variables. A pair of studies with this design were conducted over 20 weeks in groups of young (19–35 years) and older (60–75) men [33]. The results showed that lower doses of testosterone producing sub-physiological doses lead to gains of fat mass in both groups with these effects being greater in young men. Higher doses of testosterone resulted in less fat mass with the progressive effects extending into the supra-physiological range. In this set of experiments, differential testosterone dosing did not affect insulin sensitivity in the younger age group patients. Data on insulin sensitivity from the older age group has not been reported. The difference between the data from this group and the prostate cancer studies may therefore be related to the large age differential.

The Androgen Receptor in Diabetes, Obesity and the Metabolic Syndrome

The androgen receptor gene CAG repeat polymorphism (AR CAG) is discussed fully in the chapter by Zitzmann [this vol., pp. 52–61]. Long AR CAG sequences are associated with decreased transcriptional activity which leads to clinically relevant associations.

AR CAG is associated with body fat content and anthropomorphics. In a group of 106 healthy young men, longer AR CAG was associated with higher leptin levels and percentage body fat [34]. Similarly, longer AR CAG was associated with obesity and serum leptin in a group of 233 men with type 2 diabetes [35, 36]. The association of low testosterone levels and insensitive androgen receptors with obesity would be consistent with an effect of testosterone via the androgen receptor in influencing body fat distribution. Laboratory data from the testicular feminised mouse (tfm) model which has an inactive androgen receptor due to a frame shift mutation [37] supports a role of the androgen receptor in the control of weight. Feeding with a high cholesterol diet led to a marked weight gain in the tfm whereas its wild type littermate control only gained a small amount of weight [38].

Longer AR CAG sequences are also associated with higher serum insulin levels in healthy men [34]. The polymorphism was not associated with HbA_{1c} in a group of 233 men with type 2 diabetes [35], although many of these men were treated with oral hypoglycaemic agents or insulin which could confound any effects on glucose metabolism in this group. The reported association of Kennedy syndrome (a neurological syndrome caused by abnormally long AR CAG ($>$37 repeats)) with diabetes suggests that AR CAG could be relevant in the pathogenesis of diabetes in this context. The distribution of AR CAG in the male diabetic population does not differ significantly from that found in the general population which suggests that it is not a significant factor in the pathogenesis of diabetes in most cases. This may be because most individuals have an AR CAG within a relatively small range (19–24 repeats), and any changes in glucose metabolism within this range are clinically insignificant compared to other factors. It remains possible that AR CAG at the extremes of the normal range may influence glucose metabolism significantly.

Serum testosterone levels and AR CAG polymorphism lengths are both positively correlated with HDL-C in men [35, 39]. This is seemingly contradictory as it implies that a more active receptor and low testosterone levels are both associated with adverse changes in HDL-C. Data from clinical trials of testosterone replacement has also been inconsistent with some trials suggesting adverse changes in HDL-C during testosterone replacement therapy and at least one trial describing beneficial changes. Meta-analysis of data from 13 trials showed no overall change in HDL-C with testosterone replacement therapy [40]. The data may suggest that testosterone acts via separate mechanisms with opposite effects on HDL-C, for example via the androgen receptor to reduce HDL-C and after aromatisation to oestradiol to increase HDL-C. The dominant effect could be altered depending on variables such as AR CAG, obesity, age and baseline testosterone levels.

Testosterone and Body Fat: Clinical Trial Data

Interventional trials of the effects of testosterone on obesity and fat distribution in men have concerned relatively small numbers of patients and there is considerable heterogeneity in terms of study design. These differences have a potential to significantly affect results. Baseline and treatment testosterone levels are crucial factors in determining the responses to testosterone replacement. Other important variables include the length of treatment given in a study, participant age, adiposity at baseline, co-morbidities, the preparation of testosterone given and any effects this has on the availability of oestrogen and dihydrotestosterone resulting from the metabolism of testosterone.

The effect of testosterone on body fat mass have been reported in a number of trials. The longest of these involved 108 men randomized to either transdermal testosterone patches or placebo for 36 months and showed 2.3 kg greater weight reduction in the testosterone-treated group versus placebo [41]. Almost all this difference developed in the first 6 months of the study. Other trials have been of shorter duration but often show a similar magnitude of reductions in fat mass. This is confirmed by a meta-analysis of data from 16 randomised controlled trials involving a total of 970 men. Across these trials testosterone was associated with an average reduction of 1.6 kg fat mass which corresponded to a 6.2% reduction in total body fat during an average testosterone treatment duration of 9 months [40]. Further analysis suggested that similar changes in fat mass could be expected in men with relatively normal baseline testosterone levels (greater than 10 mmol/l) as in men with lower baseline testosterone levels.

Randomised controlled trial data relating to the effect of testosterone replacement on different fat depots is less consistent. The epidemiological links between testosterone and central obesity led us to believe that testosterone could act preferentially to reduce visceral fat. There is some support for this within the evidence from clinical trials and a number of investigators have found reductions in central obesity as reflected by waist-to-hip ratio or waist circumference in diabetic or obese men during testosterone treatment [42, 43]. Furthermore, one of these studies demonstrated that transdermal testosterone caused a reduction in CT-assessed visceral fat without changes in other fat depots when given to centrally obese middle-aged men [44]. Conversely, other studies have shown different changes in fat distribution during testosterone. Testosterone patches given for 36 months to men over 65 years of age lead primarily to reductions in subcutaneous limb fat [41]. A recent study showed that 24 weeks' transdermal testosterone gel treatment in HIV-infected men with central obesity led to significant reductions in subcutaneous fat including abdominal wall fat, but no change in visceral fat compared with placebo [45]. Therefore, patient characteristics may be important in determining the pattern of fat reduction during testosterone treatment. The duration of the study may also be important as changes in visceral fat may be likely to occur more quickly than changes in subcutaneous fat due to greater metabolic activity.

Testosterone, Insulin Resistance and Diabetes: Clinical Trial Data

Studies of the effects of testosterone treatment on glucose metabolism in non-diabetic men have shown varying results. A series of studies have investigated the effects of testosterone or dihydrotestosterone given for 6 weeks or 3 months to middle-aged obese men [44]. The findings were that physiological treatment doses led to improved insulin resistance as measured by euglycaemic clamp and/or serum glucose and insulin responses during glucose tolerance test. These improvements were associated with decreased central obesity, measured by computed tomography (CT) or waist-to-hip ratio, without reduced total fat mass. Insulin resistance improved more with testosterone than dihydrotestosterone treatment and beneficial effects were greater in men with lower baseline testosterone levels. Increasing testosterone levels into the supraphysiological range lead to decreased glucose tolerance. A double-blind, randomised, placebo-controlled trial of physiological testosterone or dihydrotestosterone treatment for 18 patients with low baseline serum testosterone showed improved insulin resistance measured by homeostatic model assessment (HOMA) and reduced insulin and leptin levels with testosterone and dihydrotestosterone [46]. Two other small studies have not shown these effects. An uncontrolled study of testosterone replacement in 10 men with idiopathic hypogonadatropic hypogonadism led to no significant changes in waist-to-hip ratio or insulin resistance measured by the gold standard euglycaemic clamp method [47]. A study of 30 healthy men given supraphysiological testosterone treatment for 6 weeks showed a neutral effect on waist-to-hip ratio, fasting serum glucose and insulin and responses to the oral glucose tolerance test [48].

Trials have also assessed the effects testosterone treatment on glycaemic control and insulin resistance in men with type 2 diabetes. A trial conducted in our research unit assessed the effects of 200 mg intramuscular mixed esters (Sustanon 250®) given every 2 weeks compared with placebo injections in 24 men with diabetes and hypogonadism, 10 of whom were treated with insulin [43]. The study was of randomised, double-blind crossover design with two 3-month treatment periods separated by a 1-month wash-out period. Total testosterone levels rose from an average of 8.6 nmol/l at baseline to a 12.8-nmol/l trough level, which confirms adequate testosterone replacement therapy. Testosterone led to a significant reduction in HbA_{1c} (−0.37%) and also to improved fasting glucose and insulin resistance measured by HOMA in the 14 non-insulin-treated patients (fig. 2). It is not possible to assess HOMA in patients treated with insulin but 5 of 10 of the insulin-treated men had a reduction of insulin dose during testosterone replacement. Other significant changes during testosterone treatment in this trial were reduced total cholesterol, waist circumference and leptin concentrations. Similarly, a placebo-controlled but non-blinded trial in 24 men with visceral obesity, diabetes and hypogonadism found that testosterone led to significant reductions in HbA_{1c}, fasting glucose, post-prandial glucose, weight, fat mass and waist-to-hip ratio during 3 months of treatment. Testosterone in the trial was given as a daily dose of 120 mg oral testosterone undecanoate and resulted in an increase in total testosterone levels from 9.6 to 15.5 nmol/l [42]. This study describes a reduction of HbA_{1c} from 10.4 to 8.6% in the testosterone-treated group, which is much larger than has been

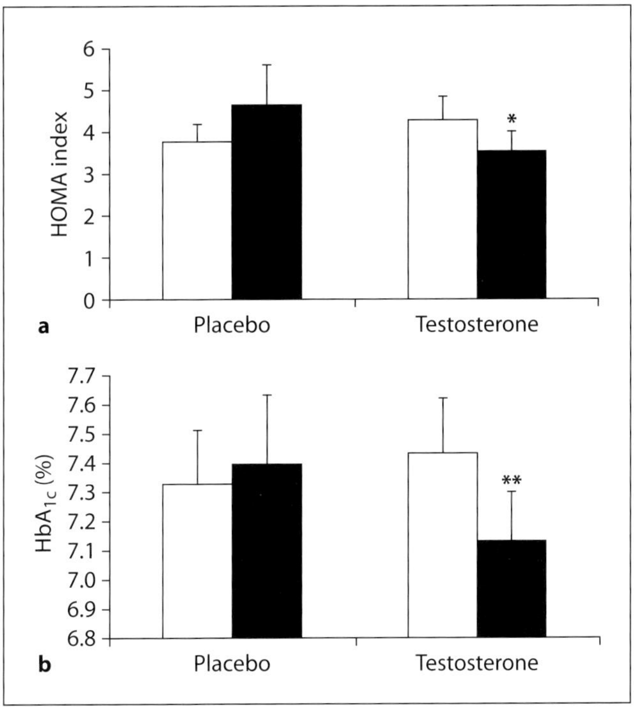

Fig. 2. Data from the Barnsley Study of the effect of testosterone replacement therapy versus placebo on HOMA index and HbA_{1c} in hypogonadal diabetic men. **a, b** Baseline data are represented by the white bar and 3-month data by the black bar. *p = 0.02, **p = 0.03. ©Society of the European Journal of Endocrinology 2006, vol. 154, pp. 899–906.

found in other studies. The non-blinded nature of the study design does call the validity of this magnitude of improvement in HbA_{1c} during testosterone replacement therapy into question.

In contrast, other small studies have not found significant effects of testosterone on glycaemic control in diabetes. An uncontrolled study of 150 mg intramuscular testosterone given to 10 patients with diabetes and hypogonadism found no significant change in diabetes control, fasting glucose or insulin levels despite increases of testosterone levels into the normal range [49]. Another uncontrolled study did not show a beneficial effect of testosterone treatment on insulin resistance measured by HOMA and the 'minimal model' of area under acute insulin response curves in 11 patients with type 2 diabetes [50]. Baseline average body mass index was within the normal range in this population and there was no change in waist-to-hip ratio or weight during testosterone treatment. Baseline testosterone levels were low at 3.85 nmol/l and patients received a relatively small dose of 100 mg intramuscular testosterone every 3 weeks. A good increase in testosterone levels during the trial is described but the average was still rather low at 10 nmol/l and it is not stated at which time during the 3-week cycle the testosterone levels were tested. Therefore, studies

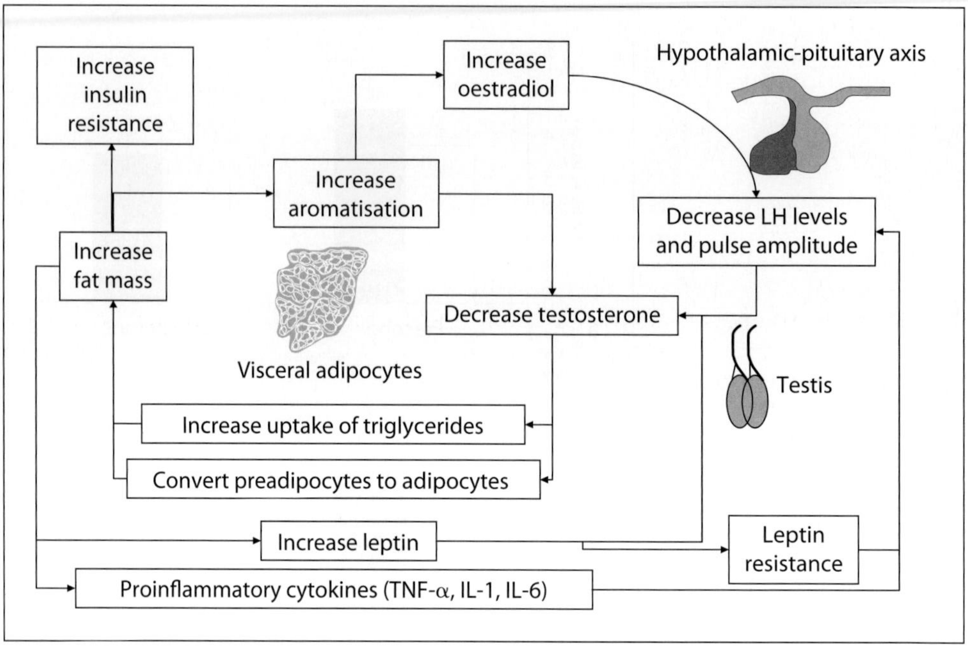

Fig. 3. Hypogonadal-obesity-adipocytokine cycle. This hypothesis describes a cycle of low testosterone levels and obesity. Normally, the negative feedback loop of the hypothalamic-pituitary-testicular axis would overcome the cycle and prevent reductions in testosterone but this response is interfered with by the actions of oestradiol, leptin and proinflammatory cytokines.

that have shown neutral effects of testosterone on glucose metabolism have not measured or shown neutral effects [47, 50] on central obesity.

Published data have therefore come from small trials of short duration. Baseline data from a 1-year placebo-controlled, double-blind, parallel group study of 215 men with type 2 diabetes and the metabolic syndrome was recently presented. On completion, this trial will confirm the effects of testosterone replacement therapy on glycaemic control, insulin resistance and other parameters in men with type 2 diabetes over an extended treatment period. It will also be the first trial to reveal the effects of testosterone replacement in men with the metabolic syndrome.

The Hypogonadal-Obesity-Adipocytokine Cycle

The link between visceral adiposity, insulin resistance and testosterone deficiency can be explained by the hypogonadal-obesity-adipocytokine hypothesis (fig. 3). The hypogonadal-obesity cycle was originally proposed by Cohen and has been developed to incorporate the effects at the hypothalamic-pituitary-testicular axis by ourselves

[51]. The hypothesis does not define whether obesity or hypogonadism is the primary change which starts the cycle, but for the purposes of explanation we shall start with obesity. Obesity leads to greater metabolism of testosterone to oestradiol via the actions of aromatase which is primarily found in adipose tissue. Visceral fat is particularly relevant here due to its greater metabolic activity and higher concentration of androgen receptors. Lower testosterone levels lead to laying down of adipose tissue due to enhanced activity of lipoprotein lipase with increased uptake of free fatty acids into fat cells and increased conversion of pre-adipocytes into adipocytes [52]. Testosterone promotes development of pluripotent stem cells to develop toward the myocyte lineage whereas testosterone deficiency promotes adipocyte generation thus increasing fat mass [53]. Greater adiposity leads to changes in adipocytokine levels such as leptin, adiponectin, IL-6 and TNF-α, exacerbates insulin resistance and drives the cycle to further reduce testosterone levels.

Normally, the homeostatic function of the hypothalamic-pituitary axis would be expected to detect reductions in testosterone levels and maintain levels via increased secretion of luteinising hormone (LH) to stimulate the testis. Inhibition of this response is possible by different mechanisms in obese hypogonadal men. Oestradiol, which is in excess from the actions of aromatase, is known to have a direct inhibitory action on LH production at the hypothalamic-pituitary axis [54]. Adverse changes in adipocytokines such as IL-6 and TNF-α also reduce pituitary responses and LH production. High leptin levels in obese men would be expected to stimulate LH production but obesity is associated with leptin resistance at the hypothalamic-pituitary axis. Leptin also reduces testicular responses to gonadotropins [55].

This hypothesis would explain the epidemiological and clinical trial data supporting a synergistic relationship between obesity and hypogonadism. It would also explain the clinical observation of a high incidence of hypogonadism with normal LH levels in obese men.

Conclusion

There are undoubted links with obesity, insulin resistance, the metabolic syndrome and diabetes to low serum testosterone levels in the human male. The findings from prospective trials, genetic studies of the AR CAG and studies in men rendered hypogonadal as part of the treatment for prostate cancer suggest that low serum testosterone may have a role to play in the pathogenesis of these conditions. Furthermore, clinical trial data are clear in demonstrating that testosterone replacement therapy produces reductions in obesity. Data from pilot studies also shows promising benefits in type 2 diabetes and results from ongoing larger trials of testosterone replacement in men with type 2 diabetes and the metabolic syndrome are awaited with great interest. The effects of testosterone on cardiovascular disease is of great importance in these populations who have a high rate of cardiovascular morbidity and mortality.

These risks may previously have led to reluctance on the part of physicians to institute testosterone replacement therapy in these patients but the realisation that testosterone may be beneficial rather than detrimental to male cardiovascular health should allay these fears.

The diagnosis of hypogonadism as defined by symptoms ± signs and evidence of biochemical testosterone deficiency remains the primary indication for treatment with testosterone in this group. We would suggest that monitoring patients with diabetes for the symptoms of hypogonadism is an important aspect of care. Hypogonadal symptoms are often found and a significant proportion of these men will prove to be hypogonadal but the condition is underdiagnosed. We have found that identification and treatment of these individuals often leads to improvements in quality of life.

This data from male patients is in contrast to females where the hyperandrogenous state is associated with polycystic ovarian syndrome, central obesity, insulin resistance, diabetes and adverse cardiovascular consequences. Therefore, there are striking similarities between the metabolic profile of the hypogonadal male and the female with androgen excess. The reason for this paradox is presently unknown but is clearly an exciting and important area for future study.

References

1 Kapoor D, Malkin CJ, et al: Androgens, insulin resistance and vascular disease in men. Clin Endocrinol (Oxf) 2005;63:239–250.

2 Seidell JC, Bjorntorp P, et al: Visceral fat accumulation in men is positively associated with insulin, glucose, and C-peptide levels, but negatively with testosterone levels. Metabolism 1990;39:897–901.

3 Couillard C, Gagnon J, et al: Contribution of body fatness and adipose tissue distribution to the age variation in plasma steroid hormone concentrations in men: the HERITAGE Family Study. J Clin Endocrinol Metab 2000;85:1026–1031.

4 Katznelson L, Rosenthal DI, et al: Using quantitative CT to assess adipose distribution in adult men with acquired hypogonadism. AJR Am J Roentgenol 1998; 170:423–427.

5 Simon D, Preziosi P, et al: Interrelation between plasma testosterone and plasma insulin in healthy adult men: the Telecom Study. Diabetologia 1992;35: 173–177.

6 Haffner SM, Valdez RA, et al: Decreased testosterone and dehydroepiandrosterone sulfate concentrations are associated with increased insulin and glucose concentrations in nondiabetic men. Metabolism 1994;43:599–603.

7 Haffner SM, Karhapaa P, et al: Insulin resistance, body fat distribution, and sex hormones in men. Diabetes 1994;43:212–219.

8 Ding EL, Song Y, et al: Sex differences of endogenous sex hormones and risk of type 2 diabetes: a systematic review and meta-analysis. JAMA 2006;295: 1288–1299.

9 Dhindsa S, Prabhakar S, et al: Frequent occurrence of hypogonadotropic hypogonadism in type 2 diabetes. J Clin Endocrinol Metab 2004;89:5462–5468.

10 Kapoor D, Aldred H, et al: Clinical and biochemical assessment of hypogonadism in men with type 2 diabetes: correlations with bioavailable testosterone and visceral adiposity. Diabetes Care 2007;30:911–917.

11 Selvin E, Feinleib M, et al: Androgens and diabetes in men: results from the Third National Health and Nutrition Examination Survey (NHANES III). Diabetes Care 2007;30:234–238.

12 Pitteloud N, Mootha VK, et al: Relationship between testosterone levels, insulin sensitivity, and mitochondrial function in men. Diabetes Care 2005;28: 1636–1642.

13 Grillo ML, Jacobus AP, et al: Testosterone rapidly stimulates insulin release from isolated pancreatic islets through a non-genomic dependent mechanism. Horm Metab Res 2005;37:662–665.

14 Laaksonen DE, Niskanen L, et al: Sex hormones, inflammation and the metabolic syndrome: a population-based study. Eur J Endocrinol 2003;149:601–608.

15 Blouin K, Despres JP, et al: Contribution of age and declining androgen levels to features of the metabolic syndrome in men. Metabolism 2005;54:1034–1040.

16 Corona G, Mannucci E, et al: Psychobiologic correlates of the metabolic syndrome and associated sexual dysfunction. Eur Urol 2006;50:595–604; discussion 604.
17 Van Pottelbergh I, Braeckman L, et al: Differential contribution of testosterone and estradiol in the determination of cholesterol and lipoprotein profile in healthy middle-aged men. Atherosclerosis 2003; 166:95–102.
18 Agledahl I, Skjaerpe PA, et al: Low serum testosterone in men is inversely associated with non-fasting serum triglycerides: The Tromso study. Nutr Metab Cardiovasc Dis 2007, in press.
19 Svartberg J, von Muhlen D, et al: Association of endogenous testosterone with blood pressure and left ventricular mass in men. The Tromso Study. Eur J Endocrinol 2004;150:65–71.
20 Tsai EC, Boyko EJ, et al: Low serum testosterone level as a predictor of increased visceral fat in Japanese-American men. Int J Obes Relat Metab Disord 2000;24:485–491.
21 Khaw KT, Barrett-Connor E: Lower endogenous androgens predict central adiposity in men. Ann Epidemiol 1992;2:675–682.
22 Stellato RK, Feldman HA, et al: Testosterone, sex hormone-binding globulin, and the development of type 2 diabetes in middle-aged men: prospective results from the Massachusetts male aging study. Diabetes Care 2000;23:490–494.
23 Haffner SM, Shaten J, et al: Low levels of sex hormone-binding globulin and testosterone predict the development of non-insulin-dependent diabetes mellitus in men. MRFIT Research Group. Multiple Risk Factor Intervention Trial. Am J Epidemiol 1996;143:889–897.
24 Oh JY, Barrett-Connor E, et al: Endogenous sex hormones and the development of type 2 diabetes in older men and women: the Rancho Bernardo study. Diabetes Care 2002;25:55–60.
25 Laaksonen DE, Niskanen L, et al: Testosterone and sex hormone-binding globulin predict the metabolic syndrome and diabetes in middle-aged men. Diabetes Care 2004;27:1036–1041.
26 Kupelian V, Page ST, et al: Low SHBG, total testosterone, and symptomatic androgen deficiency are associated with development of the metabolic syndrome in non-obese men. J Clin Endocrinol Metab 2006;91:843–850.
27 Laaksonen DE, Niskanen L, et al: The metabolic syndrome and smoking in relation to hypogonadism in middle-aged men: a prospective cohort study. J Clin Endocrinol Metab 2005;90:712–719.
28 Keating NL, O'Malley AJ, et al: Diabetes and cardiovascular disease during androgen deprivation therapy for prostate cancer. J Clin Oncol 2006;24: 4448–4456.
29 Derweesh IH, Diblasio CJ, et al: Risk of new-onset diabetes mellitus and worsening glycaemic variables for established diabetes in men undergoing androgen-deprivation therapy for prostate cancer. BJU Int 2007.
30 Smith JC, Bennett S, et al: The effects of induced hypogonadism on arterial stiffness, body composition, and metabolic parameters in males with prostate cancer. J Clin Endocrinol Metab 2001;86: 4261–4267.
31 Basaria S, Muller DC, et al: Hyperglycemia and insulin resistance in men with prostate carcinoma who receive androgen-deprivation therapy. Cancer 2006;106:581–588.
32 Yassin A, Saad F, et al: Effect of androgen deprivation on glycaemic control and on biochemical cardiovascular risk factors in men with diabetes. J Urol 2006;175(suppl):385.
33 Bhasin S, Woodhouse L, et al: Older men are as responsive as young men to the anabolic effects of graded doses of testosterone on the skeletal muscle. J Clin Endocrinol Metab 2005;90:678–688.
34 Zitzmann M, Nieschlag E: The CAG repeat polymorphism within the androgen receptor gene and maleness. Int J Androl 2003;26:76–83.
35 Stanworth R, Kapoor D, et al: HDL cholesterol levels are positively associated with testosterone and are lower with shorter androgen receptor CAG repeat lengths in men with type 2 diabetes. Society for Endocrinology BES, 2007.
36 Stanworth R, Kapoor D, et al: Serum testosterone levels and obesity are associated with androgen receptor CAG repeat polymorphism length in men with type 2 diabetes. The Endocrine Society's 89th Annual Meeting, 2007.
37 Jones RD, Pugh PJ, et al: Altered circulating hormone levels, endothelial function and vascular reactivity in the testicular feminised mouse. Eur J Endocrinol 2003;148:111–120.
38 Nettleship JE, Jones TH, et al: Physiological testosterone replacement therapy attenuates fatty streak formation and improves high-density lipoprotein cholesterol in the Tfm mouse: an effect that is independent of the classic androgen receptor. Circulation 2007;116:2427–2434.
39 Zitzmann M, Brune M, et al: The CAG repeat polymorphism in the AR gene affects high density lipoprotein cholesterol and arterial vasoreactivity. J Clin Endocrinol Metab 2001;86:4867–4873.
40 Isidori AM, Giannetta E, et al: Effects of testosterone on body composition, bone metabolism and serum lipid profile in middle-aged men: a meta-analysis. Clin Endocrinol (Oxf) 2005;63:280–293.

41 Snyder PJ, Peachey H, et al: Effect of testosterone treatment on body composition and muscle strength in men over 65 years of age. J Clin Endocrinol Metab 1999;84:2647–2653.

42 Boyanov MA, Boneva Z, et al: Testosterone supplementation in men with type 2 diabetes, visceral obesity and partial androgen deficiency. Aging Male 2003;6:1–7.

43 Kapoor D, Goodwin E, et al: Testosterone replacement therapy improves insulin resistance, glycaemic control, visceral adiposity and hypercholesterolaemia in hypogonadal men with type 2 diabetes. Eur J Endocrinol 2006;154:899–906.

44 Marin P, Holmang S, et al: Androgen treatment of abdominally obese men. Obes Res 1993;1:245–251.

45 Bhasin S, Parker RA, et al: Effects of testosterone supplementation on whole body and regional fat mass and distribution in human immunodeficiency virus-infected men with abdominal obesity. J Clin Endocrinol Metab 2007;92:1049–1057.

46 Simon D, Charles MA, et al: Androgen therapy improves insulin sensitivity and decreases leptin level in healthy adult men with low plasma total testosterone: a 3-month randomized placebo-controlled trial. Diabetes Care 2001;24:2149–2151.

47 Tripathy D, Shah P, et al: Effect of testosterone replacement on whole body glucose utilisation and other cardiovascular risk factors in males with idiopathic hypogonadotrophic hypogonadism. Horm Metab Res 1998;30:642–645.

48 Friedl KE, Jones RE, et al: The administration of pharmacological doses of testosterone or 19-nortestosterone to normal men is not associated with increased insulin secretion or impaired glucose tolerance. J Clin Endocrinol Metab 1989;68:971–975.

49 Corrales JJ, Burgo RM, et al: Partial androgen deficiency in aging type 2 diabetic men and its relationship to glycemic control. Metabolism 2004;53:666–672.

50 Lee CH, Kuo SW, et al: The effect of testosterone supplement on insulin sensitivity, glucose effectiveness, and acute insulin response after glucose load in male type 2 diabetics. Endocr Res 2005;31:139–148.

51 Jones TH: Testosterone associations with erectile dysfunction, diabetes and the metabolic syndrome. Eur Urol Suppl 2007;6:847–857.

52 Marin P, Oden B, et al: Assimilation and mobilization of triglycerides in subcutaneous abdominal and femoral adipose tissue in vivo in men: effects of androgens. J Clin Endocrinol Metab 1995;80:239–243.

53 Singh R, Artaza JN, Taylor WE, Gonzalez-Cadavid NF, Bhasin S: Androgens stimulate myogenic differentiation and inhibit adipogenesis in C3H 10T1/2 pluripotent cells through an androgen receptor-mediated pathway. Endocrinology 2003;144:5081–5088.

54 Guay AT, Bansal S, et al: Effect of raising endogenous testosterone levels in impotent men with secondary hypogonadism: double blind placebo-controlled trial with clomiphene citrate. J Clin Endocrinol Metab 1995;80:3546–3552.

55 Isidori AM, Caprio M, et al: Leptin and androgens in male obesity: evidence for leptin contribution to reduced androgen levels. J Clin Endocrinol Metab 1999;84:3673–3680.

Dr. Roger D. Stanworth
Robert Hague Centre for Diabetes and Endocrinology
Barnsley Hospital NHS Foundation Trust
Gawber Road, Barnsley S75 2EP (UK)
Tel. +44 1226 777947, Fax +44 1226 777771, E-Mail rogerstanworth@btinternet.com

Jones TH (ed): Advances in the Management of Testosterone Deficiency.
Front Horm Res. Basel, Karger, 2009, vol 37, pp 91–107

Testosterone and Coronary Artery Disease

Joanne E. Nettleship[a] · Richard D. Jones[a] · Kevin S. Channer[b,c] · T. Hugh Jones[a,d]

[a]Academic Unit of Diabetes, Endocrinology and Metabolism, University of Sheffield, [b]Department of Cardiology, Royal Hallamshire Hospital, and [c]Biomedical Research Centre, Sheffield Hallam University, Sheffield, and [d]Robert Hague Centre for Diabetes and Endocrinology, Barnsley Hospital NHS Foundation Trust, Barnsley, UK

Abstract

The strongest independent risk factors for coronary artery disease (CAD) are increasing age and male gender. Whilst a wide variation in CAD mortality exists between countries, a male to female ratio of approximately 2:1 is consistently observed. These observations have led to the assumption that testosterone may exert a detrimental influence on the cardiovascular system. Despite this, coronary atherosclerosis increases with age, whilst a marked fall in serum bioavailable testosterone levels is observed. Similarly, low testosterone levels are also associated with other cardiovascular risk factors and increased expression of mediators of the atherosclerotic process. This in itself suggests that testosterone does not promote atheroma formation. Moreover, epidemiological studies show an inverse relationship between testosterone levels and surrogate markers of atherosclerosis, which suggests that it may be a testosterone deficient state, rather than male sex which is associated with CAD. In cholesterol-fed animal models, atherosclerosis is accelerated by castration and reduced after testosterone replacement therapy. Testosterone has also been shown to improve myocardial ischemia in men with angina pectoris. Consequently, increasing evidence suggests that the process of atherosclerosis is beneficially modulated by testosterone. These studies are the focus of this chapter.

Pathophysiology of Coronary Artery Disease

Coronary artery disease (CAD) is the leading cause of death in the western world. CAD and is almost exclusively caused by atherosclerosis; indeed the two terms are often used synonymously. The great majority of ischaemic damage to the myocardium is the result of coronary atherosclerosis. Atherosclerosis is an intimal disease of the medium and large arteries including, the aorta, carotid and cerebral arteries. CAD is characterised pathologically by the atherosclerotic plaque, and is described as a focal inflammatory fibro-proliferative response to multiple forms of endothelial injury, in which a number of distinct but overlapping pathways of pathogenesis are involved.

The endothelial layer forms a complex of intercellular tight junctions, and functions as a selectively permeable barrier between blood and tissues. Among the physical forces acting on the endothelial cells, affecting endothelial cell morphology, is fluid shear stress. Cells in regions of arterial branching or curvature, where blood flow is disrupted, have a polygonal shape and no particular orientation. These areas show an increase in endothelial permeability to macromolecules such as low-density lipoprotein (LDL) cholesterol and are the preferred sites for lesion formation. In contrast, cells in the arteries of tubular regions, where blood flow is uniform and laminar exhibit ellipsoid shapes and are aligned in the direction of the flow. Therefore, due to these differences in blood flow dynamics, branched areas are the more common sites for lesion formation within the arteries. Haemodynamic forces act at these sites to influence the permeability of the endothelial barrier, allowing passive diffusion of LDL cholesterol through endothelial junctions. It is thought that the principal event initiating lesion formation is endothelial cell injury. This encourages monocyte attachment, via the expression of adhesion molecules and chemokines on the endothelial cell surface. When activated by injury, endothelial cells and the attached monocytes and macrophages generate free radicals, which oxidise LDL, resulting in lipid peroxidation and destruction of the receptor needed for normal receptor-mediated clearance of LDL. Consequently oxidised LDL (ox-LDL) accumulates in the sub-endothelial space where it is taken up by macrophages via scavenger receptors to form foam cells. Oxidised LDL is proposed to exacerbate the local inflammatory response, and has other effects, such as inhibiting the production of nitric oxide, an important chemical mediator with multiple anti-atherogenic properties, including vasorelaxation. After taking up LDL, these macrophages (now foam cells) migrate sub-endothelially. Sub-endothelial collections of foam cells form the 'fatty streaks', which presage atherosclerosis. Although the fatty streaks themselves are not clinically significant, they are now accepted to be the precursors of more advanced lesions, which may go on to become the sites of thrombosis. Atherosclerotic lesions are considered advanced by the following histological criteria: accumulations of lipid, smooth muscle cells, T lymphocytes, macrophages, necrotic cell debris and matrix components (including minerals), associated with structural disorganisation and thickening of the intima, with deformity of the arterial wall. The advanced lesion is contained within a fibrous cap, formed by extensive smooth muscle cell proliferation and vascular remodelling, the result of the unabated response to endothelial injury. The cap consists of smooth muscle cells surrounded by collagen, elastic fibres and proteoglycans. Rupture of the fibrous cap, results in the spillage of the contents of the advanced lesion into the vessel lumen. This results in the formation of a thrombus, which either heals, causing further lesion progression and further compromising flow at the local site, or occludes the coronary artery completely resulting in sudden death. Plaque rupture and thrombosis are the primary complications of the advanced lesion, which cause unstable coronary syndromes or myocardial infarction.

Testosterone and Risk Factors for Coronary Artery Disease

The strongest independent risk factors for CAD are that of increased age and the male sex. Despite a wide variance in CAD mortality between countries, a consistent male:female ratio of approximately 2:1 is observed [1]. Such data have led to the supposition that male hormones, and testosterone in particular, exert a detrimental influence upon the cardiovascular system. Coronary atherosclerosis inevitably increases with age; a longer duration of exposure to possible detrimental factors, together with impairment of endothelial function, arterial compliance and immunosuppression, conspire to make atheroma formation more likely. Serum levels of testosterone also fall markedly in relation to increasing age, and testosterone replacement therapy is an emerging therapeutic option for the aging male. The fact that testosterone levels fall with age whilst atherosclerosis increases, suggests testosterone per se does not induce atheroma formation. In addition, an inverse association is also observed between serum levels of testosterone and other risk factors for CAD. These studies are summarized below.

Effect on Inflammatory Markers

Cytokines are key players in the atherosclerotic process. Pro-inflammatory cytokines such as interleukin-1β (IL-1β) and tumor necrosis factor-α (TNF-α) are known to increase adhesion molecule expression, promote smooth muscle cell proliferation and induce matrix metalloproteinase activity; critical mechanisms in the initiation of plaque development and rupture. Observational evidence suggests that inflammatory cytokines and serum testosterone levels are interconnected. Indeed, we have recently demonstrated that serum levels of IL-1β increase significantly in a step-wise manner according to atherosclerotic burden in men with marked CAD [2]. Furthermore, when patients were classified by their serum testosterone level as either eugonadal, 'borderline' hypogonadal or hypogonadal, a step-wise increase in the IL-1β was observed. Such data suggest that the underlying testosterone status may modulate IL-1β production in men with CAD. Elderly, hypogonadal men also exhibit raised serum levels of TNF-α and interleukin-6 (IL-6) [3]. Recent studies in a cardiovascular setting have also demonstrated that testosterone therapy is able to beneficially modulate cytokine activity. Malkin et al. [4] completed a randomized, single-blind, placebo-controlled crossover study of physiological testosterone therapy in 10 men with CAD and associated hypotestosteronaemia. This level of testosterone replacement therapy was sufficient to significantly reduce serum levels of TNF-α [4]. Similar observations were also observed in a larger study by Malkin et al. [5] using the same testosterone dosing regimen and randomized, placebo-controlled crossover protocol, in 27 hypogonadal men with concomitant cardiovascular disease. Physiological testosterone replacement therapy again significantly lowered serum levels of TNF-α. Additional to the reduction in TNF-α, following physiological testosterone administration, a significant elevation was observed in serum levels of the anti-inflammatory and anti-atherogenic cytokine IL-10 [5]. In this study although the effect of testosterone on IL-1β levels was not statistically significant there was a reduction which approached significance ($p = 0.08$). There was no effect on IL-6 levels. These data overall provide evidence that testosterone is able to beneficially regulate cytokine function in men with CAD.

Effect on Adhesion Molecule Expression

Testosterone is reported to have a modulatory effect upon endothelial cell adhesion molecule expression. Dihydrotestosterone has been shown to increase monocyte adhesion to IL-1β-stimulated human umbilical vein endothelial cells (HUVECs) and human umbilical artery endothelial cells (HUVACs) obtained from male donors, and also to increase IL-1β-induced vascular cell adhesion molecule-1 (VCAM-1) expression in these cells [6], via the activation of nuclear factor kappa B (NFκB) transcription factor. Similarly, the study of Zhang et al. [7] reports that testosterone increases TNF-α-induced expression of VCAM-1 and the cell adhesion molecule E-selectin, in HUVECs. In both studies the action of testosterone was abolished by androgen receptor (AR) antagonism [6, 7]. In contrast, testosterone reduces TNF-α-induced VCAM-1 expression in HUVECs of female origin, an activity blocked by oestrogen receptor antagonism and aromatase inhibition [8]. These data suggest that testosterone has a detrimental influence upon adhesion molecule expression in males via interaction with the AR, but induces potentially beneficial reductions in adhesion molecule expression in females via aromatisation to 17β-estradiol. However, vascular specificity is also apparent. Importantly, testosterone is reported to *reduce* TNF-α-induced VCAM-1 expression in human aortic endothelial cells [9]. Clearly, this preparation is more relevant in terms of atherosclerosis compared to umbilical cells. Evidently, further study is warranted, but these data suggest that testosterone could potentially exert a beneficial effect upon adhesion molecule expression in large arteries.

Effect on Haemostatic Factors

In the majority of cases, myocardial infarction occurs as a result of coronary thrombosis, triggered by atherosclerotic plaque rupture and disruption of the vascular endothelium. The thrombotic process is complex, and dependent upon a variety of intrinsic pro- and anti-thrombotic mediators which determine the coagulation status. The anti-coagulation agents tissue plasminogen activator (tPA) and tissue factor pathway inhibitor (TFPI), and the pro-thrombotic factor plasminogen activator inhibitor-1 (PAI-1) are integral to this process. Evidence suggests that low serum testosterone is associated with a hyper-coagulable state. Serum testosterone levels and tPA are reported to be positively correlated, whilst a negative correlation exists between serum levels of testosterone and PAI-1 and clotting factor VII [10–12]. Moreover, both testosterone replacement in hypogonadal men, and androgen treatment in healthy men, leads to reduced PAI-1 levels [13, 14]. In a study of physiological testosterone therapy in men with chronic stable angina which included eugonadal as well as hypogonadal men, no effect on serum tPA or PAI activity was observed [15]. These findings are significant in that no adverse effects of testosterone on clotting have been found. This is an important observation, since an increased risk of arterial and venous thromboembolism is associated with female hormone replacement therapy (HRT) and thought to account for the increased incidence in vascular events and death associated with HRT in the Women's Health Initiative study [16]. This adverse effect on coagulation is therefore not a property which would appear to be shared with testosterone.

Effect on Lipids

Elevated serum cholesterol is a powerful risk factor for CAD. Endogenous serum levels of testosterone have been reported in a number of cross-sectional studies to be negatively correlated with serum levels of pro-atherogenic total and low-density lipoprotein (LDL) cholesterol, and positively correlated with athero-protective high-density lipoprotein (HDL) cholesterol [17–22]. These data suggest that hypogonadal men may exhibit an adverse pro-atherogenic lipid profile. Healthy and diabetic men have also been shown to exhibit a positive correlation between testosterone and HDL cholesterol levels [23, 24].

Significant reductions in total and LDL cholesterol have been reported in hypogonadal men following testosterone replacement therapy [25–28], an effect which is maintained in eugonadal individuals [29–31]. Furthermore, serum total cholesterol levels are also reported to decline following physiological testosterone replacement in hypogonadal men with either CAD or type 2 diabetes despite the majority of patients already being treated with HMG-CoA reductase inhibitors [4, 32]. In contrast, testosterone has also been demonstrated to reduce HDL cholesterol in some [16, 30], but not all [31, 33], studies. A meta-analysis of these studies suggests testosterone treatment is associated with an overall small reduction in HDL cholesterol, which is much less pronounced than the reduction observed in pro-atherogenic lipid fractions [34].

Effect on Insulin Resistance and Visceral Obesity

Insulin resistance is the hallmark feature of type 2 diabetes, which is an established risk factor for CAD. Obesity is the most common cause of insulin resistance, and is itself a powerful risk factor for CAD. Evidence suggests that testosterone, insulin sensitivity and obesity are inter-linked, with testosterone having beneficial effects upon both conditions. A number of studies demonstrate that serum levels of testosterone are lower in diabetic men or individuals with impaired glucose tolerance [24, 35–37] whilst studies in healthy men report an inverse association between serum testosterone and insulin concentrations [17, 38]. Furthermore, low testosterone levels in normal men would appear to predict the future development of insulin resistance and subsequent type 2 diabetes [39, 40]. In addition, testosterone replacement in hypogonadal men is reported to improve insulin sensitivity. Simon et al. [41] demonstrated that treatment for three months with physiological concentrations of transdermal testosterone was associated with a significantly lower fasting plasma insulin, fasting plasma insulin/fasting plasma glucose ratio, HOMA index and leptin level, compared to placebo-treated controls. This is not consistent in all studies [42, 43], although this may be a consequence of the supra-physiological concentrations utilized: Marin et al. [44] demonstrated that supra-physiological testosterone administration was associated with reduced glucose tolerance in middle-aged obese men. However, following treatment with doses achieving plasma levels of testosterone high in the physiological range, insulin levels were reduced and insulin sensitivity increased, with the greatest effect observed in men with lower baseline testosterone levels. Kapoor et al. [32] recently completed the first double-blind placebo-controlled crossover study on the effects of testosterone replacement therapy in hypogonadal men with type 2 diabetes. The study reported that testosterone replacement therapy significantly reduced insulin resistance, fasting blood glucose, HbA_{1c}, cholesterol, waist circumference and waist-to-hip ratio [32].

A physical characteristic of hypogonadism is a reduction in lean body mass and an increased fat mass. Indeed, Vermeulen et al. [45] reported in a study of 57 men aged between 70 and 80 years that testosterone levels correlated negatively with percentage of body fat, abdominal fat and insulin levels. Abdominal obesity is also reported to be inversely related to total and free testosterone [46–48], and subcutaneous fat accumulation in the truncal area is highly predictive of low plasma concentrations of free testosterone [49]. Weight loss in obese men leads to a significant increase in testosterone [50], in proportion to the degree of weight loss [51]. Similarly, correction of testosterone levels in obese men reduces their BMI and visceral fat mass [44, 52, 53] and oral testosterone therapy is reported to produce a significant reduction in body weight, body fat [54] and blood glucose in men with type 2 diabetes [32, 54].

Testosterone and Coronary Artery Disease

Testosterone in Animal Models of Atherosclerosis

A number of studies report that supplemental testosterone therapy is associated with reduced aortic accumulation of cholesterol and a reduction in plaque size in male animal models of atherosclerosis. Larsen et al. [55] examined the effects of testosterone treatment in orchidectomised male rabbits fed a pro-atherogenic diet for 17 weeks. Following cholesterol feeding, aortic cholesterol accumulation was significantly retarded in the testosterone-treated, compared to the placebo-treated, group [55]. Comparable findings have also been reported in 2 other studies [56, 57], although interestingly in the study by Bruck et al. [56], testosterone administration also resulted in an increase in plaque size in female rabbits. Physiological testosterone supplementation has also been shown to reduce atherosclerosis in orchidectomised LDL-receptor knock out, an effect was not observed in animals treated simultaneously with the aromatase inhibitor anastrazole [58], which is in contrast to the findings in the rabbit model [56]. More recently, our own research group has demonstrated that physiological testosterone supplementation reduces aortic fatty streak formation in the testosterone-deficient testicular feminised (Tfm) mouse [59]. These animals express a non-functional androgen receptor, indicating that the athero-protective action of testosterone is not mediated via an androgen receptor-dependent pathway. Furthermore, since the reduction in fatty streak formation was not prevented by treatment with either the aromatase inhibitor anastrazole or the estrogen receptor α antagonist fulvestrant, the athero-protective action of testosterone is not attributable to aromatisation to 17β-estradiol, rather a non-genomic action of testosterone.

Clinical Studies

On the basis of the above observations, it would appear that testosterone may be beneficial to the male cardiovascular system, and that a relative deficiency in circulating levels of testosterone may lead to detrimental effects. Indeed, two recent studies have highlighted a link between low testosterone and increased mortality, primarily as a result of cardiovascular and respiratory disease [60, 61]. Similarly, Keating et al. [62] report that androgen deprivation therapy via gonadotropin-releasing hormone agonism, in men with prostate carcinoma, is associated with an increased risk of diabetes, coronary heart disease, myocardial infarction and sudden cardiac death. Furthermore, review of the published cross-sectional studies which have reported the serum levels of testosterone in men with CAD, demonstrates that in the majority of cases serum levels of testosterone are *reduced* in men with CAD (table 1) [63]. Recent studies which have specifically investigated the association between endogenous sex hormones and CAD, also report a negative correlation between serum levels of testosterone and atherosclerotic burden. Hak et al. [64] investigated the relationship between androgen level decline and atherosclerosis with advancing age, in a study population of over 1,000 non-smoking men and women aged 55 years or over. They found an inverse relationship between endogenous levels of testosterone and severe aortic atherosclerosis in men, whilst in women a higher level of testosterone tended to have a positive association with aortic atherosclerosis [64]. Similarly, a study by Phillips et al. [11] of 55 men aged 39–89 years, also reported an inverse relationship between serum testosterone and the degree of CAD. Van den Beld et al. [65] examined the relationship between carotid intima-media thickening (IMT), an early marker of generalised atherosclerosis and an unfavourable cardiovascular risk profile, and serum levels of testosterone in 403 men aged 73–94. This study demonstrated that increased wall thickness of the carotid artery was related to low serum testosterone. Furthermore, higher testosterone concentrations were associated with reduced IMT of the carotid artery [65]. Similarly,

Table 1. Cross-sectional studies investigating serum testosterone levels in men with atherosclerosis

Study	Number of patients	Definition of CHD	Androgen measured	Androgen levels in CHD cohort
Mendoza et al. [123]	52	MI	TT	↓
Barth et al. [124]	20	CAD	TT	↓
Hromadova et al. [125]	67	'Coronary findings'	TT	↓
Breier et al. [126]	139	CAD	TT	↓
Aksut et al. [129]	54	MI/Angina	TT	↓
Sewdarsen et al. [130]	56	MI	TT/FT	↓/↓
Chute et al. [131]	146	CAD	TT/FT	↓/↓
Hämäläinen et al. [132]	57	CHD	TT/FT	↓/↓
Lichtenstein et al. [133]	2,512	IHD	TT	↓
Swartz and Young [134]	71	MI	TT	↓
Sewdarsen et al. [135]	20	MI	TT	↓
Sewdarsen et al. [138]	224	MI	TT/FT	↓/↓
Gray et al. [139]	1,709	CAD	TT/FT	↓/↓
Rice et al. [142]	272	MI	TT/FT	↓/↓
Phillips et al. [60]	55	CAD	TT/FT	↓/↓
Zhao and Li [146]	201	CAD	TT	↓
English et al. [150]	90	CAD	TT/FT/BT	↔/↓/↓
Pugh et al. [61]	30	MI	TT/BT	↔/↓
Zumoff et al. [118]	117	MI, CAD	TT	↔
Luria et al. [119]	50	MI	TT	↔
Labropoulos et al. [120]	144	MI	TT	↔
Phillips et al. [121]	122	CHD	TT	↔
Heller et al. [122]	295	CHD	TT	↔
Small et al. [127]	100	IHD	TT	↔
Franzen and Fex [128]	92	MI	TT	↔
Baumann et al. [136]	58	Atherosclerosis	TT	↔
Slowinska-Srzednicka et al. [137]	108	MI	TT	↔
Cengiz et al. [140]	55	MI, angina	TT	↔
Hauner et al. [141]	274	CAD	TT	↔
Hautanen et al. [143]	159	CAD	TT	↔
Mitchell et al. [144]	98	MI	TT/FT	↔/↔
Marques-Vidal et al. [145]	116	MI	TT	↔
Feldman et al. [147]	1,709	Heart disease	TT/FT	↔/↔
Kabakci et al. [148]	337	CAD	TT/FT	↔/↔
Schuler-Luttmann et al. [149]	189	CAD	TT/FT	↔/↔

This table is taken from Jones et al. [63]. The reference numbers in this table pertain to that publication. Reproduced with permission.

BT = Bioavailable testosterone; CAD = coronary artery disease; CHD = coronary heart disease; FT = free testosterone; IHD = ischemic heart disease; MI = myocardial infarction; TT = total testosterone; ↔ indicates no change; ↓ indicates decrease.

low serum testosterone is also associated with increased carotid artery IMT in men with obesity and type 2 diabetes [66, 67]. Finally, Muller et al. [68] conducted a study in elderly men, to investigate the association between carotid IMT and serum testosterone at baseline and after a 4-year follow-up period. They found that the individuals with the lowest serum testosterone at baseline had the greatest progression of carotid IMT, independent of BMI, waist-to-hip ratio, hypertension, diabetes, smoking and cholesterol [68].

These studies provide further support for the concept that testosterone plays a protective role in the development of atherosclerosis in the ageing male. There are several potential sites of action in the development of the atherosclerotic plaque where testosterone could exert a protective effect (fig. 1). However, to date no studies have specifically investigated whether testosterone therapy reduces cardiovascular events, although a number of studies have investigated the effect of testosterone therapy on measures of myocardial ischaemia in men with angina.

Testosterone and Angina

Anecdotal evidence of a beneficial effect of testosterone therapy upon angina pectoris was first reported as long ago as 1942 [69], although it was another 35 years before the first placebo-controlled study was undertaken. In 1977, Jaffe [70] reported a 32% reduction in time to 1-mm ST-segment depression on exercise treadmill testing after 1 month, and 51% after 3 months, of testosterone treatment. More recent studies also report a beneficial effect of testosterone therapy upon myocardial ischaemia. Oral testosterone treatment in a cohort of 62 elderly men with angina in a 1 month placebo crossover study led to an improvement in ischaemia and anginal symptoms [71]. A double-blind, randomised placebo-controlled, add-on trial using transdermal testosterone patches (5 mg/day for 3 months) in a group of men with chronic stable angina who were unselected for baseline hypogonadism, showed that testosterone induced a significant benefit in time to 1 mm ST-segment depression by 37% (52 s) [72]. Many of these men were already treated with two to three anti-anginal drugs, and pharmacologically an increase of 52 s is greater than that which would be expected for the addition of a third or fourth drug. The study also showed that the lower the baseline bioavailable testosterone the greater the beneficial effect of testosterone therapy on the time to ischaemia [72]. A further study involving men with angina and overt hypogonadism (mean testosterone approximately 4 nmol/l) reported that 1 month of treatment with testosterone led to a 74-second imp rovement in time to 1 mm ST-segment depression (fig. 2) [4]. Acute administration of physiological doses of testosterone directly into the coronary circulation at cardiac catheterisation produces a rapid increase in coronary artery diameter and blood flow [73]. An intravenous bolus of testosterone, which produces supraphysiological levels, prior to exercise treadmill testing, results in a significant improvement in

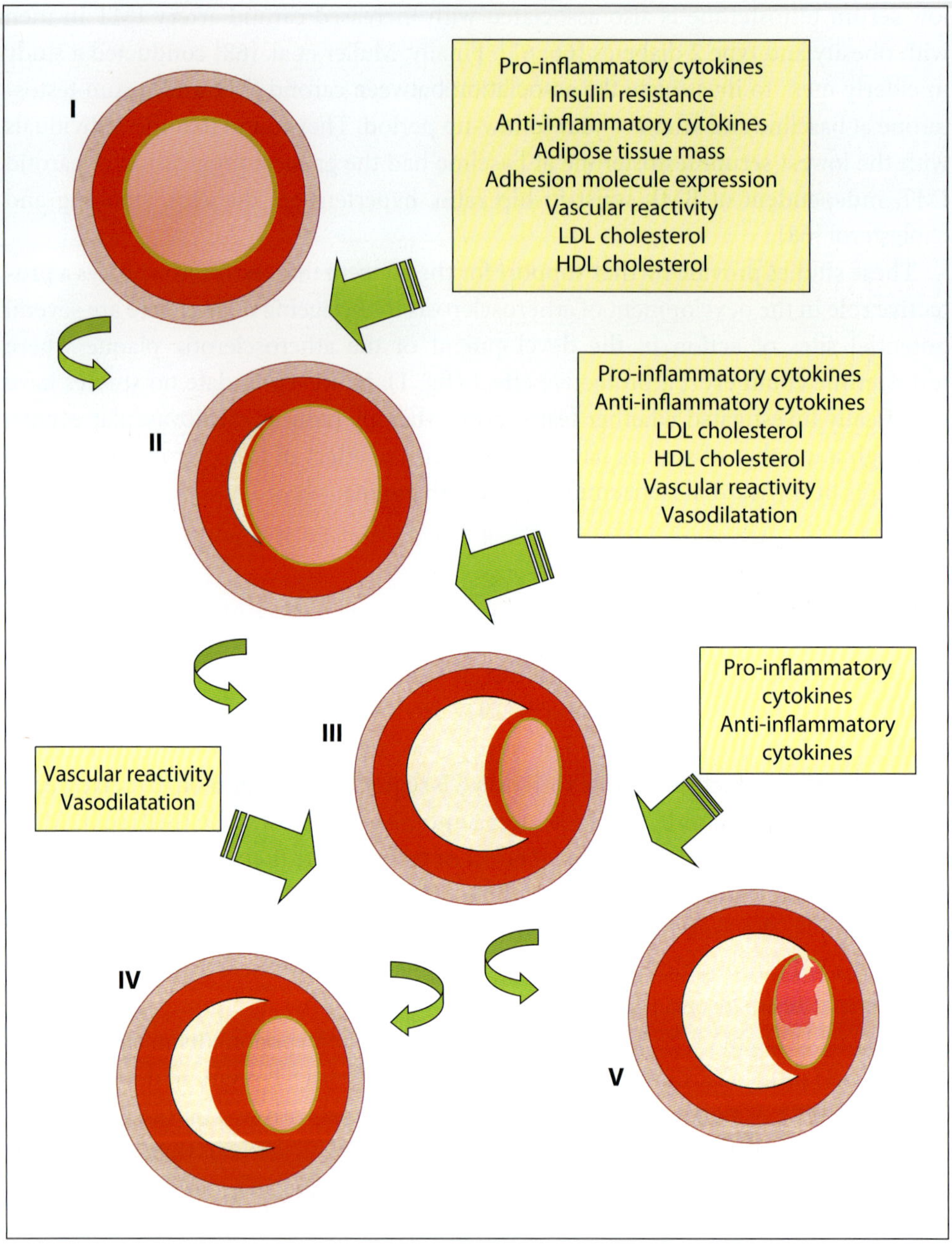

Fig. 1. Potential mechanisms by which testosterone may regulate atherosclerotic plaque development. Potential cardiovascular actions of testosterone and indication of how these responses may influence the atherosclerotic process via interaction with the normal coronary artery (I), the early atherosclerotic lesion (II), the mature unstable atherosclerotic plaque (III), the mature stable atherosclerotic plaque (IV) and the ruptured plaque (V).

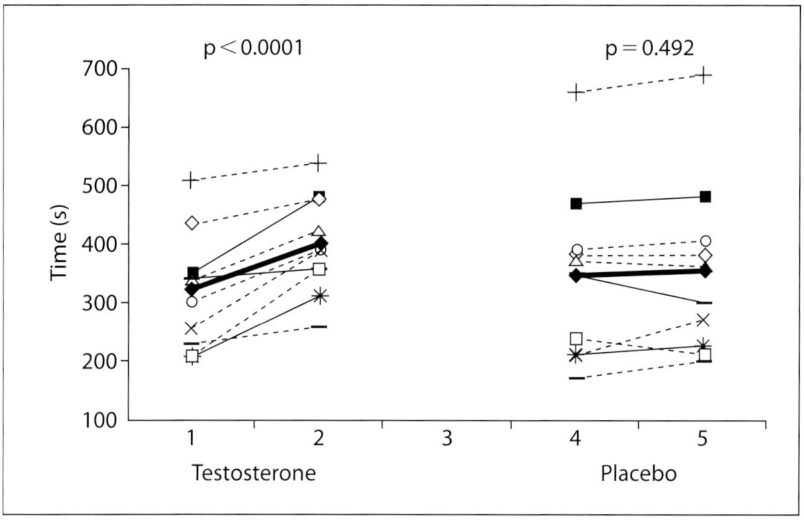

Fig. 2. Effect of testosterone replacement therapy on cardiac ischaemia threshold as assessed by time to 1 mm S-T depression during exercise treadmill testing in hypogonadal men with chronic stable angina. This was a randomised placebo controlled crossover study with intramuscular testosterone esters (Sustanon 100®) 100 mg every 2 weeks. Treatment and placebo periods each lasted 1 month with a 1-month washout in between. Bold lines depict the mean (±SEM) of all patients within each group. All other lines depict individual patient data. Reproduced with permission from Malkin et al. [4].

myocardial ischaemia in humans [73, 74]. Such observations suggest a beneficial effect of testosterone upon the coronary arterial bed, and a wealth of animal data supports the hypothesis that testosterone beneficially modulates vascular tone.

Effect on Vascular Reactivity

Maintenance of a correct response to vasoconstrictive and vasodilatory agents is essential in the control of vascular tone, especially in atherosclerosis where reduced vasodilatation and enhanced vasoconstriction further restricts coronary blood flow through the partially occluded atherosclerotic vessel. This can also lead to vasospasm, thereby exacerbating symptoms of angina. Both human and animals studies have demonstrated that testosterone elicits marked coronary vasodilatation both in vivo and in vitro an action which diminishes with aging [75, 76]. Testosterone-induced vasodilatation is rapid in onset and is unaffected by AR blockade or deficiency, and is preserved in endothelial-denuded vessels and in the presence of nitric oxide synthase inhibitors, guanylate cyclase or cyclooxygenase [reviewed in 77]. These observations demonstrate the lack of involvement of the AR, endothelial-derived mediators or dilatory prostanoids in this acute response, rather that the dilatory action of testosterone is effected by a direct action on the vascular smooth muscle. Furthermore, the

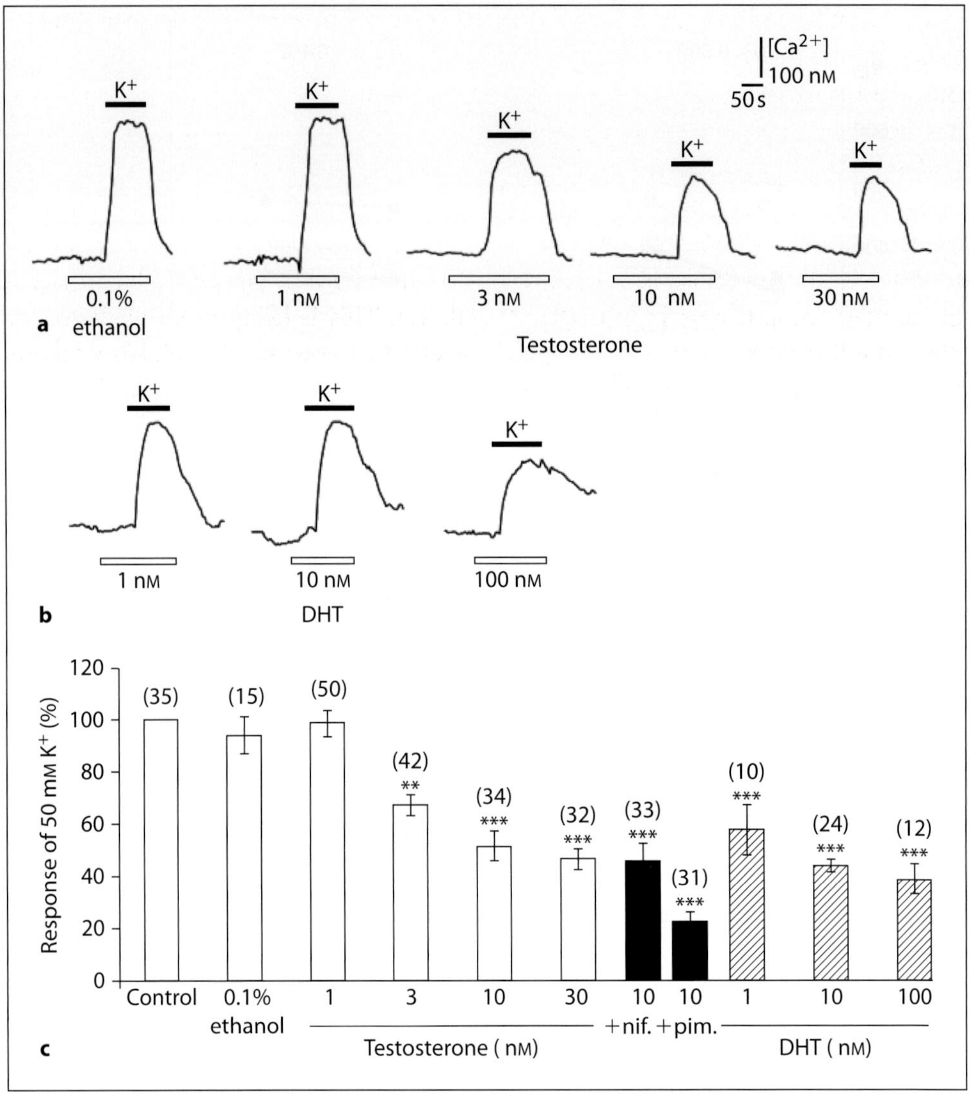

Fig. 3. Effect of testosterone and DHT on calcium channels in rat A7r5 vascular smooth muscle cells. **a** Example recordings of $[Ca^{2+}]_i$ from A7r5 cells during perfusion with 50 mM K^+-containing solution (for the periods indicated by the solid bars) in the additional presence of vehicle alone (0.1% ethanol) or increasing concentrations of testosterone (1–30 nM, as indicated), applied for the periods indicated by the open bars. **b** As **a** but cells were exposed to increasing concentrations of DHT, as indicated. Scale bars apply to traces in **a** and **b**. **c** Bar graph plotting mean percent (±SEM) response evoked by 50 mM K^+ solution in the presence of increasing concentrations of testosterone (open bars) or DHT (hatched bars), as indicated. Data are normalized to high K^+ responses evoked in the absence of steroids. Numbers in parentheses indicate the number of cells studied in each case. $^{**}p < 0.01$; $^{***}p < 0.001$ compared with control, analyzed via the Mann-Whitney U test. Also plotted is the mean response to 50 mM K^+ in the presence of both 10 nM testosterone plus 5 μM nifedipine (10 μnif; solid bar) and 10 nM testosterone plus 1 μM pimozide (10 μpim; solid bar). Reproduced with permission from Hall et al. [81].

observation that testosterone-induced dilatation is not attenuated by covalent linkage to albumin [78], which prevents its endocytosis into the smooth muscle cell, implies the dilatory signaling process is initiated at the smooth muscle cell membrane, which has been demonstrated to contain testosterone binding sites [79]. The proposed underlying mechanism of action of testosterone is thought to occur either via activation of calcium-sensitive potassium channels (K_{Ca}) or inhibition of voltage-gated calcium channels (VGCCs) [reviewed in 77]. Cellular studies have demonstrated that testosterone in physiological concentrations inhibits both L-type and T-type VGCCs in vascular smooth muscle cells (fig. 3) [80, 81]. This is likely to be mediated via direct binding to the main α_{1C} subunit of the VGCC, since a similar inhibitory action is observed in HEK 293 (human embryonic kidney) cells transfected with this channel protein [80, 81]. This is the exact site of action of deoxypyridinoline class of L-type calcium channel blocker such as nifedipine and amlodipine, which are commonly used in the treatment of angina. Additional to this direct vasodilatory action, testosterone is also reported to beneficially modulate responses induced by other vasoactive stimuli [reviewed in 82]. Both chronic exposure to physiological testosterone therapy [83] and acute exposure to supra-physiological doses of testosterone [84] are reported to increase flow-mediated brachial artery vasodilatation in men with CAD, which occurs as a result of increased nitric oxide release from the endothelium in response to changes in sheer stress. Long-term physiological testosterone therapy also improves nitrate-mediated brachial artery vasodilatation in these patients [83]. Brachial artery reactivity is recognized to correlate closely with coronary arterial responsiveness [85], and consequently such observations support a beneficial long-term effect for testosterone upon atherosclerotic coronary vasomotion. Taken together these studies provide an explanation for the observed beneficial effects of testosterone upon angina.

Conclusion

In summary, a large body of evidence suggests that physiological testosterone replacement therapy could offer cardiovascular, as well as other clinical advantages, to hypogonadal men with concomitant CAD. Recent evidence suggests that this may be a population as large as 1 in 4 of all men afflicted with the condition [86], constituting a considerable population worldwide. Large, long-term clinical trials are clearly warranted, since testosterone replacement may represent an overlooked therapeutic opportunity for this patient population.

References

1 Rayner M, Mockford C, Boaz A: Coronary Heart Disease Statistics; in: British Heart Foundation Statistics Database. London, British Heart Foundation Education Department, 1998.

2 Nettleship JE, Pugh PJ, Channer KS, Jones T, Jones RD: Inverse relationship between serum levels of interleukin-1beta and testosterone in men with stable coronary artery disease. Horm Metab Res 2007; 39:366–371.

3 Khosla S, Atkinson EJ, Dunstan CR, O'Fallon WM: Effect of estrogen versus testosterone on circulating osteoprotegerin and other cytokine levels in normal elderly men. J Clin Endocrinol Metab 2002;87: 1550–1554.

4 Malkin CJ, Pugh PJ, Morris PD, Kerry KE, Jones RD, Jones TH, Channer KS: Testosterone replacement in hypogonadal men with angina improves ischaemic threshold and quality of life. Heart 2004; 90:871–876.

5 Malkin CJ, Pugh PJ, Jones RD, Kapoor D, Channer KS, Jones TH: The effect of testosterone replacement on endogenous inflammatory cytokines and lipid profiles in hypogonadal men. J Clin Endocrinol Metab 2004;89:3313–3318.

6 McCrohon JA, Jessup W, Handelsman DJ, Celermajer DS: Androgen exposure increases human monocyte adhesion to vascular endothelium and endothelial cell expression of vascular cell adhesion molecule-1. Circulation 1999;99:2317–2322.

7 Zhang X, Wang LY, Jiang TY, Zhang HP, Dou Y, Zhao JH, Zhao H, Qiao ZD, Qiao JT: Effects of testosterone and 17-beta-estradiol on TNF-alpha-induced E-selectin and VCAM-1 expression in endothelial cells: analysis of the underlying receptor pathways. Life Sci 2002;71:15–29.

8 Mukherjee TK, Dinh H, Chaudhuri G, Nathan L: Testosterone attenuates expression of vascular cell adhesion molecule-1 by conversion to estradiol by aromatase in endothelial cells: implications in atherosclerosis. Proc Natl Acad Sci USA 2002;99:4055–4060.

9 Hatakeyama H, Nishizawa M, Nakagawa A, Nakano S, Kigoshi T, Uchida K: Testosterone inhibits tumor necrosis factor-alpha-induced vascular cell adhesion molecule-1 expression in human aortic endothelial cells. FEBS Lett 2002;530:129–132.

10 Glueck CJ, Glueck HI, Stroop D, Speirs, Hamer T, Tracy T: Endogenous testosterone, fibrinolysis, and coronary heart disease risk in hyperlipidemic men. J Lab Clin Med 1993;122:412–420.

11 Phillips GB, Pinkernell BH, Jing TY: The association of hypotestosteronemia with coronary artery disease in men. Arterioscler Thromb 1994;14: 701–706.

12 Pugh PJ, Channer KS, Parry H, Downes T, Jones TH: Bio-available testosterone levels fall acutely following myocardial infarction in men: association with fibrinolytic factors. Endocr Res 2002;28:161–173.

13 Beer NA, Jakubowicz DJ, Matt DW, Beer RM, Nestler JE: Dehydroepiandrosterone reduces plasma plasminogen activator inhibitor type 1 and tissue plasminogen activator antigen in men. Am J Med Sci 1996;311:205–210.

14 Caron P, Bennet A, Camare R, Louvet JP, Boneu B, Sie P: Plasminogen activator inhibitor in plasma is related to testosterone in men. Metabol Clin Exp 1989;38:1010–1015.

15 Smith AM, English KM, Malkin CM, Jones RD, Jones TH, Channer K: Testosterone does not adversely affect fibrinogen or tissue plasminogen activator (tPA) and plasminogen activator inhibitor-1 (PAI-1) levels in 46 men with chronic stable angina. Eur J Endocrinol 2005;152:285–291.

16 Rossouw J, Anderson G, Prentice R, LaCroix A, Kooperberg C, Stefanick M, Jackson R, Beresford S, Howard B, Johnson K, Kotchen J, Ockene J: Risks and benefits of estrogen plus progestin in healthy postmenopausal women: principal results from the Women's Health Initiative randomized controlled trial. JAMA 2002;288:321–333.

17 Barrett-Connor E, Khaw KT: Endogenous sex hormones and cardiovascular disease in men: a prospective population-based study. Circulation 1988;78: 539–545.

18 Haffner SM, Mykkanen L, Valdez RA, Katz MS: Relationship of sex hormones to lipids and lipoproteins in non-diabetic men. J Clin Endocrinol Metab 1993;77:1610–1615.

19 Simon D, Charles MA, Nahoul K, Orssaud G, Kremski J, Hully V, Joubert E, Papoz L, Eschwege E: Association between plasma total testosterone and cardiovascular risk factors in healthy adult men: The Telecom Study. J Clin Endocrinol Metab 1997; 82:682–685.

20 Dai WS, Gutai JP, Kuller LH, Laporte R, Falvo-Gerald L, Caggiula A: Relation between plasma high-density lipoprotein cholesterol and sex hormone concentrations in men. Am J Cardiol 1984; 53:1259–1263.

21 Heller RF, Wheeler MJ, Micallef J, Miller N, Lewis B: Relationship of high density lipoprotein cholesterol with total and free testosterone and sex hormone binding globulin. Acta Endocrinol 1983;104:253–256.

22 Hromadova M, Hacik T, Malatinsky E, Riecansky I: Alterations of lipid metabolism in men with hypotestosteronemia. Horm Metab Res 1991;32: 392–394.

23 Van Pottelbergh I, Braeckman L, De Bacquer D, De Backer G, Kaufman JM: Differential contribution of testosterone and estradiol in the determination of cholesterol and lipoprotein profile in healthy middle-aged men. Atherosclerosis 2003;166:95–102.
24 Barrett-Connor E: Lower endogenous androgen levels and dyslipidemia in men with non-insulin-dependent diabetes mellitus. Ann Intern Med 1992; 117:807–811.
25 Tenover JS: Effects of testosterone in the aging male. J Clin Endocrinol Metab 1992;75:1092–1098.
26 Tripathy D, Shah P, Lakshmy R, Reddy KS: Effect of testosterone replacement on whole body glucose utilisation and other cardiovascular risk factors in males with idiopathic hypogonadotrophic hypogonadism. Horm Metabol Res 1998;30:642–645.
27 Howell SJ, Radford JA, Adams JE, Smets EM, Warburton R, Shalet SM: Randomized placebo-controlled trial of testosterone replacement in men with mild Leydig cell insufficiency following cytotoxic chemotherapy. Clin Endocrinol 2001;55: 315–324.
28 Ly LP, Jimenez M, Zhuang TN, Celermajer DS, Conway AJ, Handelsman DJ: A double-blind, placebo-controlled, randomized clinical trial of transdermal dihydrotestosterone gel on muscular strength, mobility, and quality of life in older men with partial androgen deficiency. J Clin Endocrinol Metab 2001;86:4078–4088.
29 Thompson PD, Cullinane EM, Sady SP, Chenevert C, Saritelli AL, Sady MA, Herbert PN: Contrasting effects of testosterone and stanozolol on serum lipoprotein levels. JAMA 1989;261:1165–1168.
30 Bagatell CJ, Heiman JR, Matsumoto AM, Rivier JE, Bremner WJ: Metabolic and behavioral effects of high dose exogenous testosterone in healthy men. J Clin Endocrinol Metab 1994;79:561–567.
31 Uyanik BS, Ari Z, Gumus B, Yigitoglu MR, Arslan T: Beneficial Effects of testosterone undecanoate on the lipoprotein profiles in healthy elderly men. Jpn Heart J 1997;38:73–82.
32 Kapoor D, Goodwin E, Channer KS, Jones TH: Testosterone replacement therapy improves insulin resistance, glycaemic control, visceral adiposity and hypercholesterolemia in hypogonadal men with type 2 diabetes. Eur J Endocrinol 2006;154:899–906.
33 Gliczynski S, Ossowski M, Slowinska-Srzednicka J, Brzezinska A, Zgliczynski W: Effect of testosterone replacement therapy on lipids and lipoproteins in hypogonadal and elderly men. Atherosclerosis 1996; 121:35–43.
34 Whitsel EA, Boyko EJ, Matsumoto AM, Anawalt BD: Intramuscular testosterone esters and plasma lipids in hypogonadal men: a meta-analysis. Am J Med 2001;111:261–269.
35 Barrett-Connor E, Khaw KT, Yen SS: Endogenous sex hormones in older men with diabetes mellitus. Am J Epidemiol 1990;132:895–901.
36 Zietz B, Cuk A, Hugl S, Buttner R, Straub RH, Bauer B, Daffner P, Scholmerich J, Palitzsch KD: Association of increased C-peptide serum levels and testosterone in type 2 diabetes. Eur J Intern Med 2000;11: 322–328.
37 Kapoor D, Aldred H, Clark S, Channer KS, Jones TH: Clinical and biochemical assessment of hypogonadism in men with type 2 diabetes: correlations with bioavailable testosterone and visceral adiposity. Diabetes Care 2007;30:911–917.
38 Simon D, Preziosi P, Barrett-Connor E, Roger M, Saint-Paul M, Nahoul K, Papoz L: Interrelation between plasma testosterone and plasma insulin in healthy adult men. Diabetologia 1992;35:173–177.
39 Stellato RK, Feldman HA, Hamdy O, Horton ES, McKinlay JB: Testosterone, sex hormone-binding globulin, and the development of diabetes in middle-aged men: prospective results from the Massachusetts male ageing study. Diabetes Care 2000;23:490–494.
40 Haffner SM, Shaten J, Stern MP, Smith GD, Kuller L: Low levels of sex hormone binding globulin and testosterone predict the development of non insulin dependent diabetes mellitus in men. Am J Epidemiol 1996;143:889–897.
41 Simon D, Charles MA, Lahlou N, Nahoul K, Oppert JM, Gouault-Heilmann M, Lemort N, Thibult N, Joubert E, Balkau B, Eschwege E: Androgen therapy improves insulin sensitivity and decreases leptin level in healthy adult men with low plasma total testosterone. Diabetes Care 2001;24:2149–2151.
42 Singh AB, Hsia S, Alaupovic P, Sinha-Hikim I, Woodhouse L, Buchanan TA, Shen R, Bross R, Berman N, Bhasin S: The effects of varying doses of testosterone on insulin sensitivity, plasma lipids, apolipoproteins and C-reactive protein in healthy young men. J Clin Endocrinol Metab 2002;87: 136–143.
43 Friedl KE, Jones RE, Hannan CJ Jr, Plymate SR: The administration of pharmacological doses of testosterone or 19-nortestosterone to normal men is not associated with increased insulin secretion or impaired glucose tolerance. J Clin Endocrinol Metab 1989;68:971–975.
44 Marin P, Krotkiewski M, Bjorntrop P: Androgen treatment of middle-aged obese men: effects on metabolism muscle and adipose tissues. Eur J Med 1992;1: 329–336.
45 Vermeulen A, Goemaere S, Kaufman JM: Testosterone, body composition and aging. J Endocrinol Invest 1999;22:110–116.
46 Haffner SM, Valdez RA, Stern MP, Katz MS: Obesity, body fat distribution and sex hormones in men. Int J Obes 1993;17:643–649.

47 Seidell JC, Bjorntorp P, Sjostrom L, Kvist H, Sannerstedt R: Visceral fat accumulation in men is positively associated with insulin, glucose and C-peptide levels but negatively with testosterone levels. Metabolism 1990;39:897–901.
48 Phillips GB: Relationship between serum sex hormones and the glucose-insulin-lipid defect in men with obesity. Metabol 1993;42:116–120.
49 Abate N, Haffner SM, Garg A, Peshock RM, Grundy SM: Sex steroid hormones, upper body obesity and insulin resistance. J Clin Endocrinol Metab 2002;87:4522–4527.
50 Bastounis EA, Karayiannakis AJ, Syrigos K, Zbar A, Makri GG, Alexiou D: Sex hormone changes in morbidly obese patients after vertical banded gastroplasty. Eur Surg Res 1998;30:43–47.
51 Strain GW, Zumoff B, Miller LK, Rosner W, Levit C, Kalin M, Hershcopf RJ, Rosenfeld RS: Effect of massive weight loss on hypothalamic-pituitary-gonadal function in obese men. J Clin Endocrinol Metab 1988;66:1019–1023.
52 Rebuffe-Scrive M, Marin P, Bjorntrop P: Effect of testosterone on abdominal adipose tissue in men. Int J Obes 1991;15:791–795.
53 Marin P, Oden B, Bjorntrop P: Assimilation and mobilization of triglycerides in subcutaneous abdominal and femoral adipose tissue in vivo in men: effects of androgens. J Clin Endocrinol Metab 1995; 80:239–243.
54 Boyanov MA, Boneva Z, Christov VG: Testosterone supplementation in men with type 2 diabetes, visceral obesity and partial androgen deficiency. Aging Male 2003;6:1–7.
55 Larsen BA, Nordestgaard BG, Stender S, Kjeldsen K: Effect of testosterone on atherogenesis in cholesterol-fed rabbits with similar plasma cholesterol levels. Atheroscler 1993;99:79–86.
56 Bruck B, Brehme U, Gugel N, Hanke S, Finking G, Lutz C, Benda N, Schmahl FW, Haasis R, Hanke H: Gender-specific differences in the effects of testosterone and estrogen on the development of atherosclerosis in rabbits. Arterioscler Thromb Vasc Biol 1997;17:2192–2199.
57 Alexandersen P, Haarbo J, Byrjalsen I, Lawaetz H, Christiansen C: Natural androgens inhibit male atherosclerosis: a study in castrated, cholesterol-fed rabbits. Circ Res 1999;84:813–819.
58 Nathan L, Shi WB, Dinh H, Mukherjee TK, Wang XP, Lusis AJ, Chaudhuri G: Testosterone inhibits early atherogenesis by conversion to estradiol: critical role of aromatase. Proc Natl Acad Sci USA 2001;98:3589–3593.
59 Nettleship JE, Jones TH, Channer KS, Jones RD: Physiological testosterone replacement therapy attenuates fatty streak formation and improves high-density lipoprotein cholesterol in the Tfm mouse: an effects that is independent of the classical androgen receptor. Circ 2007;116:2427–2434.
60 Shores M, Matsumoto A, Slaon K, Kivlahan D: Low serum testosterone and mortality on male veterans. Arch Intern Med 2006;166:1660–1665.
61 Lauglin G, Barrett-Connor E, Bergstrom J: Low serum testosterone and mortality in older men. J Clin Endocrinol Metab 2008;93:68–75.
62 Keating N, O'Malley J, Smith M: Diabetes and cardiovascular disease during androgen deprivation therapy for prostate cancer. J Clin Oncol 2006;24: 4448–4456.
63 Jones RD, Nettleship JE, Kapoor D, Jones TH, Channer KS: Testosterone and atherosclerosis in aging men: purported association and clinical implications. Am J Cardiovasc Drugs 2005;5:141–154.
64 Hak A, Witteman J, DeJong F, Geerlings M, Hofman A, Pols H: Low levels of endogenous androgens increase the risk of atherosclerosis in elderly men: the Rotterdam Study. J Clin Endocrinol Metab 2002;87:3632–3639.
65 van den Beld A, Bots M, Janssen J, Pols H, Lamberts S: Endogenous hormones and carotid atherosclerosis in elderly men. Am J Epidemiol 2003;157:25–31.
66 De Pergola G, Pannacciulli N, Ciccone M, Tartagni M, Rizzon P, Giogino R: Free testosterone plasma levels are negatively associated with the intima-media thickness of the common carotid artery in overweight and obese glucose-tolerant young adult men. Int J Obes 2003;27:803–807.
67 Fukui M, Kitagawa Y, Nakamura N, Kadono M, Mogami S, Hirata C, Ichio N, Wada K, Hasegawa G, Yoshikawa T: Association between serum testosterone concentration and carotid atherosclerosis in men with type 2 diabetes. Diabetes Care 2003;26:1869–1873.
68 Muller M, van den Beld AW, Bots ML, Grobbee DE, Lamberts SWJ, van der Schouw YT: Endogenous sex hormones and progression of carotid atherosclerosis in elderly men. Circ 2004;109:2074–2079.
69 Hamm L: Testosterone propionate in the treatment of angina pectoris. J Clin Endocrinol 1942;2:325–328.
70 Jaffe MD: Effect of testosterone cypionate on post-exercise ST segment depression. Br Heart J 1977;39: 1217–1222.
71 Wu SZ, Weng XZ: Therapeutic effects of an androgenic preparation on myocardial ischemia and cardiac function in 62 elderly male coronary heart disease patients. Chin Med J 1993;106:415–418.

72 English KM, Steeds RP, Jones TH, Diver MJ, Channer KS: Low-dose transdermal testosterone therapy improves angina threshold in men with chronic stable angina: a randomized, double-blind, placebo-controlled study. Circulation 2000;102:1906–1911.
73 Rosano GM, Leonardo F, Pagnotta P, Pelliccia F, Panina G, Cerquetani E, della MP, Bonfigli B, Volpe M, Chierchia SL: Acute anti-ischemic effect of testosterone in men with coronary artery disease. Circulation 1999;99:1666–1670.
74 Webb CM, McNeill JG, Hayward CS, de Zeigler D, Collins P: Effects of testosterone on coronary vasomotor regulation in men with coronary heart disease. Circulation 1999;100:1690–1696.
75 Webb CM, Adamson DL, de Zeigler D, Collins P: Effect of acute testosterone on myocardial ischemia in men with coronary artery disease. Am J Cardiol 1999;83:437–439.
76 English KM, Jones RD, Jones TH, Morice AH, Channer KS: Aging reduces the responsiveness of coronary arteries from male Wistar rats to the vasodilatory action of testosterone. Clin Sci 2000;99:77–82.
77 Jones RD, Pugh PJ, Jones TH, Channer KS: The vasodilatory action of testosterone: a potassium channel opening or a calcium antagonistic action? Br J Pharmacol 2003;138:733–744.
78 Jones RD, English KM, Jones TH, Channer KS: Testosterone-induced coronary vasodilatation occurs via a non-genomic mechanism: evidence of a direct calcium antagonistic action. Clin Sci 2004;107: 149–158.
79 Jones RD, Ruban LN, Morton IE, Roberts SA, English KM, Channer KS, Jones TH: Testosterone inhibits the prostaglandin F-2-alpha mediated increase in intracellular calcium in A7r5 aortic smooth muscle cells: evidence of an antagonistic action upon store-operated calcium channels. J Endocrinol 2003;178:381–393.
80 Scragg JL, Jones RD, Channer KS, Jones TH, Peers C: Testosterone is a potent inhibitor of L-type Ca^{2+} channels. Biochem Biophys Res Commun 2004;318: 503–506.
81 Hall J, Jones RD, Jones TH, Channer KS, Peers C: Selective inhibition of L-type voltage-gated calcium channels in A7r5 cells by physiological levels of testosterone. Endocrinology 2006;147:2675–2680.
82 Jones RD, Jones TH, Channer KS: The influence of testosterone upon vascular reactivity. Eur J Endocrinol 2004;151:29–37.
83 Kang SM, Jang Y, Kim JY, Chung N, Cho SY, Chae JS, Lee JH: Effect of oral administration of testosterone on brachial arterial vasoreactivity in men with coronary artery disease. Am J Cardiol 2002; 89:862–864.
84 Ong PJ, Patrizi G, Chong WC, Webb CM, Hayward CS, Collins P: Testosterone enhances flow-mediated brachial artery reactivity in men with coronary artery disease. Am J Cardiol 2000;85:269–272.
85 Anderson TJ, Uehata A, Gerhard MD, Meredith IT, Knab S, De La Grange D, Lieberman EH, Ganz P, Creager MA, Yeung AC, Selwyn AP: Close relation of endothelial function in the human coronary and peripheral circulations. J Am Coll Cardiol 1995;26: 1235–1241.
86 Pugh PJ, Malkin CJ, Morris PD, Asif S, Jones RD, Jones TH, Channer KS: Prevalence of hypogonadism in men with coronary artery disease. J Am Coll Cardiol 2003;41:p344A.

Prof. T.H. Jones
Robert Hague Centre for Diabetes and Endocrinology
Barnsley Hospital NHS Foundation Trust
Gawber Road, Barnsley S75 2EP (UK)
Tel. +44 1226 777947, Fax +44 1226 777771, E-Mail Hugh.jones@nhs.net

Jones TH (ed): Advances in the Management of Testosterone Deficiency.
Front Horm Res. Basel, Karger, 2009, vol 37, pp 108–122

Erectile Dysfunction and Testosterone Deficiency

Michael Blute · Payam Hakimian · James Kashanian · Alex Shteynshluyger · Michael Lee · Ridwan Shabsigh

Division of Urology, Maimonides Medical Center, Brooklyn, N.Y., USA

Abstract

A definitive role of testosterone in erectile function has been controversial; however, recent evidence is becoming available which substantiates a key function for this hormone. Testosterone deficiency is associated with a decline in erectile function and testosterone levels are inversely correlated with increasing severity of erectile dysfunction. Erectile dysfunction can be caused by multifactorial pathologies. In particular, erectile dysfunction may be the first symptom of cardiovascular disease. Animal studies have demonstrated that castration causes vascular smooth muscle cell atrophy, venous leakage, adipocytes in the subtunical space, loss of elastic fibers and increase in collagen deposition. Testosterone increases the expression of nitric oxide synthase and phosphodiesterase type 5, both principal enzymes involved in the erectile process. Testosterone replacement alone in hypogonadal men can restore erectile function. A significant proportion of men who fail to respond to a PDE5 inhibitor are testosterone deficient. Testosterone replacement therapy can convert over half of these men into phosphodiesterase type 5 responders. It is now recommended that testosterone levels should be assessed in all patients with erectile dysfunction.

Testosterone is the major androgenic hormone seen in both the male and female sex. In men, it is mainly produced and released by Sertoli cells in the testes under influence of luteinizing hormone (LH) from the anterior pituitary gland (adenohypophysis) [1]. Normal levels of testosterone in males are required to maintain secondary sexual characteristics, fertility, muscle mass, hair growth, and sexual function. As part of natural male aging, there is generally a decrease in testosterone levels secondary to diminished gonadal function. The effect of reduced testosterone levels varies among subjects and has become known as androgen decline in the aging male (ADAM) [2]. In conjunction with testosterone reduction in men, a decline in erectile function is often seen. The importance of testosterone in maintaining erectile function is clinically manifested in disorders such as the metabolic syndrome in which the hypogonadal state is frequently accompanied by erectile and sexual dysfunction [3].

As testosterone levels steadily decrease in the presence of diabetes, hypercholesterolemia, and central obesity, patients will encounter and exhibit failure to achieve adequate penile tumescence and often experience a concurrent reduction in sexual desire. Outside of such disorders as the metabolic syndrome, healthy elderly males can also experience similar abnormalities. During normal aging, the increased prevalence of sexual and erectile dysfunction with hypogonadism further illustrates a possible correlation. Given the relationship between testosterone and erectile function, physiologic and pathologic, it can be determined that levels of this male androgen impact the functioning of male sexual health.

Furthermore, the effects of low testosterone levels are shown in cases of male patients undergoing androgen deprivation therapy (ADT) for prostate cancer. Along with general symptoms and signs of hypogonadism including weight gain, decreased muscle mass, loss of hair, osteoporosis, diabetes, high blood pressure, patients on ADT will often experience some degree of erectile dysfunction [4]. Still, further support for this relationship is apparent when a reproducible return of sexual function occurs in hypogonadal patients after discontinuation of ADT therapy [4] or testosterone replacement therapy [5]. In this chapter, we provide many references and evidence in the literature supporting the close relationship between hypogonadism and erectile dysfunction and lend insight into the investigation, management, and treatment of hypogonadism in men.

Hypogonadism and Erectile Dysfunction-Epidemiology

Recently, increased attention and focus has been given to the relationship between hypogonadism and erectile dysfunction. The exact mechanism by which testosterone regulates sexual function is poorly understood, however, replacement therapy has been shown to improve erectile dysfunction and heighten overall desire [6]. Low serum testosterone levels, arterial endothelial damage and psychological status are key contributing factors to erectile dysfunction [7, 8]. However, the evidence presented addressing hypogonadism in males with erectile dysfunction appears to be controversial with regards to a definitive role of testosterone in normal erectile and sexual function.

In a review, Nasser [9] found that the prevalence of hypogonadism in patients with erectile dysfunction ranged from 1.7 to 35% owing this wide variation to factors such as patient population, frequency of testosterone measurement, and definitions of erectile dysfunction and hypogonadism. In a prospective study assessing 165 male patients with erectile dysfunction, Martinez-Jabaloyas et al. [10] detected hypogonadism in 4.8% using total testosterone levels and 17.6% using free testosterone levels. The study concluded that the frequency of hypogonadism in patients with erectile dysfunction is higher when free testosterone measurements are used. There is also evidence in the literature that disputes the role of testosterone in erectile function. In a study measuring total testosterone levels in 965 patients having answered an abridged version of the International Index of Erectile Function (IIEF-5), no reliable significant correlation was demonstrated between total testosterone and erectile function ($r = 0.0163$, $p = 0.612$) [11]. Still, Tsujimura et al. [12] showed a statistical correlation between elevations in higher IIEF-5 scores and bioavailable testosterone ($r = 0.792$, $p = 0.0365$). Therefore, it is essential to further investigate a possible causal role of low testosterone levels in male erectile function [13].

Interestingly, the Massachusetts Male Aging Study (MMAS) presented the first major cross-sectional and longitudinal data on the epidemiological background of erectile dysfunction [14]. The MMAS demonstrated the prevalence of erectile dysfunction in a large community population and provided insight into the biochemical elements of impotence. The study reported that 52% of men had erectile dysfunction with 17.2% having minimal, 25.2% moderate and 9.6% complete erectile dysfunction [15]. Dehydroepiandrostenedione sulphate (DHEAS), a testosterone precursor, was the only androgen in the MMAS that showed a strong correlation to erectile dysfunction. A reduction in DHEAS from 10 to 0.5 μg/ml was associated with an increase in impotence from 3.4 to 16% after adjustment for age [15]. This study showed no association between testosterone and erectile dysfunction.

Testing for Testosterone in Patients with Chief Complaint of Erectile Dysfunction

Testosterone has been studied for its primary and secondary effects on the human body. In addition to its well-known effects on male secondary sexual characteristics, testosterone has been shown to stimulate a vasodilatory response within the cardiovascular system. Yue et al. [16] observed dilation of the coronary arteries upon administering testosterone to rabbits. Likewise, Webb et al. [17] demonstrated coronary artery vasodilation on 13 male patients during exposure to 3 min infusions of testosterone. An increase in intracoronary blood flow velocity and coronary artery diameter was noted. Therefore, the actions of testosterone, confirmed in both animal and human subjects, warrant a better understanding of patients' serum levels as part of a comprehensive clinical assessment of erectile dysfunction. With this knowledge, in addition to the importance of a history and physical exam for any diagnostic work-up, laboratory testing in patients with a chief complaint of erectile dysfunction can be performed to help diagnose hypogonadism. Studies have been conducted for this very reason to ascertain the legitimacy of said laboratory testing recommending that these values be standard of care when evaluating male impotent patients further aiding and supporting a diagnosis of hypogonadism as a probable foundation for erectile dysfunction [18–21].

In accordance with testing and analyzing testosterone levels in male patients with erectile dysfunction, Becker et al. [22] measured systemic and cavernous plasma testosterone levels in healthy patients ($n = 54$) and patients with erectile dysfunction (n = 46). They found that in healthy men, both cavernous and systemic testosterone were normal with a significant increase in levels noted from flaccidity to tumescence ($p < 0.001$ cavernous; $p = 0.001$ systemic). Patients with erectile dysfunction were classified into organogenic and psychogenic groups and demonstrated a 10 and 19% difference in testosterone levels in cavernous and systemic levels of testosterone during flaccidity, respectively. The results of this study represent a significant difference in levels of testosterone seen in healthy patients and those with erectile dysfunction. Differing levels of testosterone, as reported in this study, lend support for testing for testosterone levels in these patients, as there can clearly be opposing levels evident between healthy and erectile dysfunction patients. In a retrospective study screening for endocrine abnormalities in 1,022 patients with erectile dysfunction, the authors concluded that by testing for testosterone according to recommended screening criteria (low sexual desire, history of testes damage, or abnormal physical examination), they would have missed 40% of cases with low testosterone including 37% responding to androgen therapy [20]. This therefore evokes new thoughts on screening criteria for hypogonadal patients with erectile dysfunction in whom androgen replacement therapy may be of benefit. Does having low sexual desire, testicular trauma, or abnormalities on physical exam appropriately warrant hormonal measurement or should other factors, such as symptoms and signs of the metabolic syndrome or depressed mood, be considered and regarded as essential indicators leading to subsequent hormone evaluation?

Physiology

The penile erection is a complex physiologic process. It is dependent on a balance of neurotransmitters, vasoactive agents, endocrine factors and tissue fibroelastic properties [23]. Erectile dysfunction can be caused by an alteration in any of the previously mentioned. For instance, changes in the corpus cavernosal structure may lead to erectile dysfunction [24].

Nitric oxide (NO) is the primary non-adrenergic non-cholinergic neurotransmitter of the corpus cavernosum and is the chief mediator of arterial smooth muscle relaxation and dilation [25]. NO is released from cavernosal nerves and endothelial cells of the corpora cavernosum in response to sexual stimulation [26]. NO acts by increasing cyclic GMP which in turn modulates corporal relaxation. cGMP activates various protein kinases leading to increased intracellular KCl and decreased intracellular Ca^{2+} [25]. This results in smooth muscle relaxation and causes rapid influx of blood into the cavernosal bodies promoting filling and engorgement of the subtunical space. This expansion results in the compression of the subtunical venous plexus and the emissary veins on the tunica albuginea restricting venous outflow. This process traps the blood within the corpora cavernosum thus erecting the penis [26]. NO derived from cavernosal nerve terminals is known to initiate relaxation of the cavernosal tissue while endothelial derived NO facilitates attainment and maintenance of the full erection [27].

Testosterone and Erectile Dysfunction

Testosterone is known to be vital in the development and maintenance of male secondary sex characteristics. Testosterone has also been proven to play an integral role in the development of male sexuality and the male penile erection, such that hypogonadism is known to have a detrimental affect on the frequency of sexual desires, fantasies and intercourse [28]. Furthermore, androgen deprivation, irrespective of mode, is also proven to significantly reduce erectile function [29]. Many studies show that erectile function and sexual activity were lost in men receiving androgen deprivation therapy (ADT) with LHRH agonist leuprolide [30, 31]. The frequency, magnitude, duration and rigidity of nocturnal erections [31] and libido [30] were also markedly decreased in patients on ADT concluding that testosterone depletion by LHRH agonist 'severely suppresses erectile function and sexual activity' [31].

Low testosterone is seen in at least about 6% of all patients with erectile dysfunction. Many cases of erectile dysfunction occur in the setting of decreased plasma testosterone, where there is not complete lack of testosterone [32]. Patients with low free testosterone usually suffer from organic erectile dysfunction (i.e. vasculogenic) versus psychogenic erectile dysfunction. This may be due to alterations in corpus cavernosal structure and function at the cellular level caused by testosterone deficiency. In fact in one study, organic patients had a 40% decrease in free testosterone.

Many of the original studies performed on the relationship between testosterone and erectile dysfunction were performed on castrated rats and rabbits. Using these two experimental models we now have a better understanding of the effect of hypogonadism on the male erection. In several studies, intracavernosal pressures (ICP) were used to assess erectile function. Following stimulation of the pelvic nerve, ICP was significantly reduced in the castrated rabbit compared to the control [23]. Testosterone treatment helped restore erectile function to the baseline [23]. In another study, there was an appreciable decline in the intracavernous to systemic arterial pressure ratio in castrated rabbits without significant changes to systemic systolic and diastolic blood pressures [29]. Of note, castration did not affect rabbit ICP in the flaccid state compared to control [23].

The changes in ICP may be related to alterations in penile corpus cavernosal structure causing venous leakage. Venous leakage is a common final pathway in erectile dysfunction due to smooth muscle atrophy [24]. It is known that there is a change in the activation and maintenance of the veno-occlusive mechanism in castrated subjects. In animal models, androgen ablation (castration/deprivation) predisposes smooth muscle changes and cavernosal atrophy compromising erectile function [29]. It was shown that castration reduced smooth muscle tissue content and increased connective tissue content in the rabbit corpus cavernosum ($p < 0.02$) [23]. In another study, cavernosal tissue samples from orchiectomized animals showed clusters of 'empty' cellular structures that resembled adipocytes [24]. Androgen deprivation caused a decrease in smooth muscle and an increase in the extracellular matrix of the corporus cavernosum causing a resulting decrease in cavernosal compliance and preventing penile engorgement and venous occlusion [23, 24]. It was suggested in the previously mentioned study, that the presence of adipocytes in the subtunical space interfered with the proper veno-occlusive mechanism and contributed to venous leakage resulting in erectile dysfunction in the androgen-deprived animal. It is hypothesized that in the penis, testosterone plays a role in promoting the differentiation of progenitor stroma cells into myogenic cells and the absence of androgens redirects the pathway toward the production of adipocytes and fat accumulation [24, 33]. Interestingly, androgen replacement in the castrated rabbit prevented smooth muscle changes in the corpus cavernosum ($p < 0.02$) [24]. Testosterone replacement also induced vascular smooth muscle growth [24].

There is also a strong positive correlation between testosterone concentrations and the degree of trabecular smooth muscle relaxation in the penis [22]. Free T was proven to be positively related to peak systolic velocity and resistance index and negatively related to end-diastolic volume. This suggested a positive correlation between free T with vessel dilation and penile elasticity/cavernous artery compliance [22]. Furthermore, the graphical representation of the relationship between free T and resistance index suggested that a threshold level of free T is necessary to obtain an adequate erection secondary to smooth muscle relaxation [22].

Testosterone's role in penile erections in cellular level is supplemented by data showing its influence at the biochemical level. Testosterone is known to affect the production of two enzymes; nitric oxide synthase (NOS) and phoshodiesterase 5 (PDE5). Nitric oxide synthase (NOS) catalyzes the production of NO from L-arginine. Several studies showed that androgen deprivation reduced nitric oxide synthase expression and activity (rabbit models do not concur) [24, 34, 35]. In the rat penis, NOS activity decreased 45% after castration. This change was prevented by testosterone replacement [35]. In one study there was a close relationship between testosterone and NO in the body [36]. In this study, NOS-containing nerve fibers were decreased and erectile function was lost in orchiectomized rats [36]. And although the presence of NOS-containing nerve fibers was not completely eliminated in the castrated rat, it was severely diminished. Furthermore, immediate testosterone replacement following castration preserved NOS-containing nerve fibers and erectile function in these rats. Likewise, rats that received testosterone therapy 8 weeks after castration showed little change in the number of NOS-positive nerve fibers and no change in erectile response compared to the noncastrated controls [36]. This reduction in NOS nerve fibers is postulated to be one of the contributing factors to a decreased ICP and a longer latency period in response to pelvic nerve electrostimulation [36].

As previously stated, testosterone also affects the transcription of PDE5. PDE5 is a cGMP-binding enzyme that hydrolyzes cGMP to 5′-GMP. PDE5 gene expression is 10 to 100 times more abundant in male corpora cavernosum tissue than in any tissue of the male or female body [37]. In the study by Morelli et al. [37], PDE5 mRNA and protein levels in the rabbit corpora cavernosum were decreased in hypogonadal rabbits in comparison to eugonadal rabbits. As might be expected, PDE5 levels were restored to that of the control group with testosterone administration. This association helps explain the lower level of erectile responsiveness of hypogonadal men to PDE5 inhibitors [37].

In conclusion, Androgens maintain proper synthesis and/or release of neurotransmitters, receptor function and tissue structure and function in the corpus cavernosum. Androgens are critical in the maintenance of neural and smooth muscle functionality – shown by a diminution in erectile response to cavernosal nerve stimulation in the castrated animal [23]. Androgens are crucial in the initiation and maintenance of the male penile erection.

Testosterone Thresholds

Previous animal studies pointed to a dose-response relationship between testosterone and erectile function. In a study of castrated rats started on testosterone replacement, Armagan et al. [38] showed that erectile function in rats, as measured by intracavernosal pressures, was maintained by different testosterone levels as low as 10–12% of normal physiological concentrations. Below these concentrations, erectile function was significantly and positively associated with testosterone levels in dose-dependent manner. The protein expression of neural NO and phosphodiesterase type 5 was reduced in penile tissue from castrated rats and increased in rats on testosterone replacement.

There are also few human studies that support the notion of testosterone threshold and dose-dependent effects of testosterone on sexual function in men. In a large cross-sectional study of 434 men between age 50 and 86, the incidence of psychosomatic symptoms increased with decreasing androgen levels. The incidence of loss of libido and vigor increased below threshold testosterone level of 15 nmol/l, obesity below 12 nmol/l, diabetes mellitus type II, depression, sleep disturbances and lack of concentration below 10 nmol/l, and hot flushes and erectile function below threshold testosterone level of 8 nmol/l [7]. This study suggests that some symptoms of late-onset hypogonadism might start at higher testosterone levels than other symptoms.

Furthermore, in a study of hypogonadal men on long-acting testosterone depot injection, patients began to have symptoms of androgen deficiency leading them to request reimplantation of testosterone depot at mean total testosterone of 309 ng/dl (10.7 nm/l) [39]. Although individual threshold level for androgen deficiency symptoms varied markedly from less than 100–450 ng/dl, they occurred at highly reproducible serum testosterone levels in each patient. In another study of hypogonadal men on parenteral testosterone esters, the individual threshold levels varied from 150 to 320 ng/dl [40]. A threshold serum testosterone of 150–200 ng/dl has been described below which sleep-related erections are almost always effected [41, 42]. Unlike reflexive and psychogenic erections, sleep-related erections have been shown to be strongly androgen dependent least effected by external factors [41, 43]. In the Massachusetts Male Aging Study, total testosterone and bioavailable testosterone were significantly associated with sexual desire [44]. The prevalence of low sexual desire was 50 and 37%, respectively, in men with total testosterone <200 and 300 ng/dl and 52 and 43% in those with bioavailable testosterone <100 and 120 ng/dl. Nevertheless, while different symptoms of hypogonadism have been shown to occur at different testosterone levels, there is no clear-cut threshold for late-onset hypogonadism in the literature.

Testosterone in Patients with Erectile Dysfunction

As more evidence is produced relating to the association between testosterone and erectile and or sexual dysfunction, testosterone replacement therapy, especially in hypogonadal patients, has become a safe and efficacious treatment for improvement of male sexual performance. In many studies, testosterone replacement therapy additionally offered improvement in lean muscle mass, a decrease in body fat, and an increase in bone mass [45, 46]. As in erectile function, these improvements were seen in hypogonadal men. From this evidence, it is has become generally accepted that testosterone monotherapy is effective for treatment of erectile dysfunction in hypogonadal men who have no further contributing pathology. Erectile dysfunction has been shown to be the result of multifactorial pathologies and thus testosterone monotherapy is not the sole treatment option for all patients with erectile dysfunction. Nevertheless, treatment is aimed at restoring normal testosterone levels in hypogonadal men to achieve erectile function and may be useful in combination therapy with phosphodiesterase-5 inhibitors in a broader range of patients.

Studies have been conducted to ascertain a relationship between levels of endogenous testosterone and the severity of erectile function with concluding remarks stating that no evident correlation was identified [12, 47]. A recent study however has shown an inverse correlation with testosterone levels in men with type 2 diabetes and a positive correlation with waist circumference relationship with severity of erectile dysfunction [48]. Other studies have been shown a distinct improvement in erectile function in hypogonadal men receiving testosterone replacement therapy. In a randomized, double-blind, placebo-controlled trial conducted to evaluate the efficacy of transdermal testosterone gel in hypogonadal men, there was a significant increase initially in total testosterone at 1 month ($p = 0.024$) and 2 months ($p = 0.025$) with a concurrent significant increase in IIEF scores at 3 months ($p = 0.01$) [49]. Free testosterone levels paralleled the increases seen in total testosterone levels while the placebo group revealed no significant change in T and a decline in IIEF scores. The study concluded that transdermal testosterone gel acts to restore testosterone levels to physiologic levels with resultant improvement in sexual function. Similarly, Mulhall et al. [50] evaluated the normalization of testosterone levels in hypogonadal men and the short- and long-term effect on erectile function. All patients in the study ($n = 32$) reached physiologic testosterone levels with supplementation and analysis of IIEF scores illustrated a significant improvement in IIEF score after 1 month of treatment ($p < 0.01$). However, the improvement was not maintained at 3- and 6-month follow-up visits. The authors concluded that the failure to achieve a long-term and sustained improvement may have resulted from a placebo effect or that the etiology of erectile dysfunction may have derived from a nonendocrine source and thus use of testosterone in the study patient population as a sole treatment modality was questionable [50]. Finally, in a meta-regression analysis, testosterone replacement resulted in significant improvement in sexual function in studies on men with low and low-normal testosterone levels, and the effect of testosterone on erectile function was inversely related to the baseline serum testosterone level [51].

Still, further studies support the use of testosterone replacement therapy to ameliorate erectile dysfunction and interestingly show improvements in other deleterious health issues such as those germane to the metabolic syndrome. The metabolic syndrome is described in patients who exhibit derangements in blood pressure, cholesterol levels, insulin sensitivity, and central adipose tissue accumulation. Recently, due to the presence of features of the metabolic syndrome, further metabolic alterations in hormones, specifically testosterone, render many of these patients impotent. Therefore, hypogonadism may be a pertinent feature of the metabolic syndrome and testosterone replacement therapy lends evidence to improvements in not just the metabolic syndrome but erectile dysfunction. Multiple interventional studies have shown the improving affects of testosterone replacement on central obesity, glucose regulation, serum lipid levels, and blood pressure in patients diagnosed with the metabolic syndrome [52–56]. In their randomized, no-treatment controlled study on testosterone supplementation in men with type II diabetes, obesity, and partial hypogonadism, Boyanov et al. [52] investigated the effects of oral testosterone on the components of the metabolic syndrome and androgen deficiency. Their results from a patient population of forty-eight men with type II diabetes revealed that there was a significant improvement in body weight and BMI, body fat, sexual function, glucose insensitivity, and serum testosterone when oral testosterone was administered to their study population and when compared to the control group. For each category measured in this study, the following alterations occurred: body weight reduced by 2.66%; BMI by 3.2%; waist-to-hip ratio decreased by 3.96%; body fat by 5.6%; and blood glucose levels reduced with a decrease in HbA1c by 1.73% [52]. For all categories, the control group showed negligible changes. In a double-blind placebo controlled study using testosterone esters administered intramuscularly Kapoor et al. [53] found that testosterone improved insulin resistance, glycemic control (−0.37% over 3 months), cholesterol levels and waist circumference. Additional studies have shown the beneficial effects of testosterone replacement in hypogonadal men with regard to increasing muscle mass, strength, sexual function, energy, and a decrease in fat mass [45, 57].

The aforementioned studies reveal the importance of considering testosterone as therapy for the male patient with erectile dysfunction. In all, testosterone replacement was shown to have some effect on erectile function; however, it is also necessary to select the appropriate patient population when choosing testosterone for treatment. It is important to understand that erectile dysfunction can be the result of multiple contributing factors and testosterone may be effective in combination therapy with such agents as PDE5 inhibitors.

Combination Therapy with Testosterone and PDE5 Inhibitor

PDE5 inhibitors are first line agents in treatment of erectile dysfunction due to their safety and efficacy profile. However, about 23–50% of patients do not respond PDE5 inhibitors alone [58]. Since testosterone plays a key role in the nitric oxide pathway for erectile function, there has been a growing interest in the combined use of testosterone and PDE5 inhibitors in treatment of patients with hypogonadism and erectile dysfunction. Using multivariable analysis, hypogonadism has been shown as an independent prognostic factor for poor response to sildenafil [59].

Many studies have shown that combination therapy increases the International Index of Erectile Function (IIEF) scores, a validated tool for erectile function.

In a small randomized, placebo-controlled crossover study of 24 hypogonadal men, Rochira et al. [60] demonstrated that combination therapy with sildenafil and testosterone resulted in maximum improvement in sleep-related penile erections as measured by nocturnal penile tumescence and rigidity monitoring. The combination therapy was more effective than the sum of the effects of sildenafil alone and of testosterone alone suggesting a synergic effect.

In a recent observational study, 34% of hypogonadal patients who were unresponsive to 100 mg sildenafil monotherapy achieved satisfactory erectile function after 8 weeks of oral testosterone undecanoate monotherapy [61]. Another 38% achieved satisfactory erectile function with combination of oral testosterone undecanoate and sildenafil. Both testosterone alone and combination of testosterone and sildenafil resulted in significant improvement in mean IIEF score.

In a small prospective study of men with hypogonadal symptoms having partial or no response to sildenafil monotherapy, combination therapy consisting of sildenafil and oral testosterone undecanoate was initiated. The mean erectile function, as measured by IIEF, increased significantly following combination therapy in all patients who previously had partial or no response to sildenafil monotherapy [62]. In a similar study, 49 hypogonadal (total testosterone <400 ng/dl) men with erectile dysfunction were started on testosterone replacement with or without sildenafil. After 3 months,

31 patients had significant improvement in erectile function with testosterone replacement alone [63]. The remaining 17 men received combined T-gel and sildenafil, after which all reported significant improvement in erectile function and sexual desire domains of IIEF. Furthermore, in an open-label study of combined therapy with transdermal testosterone and tadalafil in hypogonadal nonresponders to tadalafil monotherapy, mean IIEF score increased by 11 points at the 10-week interval compared to the baseline [64].

In a small prospective observational study of 24 hypogonadal patients (total serum testosterone <400 ng/dl) unresponsive to three months of sildenafil monotherapy, 1% testosterone gel treatment was started and continued for 4 weeks and subsequently combined with sildenafil for 12 weeks. Although all men had achieved normalized serum testosterone levels after 4 weeks, none had regained erectile function. However, with combination therapy consisting of testosterone and sildenafil, 92% of men reported improved potency [65]. In another small prospective randomized placebo-controlled study of patients with erectile dysfunction and low-normal testosterone, a 1-month course of transdermal testosterone replacement resulted in improved response to sildenafil as measured by penile dynamic color duplex ultrasound [66]. There was a significant increase in arterial inflow to cavernous arteries and also a significant improvement of erectile function domain of IIEF in the testosterone arm compared to placebo arm of the study.

Finally, in a randomized, double-blinded, placebo-controlled multicenter study of 75 hypogonadal men (total serum testosterone <400 ng/dl) who failed sildenafil monotherapy, the addition of daily 1% testosterone gel to 100 mg sildenafil resulted in improvement of erectile function as measured by IIEF compared to the placebo group [67]. The mean change in IIEF score from baseline was 2.1 in the placebo group versus 4.4 in the testosterone group at 4 weeks ($p = 0.029$). In addition, quality-of-life scores were significantly improved at 12 weeks compared to the placebo.

Combination therapy with testosterone replacement and PDE5 inhibitor has also been studied in different subgroups of patients with various comorbidities including diabetes and renal insufficiency. Combination of oral testosterone undecanoate and sildenafil was effective in restoring erectile function in 70% of diabetic patients with low serum testosterone who were unresponsive to sildenafil monotherapy [68]. Similarly, Chatterjee et al. [69] showed that combination therapy with sildenafil and intramuscular injections of testosterone cypionate for 12 months in hypogonadal patients with erectile dysfunction on renal dialysis or post-transplant resulted in good response in erectile function in all patients and overall improvement of sexual performance as measured by IIEF.

In conclusion, combination therapy with testosterone and PDE5 inhibitors is indicated in patients with erectile dysfunction and hypogonadism who fail PDE5 inhibitor therapy alone. Between 10 and 20% of erectile dysfunction cases may be attributed to low testosterone levels [70]. Furthermore, in a subset of patients at high risk for hypogonadism, such as patients with diabetes mellitus type 2, chronic renal failure, metabolic syndrome and other chronic diseases may benefit from combination therapy if monotherapy with PDE5 inhibitors is inadequate.

Conclusion

Erectile dysfunction has been demonstrated to be multifactorial in nature thus requiring a multi-modality approach towards treatment. Erectile dysfunction often occurs secondary to a pathological process frequently associated with aging. These two origins commonly involve a reduction in levels of testosterone and it has been proposed that this hypogonadism perpetuates erectile dysfunction. Testosterone performs multiple normal physiologic functions throughout life from promoting male maturation to supporting spermatogenesis and finally affording men habitual sexual behavior and function. Hypogonadism is a common ailment effecting men as they age. In conjunction with an unhealthy lifestyle accompanied by weight gain, dyslipidemia, and type 2 diabetes, it is not uncommon for the male to experience not only erectile dysfunction but problems with overall mood and sexual desire. Therefore, testosterone replacement therapy is a likely choice to restore testosterone to normal levels to promote a patient's ability to achieve erectile function. As previously established, erectile dysfunction may manifest from a number of secondary causes and testosterone monotherapy may not suffice. Therefore, testosterone is often used in combination therapy with such agents as PDE5 inhibitors to re-establish erectile function. Moreover, erectile dysfunction often points to additional deleterious cardiovascular pathology, and with its beneficial metabolic effects, testosterone may offer greater protection against devastating cardiac and vascular episodes as well as return erectile and sexual function. Several limitations of our knowledge of the benefit/risk ratio of testosterone therapy make great need for large randomized controlled clinical trials.

References

1 Schlegel PN, Hardy MP, Goldstein M, Wein AJ: Campbell-Walsh Urology, ed 9. Male Reproductive Physiology. Philadelphia, Saunders, 2007, vol 1, chap. 18.

2 Spetz AC, Palmefors L, Skobe RS, Strömstedt MT, Fredriksson MG, Theodorsson E, Hammar ML: Testosterone correlated to symptoms of partial androgen deficiency in aging men (PADAM) in an elderly Swedish population. Menopause 2007;14:999–1005.

3 Kupelian V, Shabsigh R, Araujo AB, O'Donnell AB, McKinlay JB: Erectile dysfunction as a predictor of the metabolic syndrome in aging men: results from the Massachusetts Male Aging Study. J Urol 2006; 176:222–226.

4 Braga-Basaria M, Dobs AS, Muller DC, Carducci MA, John M, Egan J, Basaria S: Metabolic syndrome in men with prostate cancer undergoing long-term androgen-deprivation therapy. J Clin Oncol 2006; 24:3979–3983.

5 Seftel AD, Mack RJ, Secrest AR, Smith TM: Restorative increases in serum testosterone levels are significantly correlated to improvements in sexual functioning. J Androl 2004;25:963–972.

6 Wang C, Swerdloff RS, Iranmanesh A, Dobs A, Snyder PJ, Cunningham G, Matsumoto AM, Weber T, Berman N, Testosterone Gel Study Group: Transdermal testosterone gel improves sexual function, mood, muscle strength, and body composition parameters in hypogonadal men. J Clin Endocrinol Metab 2000;85:2839–2853.
7 Zitzmann M, Faber S, Nieschlag E: Association of specific symptoms and metabolic risks with serum testosterone in older men. J Clin Endocrinol Metab 2006;91:4335–4343.
8 Kshirsagar A, Seftel A, Ross L, Mohamed M, Niederberger C: Predicting hypogonadism in men based upon age, presence of erectile dysfunction, and depression. Int J Impot Res 2006;18:47–51.
9 Nasser M: Does testosterone have a role in erectile function? Am J Med 2006;119:373–382.
10 Martínez-Jabaloyas JM, Queipo-Zaragozá A, Pastor-Hernández F, Gil-Salom M, Chuan-Nuez P: Testosterone levels in men with erectile dysfunction. BJU Int 2006;97:1278–1283.
11 Rhoden EL, Telöken C, Sogari PR, Souto CA: The relationship of serum testosterone to erectile function in normal aging men. J Urol 2002;167:1745–1748.
12 Tsujimura A, Matsumiya K, Matsuoka Y, Takahashi T, Koga M, Iwasa A, Takeyama M, Okuyama A: Bioavailable testosterone with age and erectile dysfunction. J Urol 2003;170:2345–2347.
13 Korenman SG: Epidemiology of erectile dysfunction. Endocrine 2004;23:87–91.
14 McKinlay JB: The worldwide prevalence and epidemiology of erectile dysfunction. Int J Impot Res 2000;12(suppl 4):S6–S11.
15 Feldman HA, Goldstein I, Hatzichristou DG, Krane RJ, McKinlay JB: Impotence and its medical and psychological correlates: results of the Massachusetts male aging study. J Urol 1994;151:54–61.
16 Yue P, Chatterjee K, Beale C, Poole-Wilson PA, Collins P: Testosterone relaxes rabbit coronary arteries and aorta. Circulation 1995;91:1154–1160.
17 Webb CM, McNeill JG, Hayward CS, de Zeigler D, Collins P: Effects of testosterone on coronary vasomotor regulation in men with coronary heart disease. Circulation 1999;100:1690–1696.
18 Bodie J, Lewis J, Schow D, Monga M: Laboratory evaluations of erectile dysfunction: an evidence based approach. J Urol 2003;169:2262–2264.
19 Earle CM, Stuckey BG: Biochemical screening in the assessment of erectile dysfunction: what tests decide future therapy? Urology 2003;62:727–731.
20 Buvat J, Lemaire A: Endocrine screening in 1,022 men with erectile dysfunction: clinical significance and cost-effective strategy. J Urol 1997;158:1764–1767.
21 Gore J, Rajfer J: The role of serum testosterone testing: routine hormone analysis is an essential part of the initial screening of men with erectile dysfunction. Rev Urol 2004;6:207–210.
22 Becker AJ, Uckert S, Stief CG, Scheller F, Knapp WH, Hartmann U, Jonas U: Cavernous and systemic testosterone plasma levels during different penile conditions in healthy males and patients with erectile dysfunction. Urology 2001;58:435–440.
23 Traish AM, Park K, Dhir V, Kim NN, Moreland RB, Goldstein I: Effects of castration and androgen replacement on erectile function in a rabbit model. Endocrinology 1999;140:1861–1868.
24 Traish AM, Toselli P, Jeong SJ, Kim NN: Adipocyte accumulation in penile corpus cavernosum of the orchiectomized rabbit: a potential mechanism for veno-occlusive dysfunction in androgen deficiency. J Androl 2005;26:242–248.
25 Azadzoi KM, Kim N, Brown ML, Goldstein I, Cohen RA, Saenz de Tejada I: Endothelium-derived nitric oxide and cyclooxygenase products modulate corpus cavernosum smooth muscle tone. J Urol 1992; 147:220–225.
26 Lue TF: Erectile dysfunction. N Engl J Med 2000; 342:1802–1813.
27 Burnett AL: Novel nitric oxide signaling mechanisms regulate the erectile response. Int J Impot Res 2004;16(suppl 1):S15–S19.
28 Bancroft J, Wu FC: Changes in erectile responsiveness during androgen replacement therapy. Arch Sex Behav 1983;12:59–66.
29 Traish AM, Munarriz R, O'Connell L, Choi S, Kim SW, Kim NN, Huang YH, Goldstein I: Effects of medical or surgical castration on erectile function in an animal model. J Androl 2003;24:381–387.
30 Eri LM, Tveter KJ: Safety, side effects and patient acceptance of the luteinizing hormone releasing hormone agonist leuprolide in treatment of benign prostatic hyperplasia. J Urol 1994;152:448–452.
31 Marumo K, Baba S, Murai M: Erectile function and nocturnal penile tumescence in patients with prostate cancer undergoing luteinizing hormone-releasing hormone agonist therapy. Int J Urol 1999; 6:19–23.
32 Aversa A, Isidori AM, De Martino MU, Caprio M, Fabbrini E, Rocchietti-March M, Frajese G, Fabbri A: Androgens and penile erection: evidence for a direct relationship between free testosterone and cavernous vasodilation in men with erectile dysfunction. Clin Endocrinol 2000;53:517–22.33.
33 Bhasin S, Taylor WE, Singh R, Artaza J, Sinha-Hikim I, Jasuja R, Choi H, Gonzalez-Cadavid NF: The mechanisms of androgen effects on body composition: mesenchymal pluripotent cell as the target of androgen action. J Gerontol [A] 2003;58: M1103–M1110.

34 Chamness SL, Ricker DD, Crone JK, Dembeck CL, Maguire MP, Burnett AL, Chang TS: The effect of androgen on nitric oxide synthase in the male reproductive tract of the rat. Fertil Steril 1995;63:1101–1107.
35 Garban H, Marquez D, Cai L, Rajfer J, Gonzalez-Cadavid NF: Restoration of normal adult penile erectile response in aged rats by long-term treatment with androgens. Biol Reprod 1995;53:1365–1372.
36 Baba K, Yajima M, Carrier S, Morgan DM, Nunes L, Lue TF, Iwamoto T: Delayed testosterone replacement restores nitric oxide synthase-containing nerve fibres and the erectile response in rat penis. BJU Int 2000;85:953–958.
37 Morelli A, Filippi S, Mancina R, Luconi M, Vignozzi L, Marini M, Orlando C, Vannelli GB, Aversa A, Natali A, Forti G, Giorgi M, Jannini EA, Ledda F, Maggi M: Androgens regulate phosphodiesterase type 5 expression and functional activity in corpora cavernosa. Endocrinology 2004;145:2253–2263.
38 Armagan A, Kim NN, Goldstein I, Traish AM: Dose-response relationship between testosterone and erectile function: evidence for the existence of a critical threshold. J Androl 2006;27:517–526.
39 Kelleher S, Conway AJ, Handelsman DJ: Blood testosterone threshold for androgen deficiency symptoms. J Clin Endocrinol Metab 2004;89:3813–3817.
40 Gooren LJ: Androgen levels and sex functions in testosterone-treated hypogonadal men. Arch Sex Behav 1987;16:463–473.
41 Granata AR, Rochira V, Lerchl A, Marrama P, Carani C: Relationship between sleep-related erections and testosterone levels in men. J Androl 1997;18:522–527.
42 Carani C, Granata AR, Fustini MF, Marrama P: Prolactin and testosterone: their role in male sexual function. Int J Androl 1996;19:48–54.
43 Cunningham GR, Hirshkowitz M, Korenman SG, Karacan I: Testosterone replacement therapy and sleep-related erections in hypogonadal men. J Clin Endocrinol Metab 1990;70:792–797.
44 Travison TG, Morley JE, Araujo AB, O'Donnell AB, McKinlay JB: The relationship between libido and testosterone levels in aging men. J Clin Endocrinol Metab 2006;91:2509–2513.
45 Wang C, Swerdloff RS: Androgen replacement therapy. Ann Med 1997;29:365–370.
46 Wand C, Swerdloff RS: Androgen replacement therapy, risks and benefits; in Wang C (ed): Male Reproductive Function. Boston, Kluwer, 1999, pp 157–172.
47 Rhoden EL, Telöken C, Mafessoni R, Souto CA: Is there any relation between serum levels of total testosterone and the severity of erectile dysfunction? Int J Impot Res 2002;14:167–171.
48 Kapoor D, Clarke S, Chaner KS, Jones TH: Erectile dysfunction is associated with low bioactive testosterone levels and visceral adiposity in men with type 2 diabetes. Int J Androl 2007;30:500–507.
49 Chiang HS, Hwang TI, Hsui YS, Lin YC, Chen HE, Chen GC, Liao CH: Transdermal testosterone gel increases serum testosterone levels in hypogonadal men in Taiwan with improvements in sexual function. Int J Impot Res 2007;19:411–417.
50 Mulhall JP, Valenzuela R, Aviv N, Parker M: Effect of testosterone supplementation on sexual function in hypogonadal men with erectile dysfunction. Urology 2004;63:348–352; discussion 352–353.
51 Isidori AM, Giannetta E, Gianfrilli D, Greco EA, Bonifacio V, Aversa A, Isidori A, Fabbri A, Lenzi A: Effects of testosterone on sexual function in men: results of a meta-analysis. Clin Endocrinol (Oxf) 2005;63:381–394.
52 Boyanov MA, Boneva Z, Christov VG: Testosterone supplementation in men with type 2 diabetes, visceral obesity and partial androgen deficiency. Aging Male 2003;6:1–7.
53 Kapoor D, Goodwin E, Channer KS, Jones TH: Testosterone replacement therapy improves insulin resistance, glycaemic control, visceral adiposity and hypercholesterolaemia in hypogonadal men with type 2 diabetes. Eur J Endocrinol 2006;154:899–906.
54 Kaplan N: The deadly quartet: upper body obesity, glucose intolerance, hypertriglyceridemia, and hypertension. Arch Intern Med 189;149:1514–1520.
55 Marin P, Krotkiewski M, Bjorntorp P: Androgen treatment of middle-aged, obese men: effects on metabolism, muscle and adipose tissues. Eur J Med 1992;1:329–336.
56 Marin P, Holmang S, Gustafsson C, Bjorntorp P: Androgen treatment of abdominally obese men. Obes Res 1993;1:245–251.
57 Snyder PJ, Peachey H, Berlin JA, Hannoush P, Haddad G, Dlewati A, Santanna J, Loh L, Lenrow DA, Holmes JH, Kapoor SC, Atkinson LE, Strom BL: Effects of testosterone replacement in hypogonadal men. J Clin Endocrinol Metab 2000;85:2670–2677.
58 Salonia A, Rigatti P, Montorsi F: Sildenafil in erectile dysfunction: a critical review. Curr Med Res Opin 2003;19:241–262.
59 Park K, Ku JH, Kim SW, Paick JS: Risk factors in predicting a poor response to sildenafil citrate in elderly men with erectile dysfunction. BJU Int 2005;95:366–370.
60 Rochira V, Balestrieri A, Madeo B, Granata AR, Carani C: Sildenafil improves sleep-related erections in hypogonadal men: evidence from a randomized, placebo-controlled, crossover study of a synergic role for both testosterone and sildenafil on penile erections. J Androl 2006;27:165–175.

61 Hwang TI, Chen HE, Tsai TF, Lin YC: Combined use of androgen and sildenafil for hypogonadal patients unresponsive to sildenafil alone. Int J Impot Res 2006;18:400–404.
62 Shamloul R, Ghanem H, Fahmy I, El-Meleigy A, Ashoor S, Elnashaar A, Kamel I: Testosterone therapy can enhance erectile function response to sildenafil in patients with PADAM: a pilot study. J Sex Med 2005;2:559–564.
63 Greenstein A, Mabjeesh NJ, Sofer M, Kaver I, Matzkin H, Chen J: Does sildenafil combined with testosterone gel improve erectile dysfunction in hypogonadal men in whom testosterone supplement therapy alone failed? J Urol 2005;173:530–532.
64 Yassin AA, Saad F, Diede HE: Testosterone and erectile function in hypogonadal men unresponsive to tadalafil: results from an open-label uncontrolled study. Andrologia 2006;38:61–68.
65 Rosenthal BD, May NR, Metro MJ, Harkaway RC, Ginsberg PC: Adjunctive use of AndroGel (testosterone gel) with sildenafil to treat erectile dysfunction in men with acquired androgen deficiency syndrome after failure using sildenafil alone. Urology 2006;67:571–574.
66 Aversa A, Isidori AM, Spera G, Lenzi A, Fabbri A: Androgens improve cavernous vasodilation and response to sildenafil in patients with erectile dysfunction. Clin Endocrinol (Oxf) 2003;58:632–638.
67 Shabsigh R, Kaufman JM, Steidle C, Padma-Nathan H: Randomized study of testosterone gel as adjunctive therapy to sildenafil in hypogonadal men with erectile dysfunction who do not respond to sildenafil alone. J Urol 2004;172:658–663.
68 Kalinchenko SY, Kozlov GI, Gontcharov NP, Katsiya GV: Oral testosterone undecanoate reverses erectile dysfunction associated with diabetes mellitus in patients failing on sildenafil citrate therapy alone. Aging Male 2003;6:94–99.
69 Chatterjee R, Wood S, McGarrigle HH, Lees WR, Ralph DJ, Neild GH: A novel therapy with testosterone and sildenafil for erectile dysfunction in patients on renal dialysis or after renal transplantation. J Fam Plann Reprod Health Care 2004;30: 88–90.
70 Shabsigh R: Hypogonadism and erectile dysfunction: the role for testosterone therapy. Int J Impot Res 2003;15(suppl 4):S9–S13.

Prof. Ridwan Shabsigh
Division of Urology, Maimonides Medical Center
Columbia University
904 49th St, Brooklyn, NY 11219 (USA)
Tel. +1 718 283 7746, Fax +1 718 635 7424, E-Mail rshabsigh@maimonidesmed.org

Jones TH (ed): Advances in the Management of Testosterone Deficiency.
Front Horm Res. Basel, Karger, 2009, vol 37, pp 123–132

Testosterone, Bone and Osteoporosis

Stephen P. Tuck[a] · Roger M. Francis[b]

[a]Department of Rheumatology, James Cook University Hospital, Middlesbrough, and
[b]School of Clinical Medical Sciences, University of Newcastle upon Tyne, Medical School, Newcastle upon Tyne, UK

Abstract

Osteoporosis and osteoporotic fractures are generally considered to mainly affect older postmenopausal women, but up to 20% of symptomatic vertebral fractures and 30% of hip fractures occur in men. Osteoporotic fractures in men are associated with substantial morbidity, greater excess mortality than in women and account for almost 25% of the cost of osteoporotic fractures in the UK. One of the major secondary causes of osteoporosis in men is hypogonadism, which is found in up to 20% of men with symptomatic vertebral fractures and 50% of elderly men with hip fractures. This chapter outlines the pathogenesis of osteoporosis in men, placing particular emphasis on the importance of sex steroids in the maintenance of bone health. The effects of hypogonadism on the skeleton are described, as well as the consequences of androgen deprivation therapy in men with prostate cancer. Finally, we review the effects of testosterone replacement in hypogonadism and explore other options for the treatment of osteoporosis secondary to loss of sex steroids in men.

Introduction

Osteoporosis is a skeletal disorder characterized by compromised bone strength, predisposing a person to an increased risk of low trauma fracture. The major osteoporotic fractures are those of the vertebral body, hip and forearm, but fractures of the humerus, tibia, pelvis and ribs are also common. Although osteoporosis and osteoporotic fractures are widely considered to mainly affect older postmenopausal women, up to 20% of symptomatic vertebral fractures and 30% of hip fractures occur in men [1]. Osteoporotic fractures in men are associated with substantial morbidity, greater excess mortality than in women and account for almost 25% of the cost of osteoporotic fractures in the UK. The number of men presenting with these fractures is rising, because of increased life expectancy and a doubling of the age-specific incidence of fractures over the past three decades [1]. Despite the importance of male osteoporosis, it is currently both under-diagnosed and under-treated. A retrospective cohort study from the US in 1,171 men with osteoporotic fractures showed that only

1.1% underwent bone mineral density (BMD) measurement and 7.1% received treatment for osteoporosis [2].

The risk of fracture is determined by skeletal and non-skeletal risk factors. The skeletal risk factors comprise BMD, bone turnover, trabecular architecture, bone size, and skeletal geometry, whereas non-skeletal risk factors include postural instability and propensity for falling [1]. There is an inverse relationship between BMD and the incidence of vertebral and hip fractures in men, which is similar to that observed in women. Case-control studies also demonstrate that men with distal forearm, symptomatic vertebral and hip fractures have lower BMD than age-matched control subjects [1]. BMD in adults is influenced by the peak bone mass achieved during childhood and adolescence and by the subsequent rate of bone loss. Underlying secondary causes of osteoporosis, such as hypogonadism may lead to the acquisition of a suboptimal peak bone mass and accelerated bone loss in adult life, depending when the testosterone deficiency develops.

Bone Mass throughout Life

In growth there is a rapid increase in bone size and total bone mass as assessed by bone mineral content (BMC), such that 80–90% of peak values are achieved by late adolescence [3]. The peak areal BMD (g/cm^2) is higher in young men than women because of greater bone size, but the volumetric BMD (g/cm^3) is similar. The increase in volumetric BMD during adolescence is also more modest than the changes in BMC. Skeletal consolidation in early adult life is associated with further increases in bone size and BMC, but little change in volumetric BMD [3].

Skeletal growth is regulated by genetic, endocrine, nutritional and mechanical factors, but the interaction of sex steroids, growth hormone and insulin-like growth factor 1 (IGF-1) is particularly important. Testosterone increases periosteal and endosteal apposition, bone size and cortical and trabecular thickness in adolescent males [4]. Young men with constitutionally delayed puberty have reduced areal BMD, but bone turnover and volumetric BMD are normal [5]. Nevertheless, these men have a thin cortex because of reduced endosteal apposition, which may place them at increased risk of fractures in later life [4].

Bone loss begins between the ages of 35 and 50 years and continues into old age in both sexes, but there is accelerated bone loss in the decade after menopause in women [1]. There are also gender differences in the changes in cortical and trabecular bone with advancing age (figs. 1, 2). Periosteal apposition continues in cortical bone in both sexes, but is greater in men than women. This results in greater expansion of bone width with age in men, which in part compensates for any bone loss that occurs. Endosteal resorption on the inner surface of the cortex is greater in women than men, resulting in thinner cortices (fig. 1). Trabecular bone loss in men is generally associated with thinning of the trabecular bars but maintenance of their connectivity (fig. 2), whereas in women there is

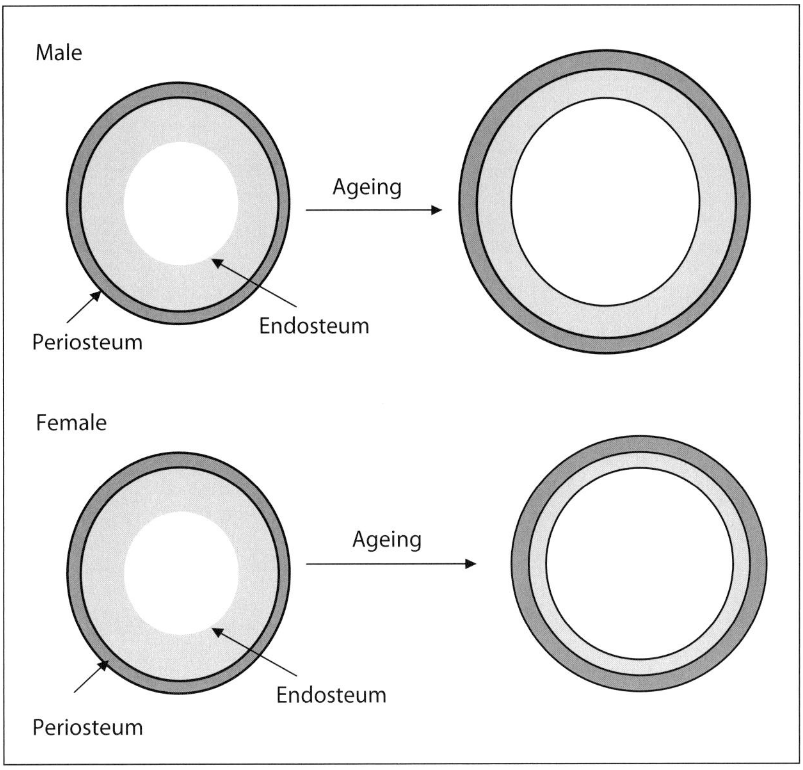

Fig. 1. Schematic representation of the changes in cortical bone with advancing age. In males, endosteal resorption is compensated by periosteal apposition which helps maintain the cortical shell and results in bone expansion. In females, there is less periosteal apposition and greater endosteal resorption, resulting in a thinner cortex and less bone expansion.

a loss of connectivity and disruption of the trabecular architecture, which further reduces bone strength [4]. Age-related bone loss in men may be influenced by low body mass index, smoking, physical inactivity, impaired vitamin D production and metabolism and secondary hyperparathyroidism [1]. The age-related decrease in circulating free testosterone, adrenal androgens, growth hormone and IGF1 may all contribute to the observed reduction in bone formation and continuing bone loss with age in men.

Sex Steroids and Bone Metabolism

One of the major causes of osteoporosis in women is the loss of sex steroids at the menopause, which leads to increased bone turnover and bone loss. Sex steroids also play an important role in the maintenance of bone density in men, as demonstrated by the rapid bone loss seen after castration or androgen deprivation therapy (ADT)

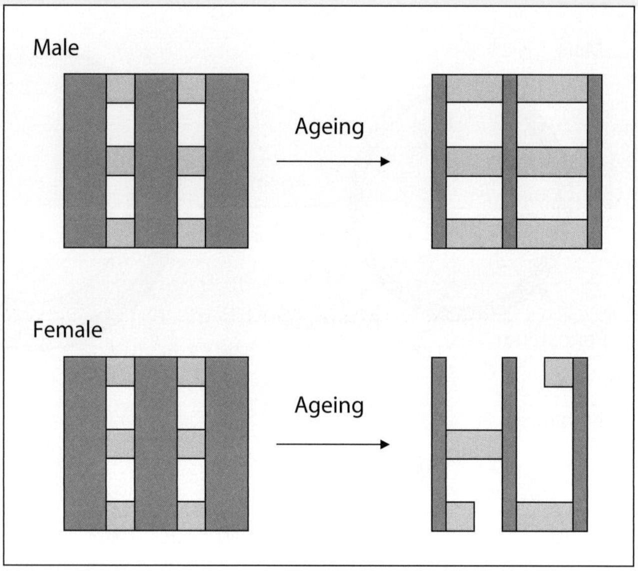

Fig. 2. Schematic representation of the changes in trabular bone with advancing age. In males, there is thinning of the individual trabeculae, but maintenance of trabecular connectivity. In females, there is reduction in tabecular number and loss of trabecular connectivity.

[6, 7]. Furthermore, up to 20% of men with symptomatic vertebral fractures and 50% of men with hip fractures have evidence of hypogonadism [1].

The major carrier of sex steroids in serum is sex hormone-binding globulin (SHBG). The circulating concentration of SHBG rises with age and results in lower free levels of testosterone and oestradiol, both of which may play a role in the pathogenesis of osteoporosis in men. SHBG is higher in men with vertebral fractures and/or osteoporosis than in control subjects [8, 9]. In men with primary and secondary osteoporosis, SHBG is correlated with bone turnover markers, BMD and the risk of vertebral fractures [9].

The actions of testosterone on the male skeleton are mediated in part by aromatization to oestradiol, so that oestrogen deficiency may contribute to age-related bone loss in men [1]. Case reports have described osteoporosis in men with mutations in the oestrogen receptor or aromatase genes. Studies also show that BMD and the prevalence of vertebral fracture in men are more closely related to serum oestradiol than to serum testosterone [1]. Furthermore, oestradiol appears to be the dominant sex hormone-regulating bone resorption in men [10].

Hypogonadism and Osteoporosis

Hypogonadism is widely considered to be a major risk factor for osteoporosis in men. A study from Eastern Europe of men castrated for 'sexual delinquency' showed rapid bone loss, particularly in the first five years after surgery [6]. Up to 20% of men with symptomatic vertebral fractures and 50% of elderly men with hip fractures are also reported to have hypogonadism [1]. However, a case-control study of 91 men with symptomatic vertebral fractures showed no increased risk of fracture with hypogonadism [8]. Furthermore, serum total testosterone was similar in patients with vertebral fractures and in the control group. Nevertheless, SHBG was significantly higher in the patients with vertebral fractures than the control group, leading to a reduction in the free androgen index and free oestrogen index.

A case-control study of men with hip fractures showed a marked reduction in serum testosterone compared to the control group [11]. Nevertheless, over the 12 months of follow-up, the serum testosterone increased in the men with fractures, but was still significantly lower than in the control group. Although low serum testosterone concentrations in men with hip fractures may be due in part to disturbance of the hypothalamic-pituitary-gonadal axis related to the fracture and subsequent surgery, this study suggests that hypogonadism is a risk factor for hip fractures in men [11].

An early study of the pathogenesis of osteoporosis in hypogonadal men showed not only low serum testosterone concentrations, but also reduced serum oestradiol [12]. Serum 1,25-dihydroxyvitamin D (1,25$(OH)_2$D) and radiocalcium absorption were also reduced in this group of men with hypogonadism. Treatment with intramuscular testosterone esters led to a correction of the hypogonadism and significant increases in serum oestradiol, total and free 1,25$(OH)_2$D and radiocalcium absorption. Metabolic balance studies also showed an increase in urine calcium, net absorption and calcium balance with testosterone replacement.

Follicle-stimulating hormone (FSH) has been shown to stimulate tumour necrosis factor (TNF) production from immune cells, which enhances osteoblast and osteoclast formation and may directly influence bone mass in postmenopausal women [13]. Nevertheless, osteoporosis has been reported in hypogonadotrophic and hypergonadotrophic hypogonadism in men, suggesting that FSH is not an important determinant of bone loss in hypogonadal males [14]. Other work shows that testosterone replacement in hypogonadal men suppresses circulating concentrations of TNF and other pro-inflammatory cytokines [15], which may contribute to the beneficial effects of testosterone on the skeleton.

Elderly men with hypogonadism have increased bone resorption, reduced muscle strength, impaired static and dynamic balance, a higher risk of falls and a lower BMD [16], which may contribute to an increased risk of fracture. Male hypogonadism is associated with more marked deterioration of trabecular architecture than is apparent from bone density measurements [17].

Androgen Deprivation Therapy in Prostate Cancer

ADT results in a high annual rate of bone loss, with BMD falling between 2 and 10% depending on region and study [7]. During ADT there is a dramatic decrease in the circulating levels of both testosterone and oestradiol. This causes a decrease in osteoblastic bone formation, an increase in osteoclastic bone resorption and hence accelerated bone loss. It has recently been suggested that ADT induced suppression of sex steroids in elderly men increases the skeletal responsiveness to the bone resorbing effects of parathyroid hormone (PTH), but does not affect the response of bone formation markers or $1,25(OH)_2D$ to PTH [18]. Reduction in muscle mass may also contribute to bone loss by decreasing mechanical loading, as well as increasing the risk of falls and fractures.

There is a high prevalence of osteoporosis prior to initiating therapy [19], which may be due to a number of factors, including age, frailty and the physical effects of the disease. However, bone loss and increased risk of fractures after starting ADT has been well documented [7]. In a US study from the Medicare database, 19% of men with prostate cancer who received ADT sustained a fracture, compared with 13% of those who did not receive androgen-deprivation therapy [20]. Bilateral orchidectomies have also been shown to be associated with increased fracture risk in men with prostate cancer [21].

Testosterone Replacement in Hypogonadal Men

Early studies of the effect of testosterone supplementation in hypogonadal men showed improvement in bone density in the forearm and lumbar spine, although the increase in spine BMD was greater in men with open epiphyses [22]. An observational study investigated the long-term effects of testosterone replacement on bone density in 72 hypogonadal men [23]. Trabecular BMD of the spine was measured annually using quantitative computerised tomography (QCT). In men who had received no previous treatment, testosterone replacement increased spine BMD by 25%. In men who had already received treatment previously, there was a further increase in BMD of 15% [23].

Another study compared body composition and BMD measurements in hypogonadal men and age-matched control subjects [24]. The hypogonadal men had a significantly higher body fat and lower spine BMD than the eugonadal control subjects. Treatment of the hypogonadal men with intramuscular testosterone enanthanate increased muscle mass by 17%, spine BMD by 5% and trabecular BMD by 14%, and decreased body fat by 13% over 18 months. Testosterone replacement also decreased bone turnover, as reflected by the reduction in bone specific alkaline phosphatase and urine deoxypyridinoline.

A randomised controlled cross-over study compared the effects of treatment with intramuscular injections of testosterone enanthanate and placebo injections for three months each on sex steroid concentrations, biochemical markers of bone turnover and body composition [25]. The study participants were otherwise healthy older men, all of whom had a low normal serum testosterone. During the treatment with testosterone there was an increase in serum testosterone of 70% and serum oestradiol of 127%, associated with a significant reduction in urine hydroxyproline, indicating a decrease in bone resorption. Testosterone treatment also decreased body fat and increased muscle mass.

A randomised controlled trial in 108 healthy men aged above 65 years with a serum testosterone <16.5 nmol/l, compared the effects of 36 months' treatment with testosterone or placebo patch on BMD and biochemical markers of bone turnover [26]. Treatment with testosterone increased the serum concentrations from 4.7–21.7 nmol/l. There was an increase in spine BMD of 4.2% in the testosterone treated group and 2.5% in the placebo group, although the differences were not statistically significant. There was also no significant change in bone-specific alkaline phosphatase or N-telopeptide in either group. Sub-group analysis showed an inverse relationship between the increase in BMD and the basal serum testosterone concentration.

More recent work suggests that testosterone replacement in men with hypogonadism not only increases BMD, but also improves trabecular architecture [27]. A cross-sectional study of men with hypogonadism receiving long-term testosterone replacement therapy showed that BMD was not different from the age-matched reference range for normal men [28]. In contrast, another study in men with hypergonadotrophic hypogonadism receiving long-term testosterone replacement therapy reported lower forearm bone mass than in control subjects [29].

Other Treatments for Hypogonadal Osteoporosis

A randomised controlled trial investigated the effect of alendronate treatment in 241 men with osteoporosis aged between 31 and 87 years, 37% of whom were hypogonadal. This showed a mean increase in BMD of 7.1% at the lumbar spine and 2.5% at the femoral neck, compared with changes in the control group of 1.8 and −0.1%, respectively [30]. There were similar increases in BMD in eugonadal and hypogonadal men treated with alendronate. A recent study shows that the addition of alendronate treatment to hypogonadal men on testosterone replacement therapy increases BMD more than testosterone alone, supporting the concomitant use of a bisphosphonate [31].

There is growing interest in the potential use of selective estrogen receptor modulators (SERMs) and selective androgen receptor modulators (SARMs) in hypogonadal men with osteoporosis. In an open-label study, men with non-metastatic prostate cancer receiving ADT were randomised to receive the SERM raloxifene or to no treatment. Raloxifene significantly increased BMD at the hip and tended to increase spine BMD [32]. Another SERM (toremifene) increases BMD in men on ADT and is currently undergoing further clinical trials [33]. Studies in orchidectomised rats suggest that SARMs may prevent bone loss, improve bone formation and muscle mass, without adverse effects on the prostate [34].

Prevention of Androgen Deprivation Therapy-Induced Bone Loss

There are relatively few studies of potential treatments for the bone loss induced by androgen deprivation therapy (ADT) in men with prostate cancer, as most work has concentrated on metastatic disease. There are also no data available on whether or not there is recovery of bone density after cessation of ADT. The only oral bisphosphonate to have been investigated is alendronate, which increases BMD in eugonadal and hypogoadal men with osteoporosis [30]. Greenspan et al. [35] used oral alendronate 70 mg weekly in a case-control study of men with prostate cancer and after 12 months there was a 5.1% difference at the lumbar spine and 2.3% at the femoral neck between the two groups. However, only approximately 1% of oral bisphosphonate therapy is absorbed and they are associated with poor compliance. A small randomised, placebo-controlled crossover study suggested that intravenous pamidronate decreased bone turnover and increased BMD in men on ADT [36]. Two subsequent studies demonstrated that intravenous zoledronate 4 mg given either every 3 months or annually prevents bone loss in patients with prostate cancer receiving ADT [37, 38]. There have been no studies large enough to demonstrate a reduction in fracture rate.

In addition, all patients who require hormone therapy for prostate cancer are given the option of using bicalutamide 150 mg daily as monotherapy. This allows the preservation of sexual function. There is some evidence that bicalutamide can increase BMD [39, 40].

Conclusions

Osteoporotic fractures are less common in men than women, as they have a larger skeletal size and do not experience the accelerated phase of bone loss associated with the menopause. The gender differences in the changes in cortical and trabecular bone with advancing age, which are mediated by sex steroids, also confers mechanical advantages to the male skeleton. Both testosterone and oestradiol are important for skeletal health and these sex steroids have profound direct and indirect effects on bone cells and bone metabolism. Hypogonadism is an important cause of osteoporosis in men, as demonstrated by the rapid bone loss seen after castration or treatment with ADT for prostate cancer. This is also accompanied by loss of muscle mass and increase in fat mass. These changes in body composition reduce the forces applied to the bones and may cause further bone loss and increase the risk of falls. Hypogonadal men can be effectively treated with testosterone supplementation, which results in substantial improvements in bone density and body composition. Alternatively, bisphosphonates such as oral alendronate can be used. A variety of novel therapies are still under evaluation such as SARMS. ADT-induced bone loss can be prevented by the use of oral and intravenous bisphosphonates, but further work is required to confirm that this reduces the risk of fractures.

References

1 Tuck SP, Francis RM: Osteoporosis in men; in Arden NK (ed): Osteoporosis. London, Remedica, 2006, pp 163–183.

2 Feldstein AC, Nichols G, Orwoll E, Elmer PJ, Smith DH, Herson M, Aicklin M: The near absence of osteoporosis treatment in older men with fractures. Osteoporos Int 2005;16:953–962.

3 Henry YM, Fatayerji D, Eastell R: Attainment of peak bone mass at the lumbar spine, femoral neck and radius in men and women: relative contributions of bone size and volumetric bone density. Osteoporos Int 2004;15:263–273.

4 Seeman E: Pathogenesis of bone fragility in women and men. Lancet 2002;359:1841–1850.

5 Bertelloni S, Baroncelli GI, Ferdeghini M, Perri G, Saggese G: Normal volumetric bone mineral density and bone turnover in young men with histories of constitutional delay of puberty. J Clin Endocrinol Metab 1998;83:4280–4283.

6 Stepan JJ, Lachman M, Zverina J, Pacovsky V, Baylink DJ: Castrated men exhibit bone loss: effect of calcitonin treatment on biochemical indices of bone remodelling. J Clin Endocrinol Metab 1989;69: 523–527.

7 Alibhai SMH, Gogov S, Allibhai Z: Long-term side effects of androgen deprivation therapy in men with non-metastatic prostate cancer: a systematic literature review. Clin Rev Oncol Haematol 2006;60: 201–215.

8 Scane AC, Francis RM, Sutcliffe AM, Francis MJD, Rawlings DJ, Chapple CL: Case-control study of the pathogenesis and sequelae of symptomatic vertebral fractures in men. Osteoporos Int 1999;9:91–97.

9 Legrand E, Hedde C, Gallois Y, Degasne I, Boux de Casson F, Mathieu E, Basle MF, Chappard D, Audran M: Osteoporosis in men: a potential role for the sex hormone binding globulin. Bone 2001;29: 90–95.

10 Falahati-Nini A, Riggs BL, Atkinson EJ, O'Fallon WM, Eastell R, Khosla S: Relative contributions of testosterone and oestrogen in regulating bone reorption and formation in normal men. J Clin Invest 2000;106:1553–1560.

11 Pande I: Causes and consequences of hip fracture in men; PhD thesis, University of London, 2000.

12 Francis RM, Peacock M, Aaron JE, Selby PL, Taylor GA, Thompson J, Marshall DH, Horsman A: Osteoporosis in hypogonadal men: role of decreased plasma 1,25-dihydroxyvitamin D, calcium malabsorption and low bone formation. Bone 1986;7: 261–268.

13 Sun L, Peng Y, Sharrow AC, Iqbal J, Zhang Z, Papachristou DJ, Zaidi S, Zhu LL,Yaroslavskiy BB, Zhou H, Zallone A, Sairam MR, Kumar TR, Bo W, Braun J, Cardoso-Landa L, Schaffler MB, Moonga BS, Blair HC, Zaidi M: FSH directly regulates bone mass. Cell 2006;125:247–260.

14 De Rosa M, Paesano L, Nuzzo V, Zarrilli S, Del Puente A, Oriente P, Lupoli G: Bone mineral density and bone markers in hypogonadotropic and hypergonadotropic hypogonadal men after prolonged testosterone treatment. J Endocrinol Invest 2001;24: 246–252.

15 Malkin CJ, Pugh PJ, Jones RD, Kapoor D, Channer KS, Jones TH: The effect of testosterone replacement on endogenous inflammatory cytokines and lipid profiles in hypogonadal men. J Clin Endocrinol Metab 2004;89:3313–3318.

16 Szulc P, Claustrat B, Marchand F, Delmas PD: Increased risk of falls and increased bone resorption in elderly men with partial androgen deficiency: the MINOS study. J Clin Endocrinol Metab 2003;88: 5240–5247.

17 Benito M, Vasilic B, Wehrli FW, Bunker B, Wald M, Gomberg B, Wright AC, Zemel B, Cucchiara A, Snyder PJ: Deterioration of trabecular architecture in hypogonadal men. J Clin Endocrinol Metab 2003; 88:1497–1502.

18 Leder BZ, Smith MR, Fallon MA, Lee ML, Finkelstein JS: Effects of gonadal steroid suppression on skeletal sensitivity to parathyroid hormone in men. J Clin Endocrinol Metab 2001;86:511–516.

19 Smith MR, McGovern FJ, Fallon MA, Schoenfield D, Kantoff PW, Finkelstein JS: Low bone mineral density in hormone-naïve men with prostate carcinoma. Cancer 2001;91:2238–2245.

20 Shahinian VB, Kuo YF, Freeman JL, Goodwin JS: Risk of fracture after androgen deprivation for prostate cancer. N Engl J Med 2005;352:154–164.

21 Melton LJ III, Alotham KI, Khosla S, Achenbach SJ, Oberg AL, Zincke H: Fracture risk following bilateral orchiectomy. J Urol 2003;169:1747–1750.

22 Francis RM: The effects of testosterone on osteoporosis in men. Clin Endocrinol 1999;50:411–414.

23 Behre HM, Kliesch S, Leifke E, Link TM, Nieschlag E: Long-term effect of testosterone therapy on bone mineral density in hypogonadal men. J Clin Endocrinol Metab 1997;82:2386–2390.

24 Katznelson L, Finkelstein JS, Schoenfield DA, Rosenthal DI, Anderson EJ, Klibanski A: Increase in bone density and lean body mass during testosterone administration in men with acquired hypogonadism. J Clin Endocrinol Metab 1996;81:4358–4365.

25 Tenover J: Effects of testosterone supplementation in the aging male. J Clin Endocrinol Metab 1992; 75:1092–1098.
26 Snyder PJ, Peachey H, Hannoush P, Beirlin JA, Loh L, Holmes JH, Dlewati A, Staley J, Santanna J, Kapoor SC, Attie MF, Haddad JG, Strom BL: Effect of testosterone treatment on bone mineral density in men over 65 years of age. J Clin Endocrinol Metab 1999;84:1966–1972.
27 Benito M, Vasilic B, Wehrli FW, Bunker B, Wald M, Gomberg B, Wright AC, Zemel B, Cucchiara A, Snyder PJ: Effect of testosterone replacement on trabecular architecture in hypogonadal men. J Bone Miner Res 2005;20:1785–1791.
28 Zacharin MR, Pua J, Kanumakala S: Bone mineral density outcomes following long-term treatment with subcutaneous testosterone pellet implants in male hypogonadism. Clin Endocrinol 2003;58: 691–695.
29 Medras M, Jankowska EA, Rogucka E: Effects of long-term testosterone substitutive therapy on bone mineral content in men with hypergonadotrophic hypogonadism. Andrologia 2001;33:47–52.
30 Orwoll E, Ettinger M, Weiss S, Miller P, Kendler D, Graham J, Adami S, Weber K, Lorenc R, Pietschmann P, Vandormel K, Lombardi A: Alendronate treatment of osteoporosis in men. N Engl J Med 2000; 343:604–610.
31 Shimon I, Eshed V, Doolman R, Sela BA, Karasik A, Vered I: Alendronate for osteoporosis in men with androgen-repleted hypogonadism. Osteoporos Int 2005;16:1591–1596.
32 Smith MR, Fallon MA, Lee H, Finkelstein JS: Raloxifene to prevent gonadotropin-releasing hormone agonist-induced bone loss in men with prostate cancer: a randomized controlled trial. J Clin Endocrinol Metab 2004;89:3841–3846.
33 Smith MR: Therapy Insight: osteoporosis during hormone therapy for prostate cancer. Nat Clin Pract Urol 2005;2:608–615.
34 Rosen J, Negro-Vilar A: Novel, non-steroidal, selective androgen receptor modulators (SARMs) with anabolic activity in bone and muscle and improved safety profile. J Musculoskelet Neuronal Interact 2002;2:222–224.
35 Greenspan SL, Nelson JB, Trump DL, Resnick NM: Effect of oral alendronate on bone loss in men receiving androgen deprivation therapy for prostate cancer. Ann Intern Med 2007;146:416–424.
36 Diamond TH, Winters J, Smith A, De Souza P, Kersley JH, Lynch WJ, Bryant C: The antiosteoporotic efficacy of intravenous pamidronate in men with prostate carcinoma receiving combined androgen blockade: a double blind, randomized, placebo-controlled crossover study. Cancer 2001;92: 1444–1450.
37 Smith MR, Eastham J, Gleason DM, Shasha D, Tchekmedvian S, Zinner N: Randomized controlled trial of zoledronic acid to prevent bone loss in men undergoing androgen deprivation therapy for nonmetastatic prostate cancer. J Urol 2003;169: 2008–2012.
38 Michaelson MD, Kaufman DS, Lee H, McGovern FJ, Kantoff PW, Fallon MA, Finkelstein JS, Smith MR: Randomized control trial of annual zoledronic acid to prevent gonadotropin-releasing hormone agonist-induced bone loss in men with prostate cancer. J Clin Oncol 2007;25:1038–1042.
39 Sieber PR, Keiller DL, Kahnoski RJ, Gallo J, McFadden S: Bicalutamide 150 mg maintains bone mineral density during monotherapy for localised or locally advanced prostate cancer. J Urol 2004;171: 2272–2276.
40 Smith MR, Goode M, Zietman AL, et al: Bicalutamide monotherapy versus leuprolide monotherapy for prostate cancer: effects on bone mineral density and body composition. J Clin Oncol 2004; 22:2546–2553.

Prof. Roger M. Francis
Musculoskeletal Unit
Freeman Hospital
Newcastle upon Tyne, NE7 7DN (UK)
Tel. +44 191 223 1160, Fax +44 191 223 1161, E-Mail RMFrancis@compuserve.com

Jones TH (ed): Advances in the Management of Testosterone Deficiency.
Front Horm Res. Basel, Karger, 2009, vol 37, pp 133–149

Frailty and Muscle Function: Role for Testosterone?

U. Srinivas-Shankar · Frederick C.W. Wu

Department of Endocrinology, University of Manchester, Manchester Royal Infirmary, Manchester, UK

Abstract

Frailty is a clinical syndrome characterised by reduced physiologic reserve affecting multiple organ systems and is associated with increased risk of falls, fractures, hospitalisation and death. The impact of age-related physical frailty on well-being and health in older men and the potential for prevention and treatment are beginning to be explored. Frailty is multifactorial with aging, comorbidity, sarcopenia, and endocrine immune dysfunction contributing to the condition. Falling testosterone levels with advancing age are associated with muscle loss (sarcopenia) and strength. Among the various therapeutic options being considered, testosterone supplementation offers promise due to its anabolic effects on muscle. In this review, we discuss the syndrome of frailty, its relationship with low testosterone and the effects of testosterone supplementation in healthy and unhealthy/frail older men on muscle mass, strength and physical performance.

Faced with an ageing population, physical frailty is increasingly being recognised as an important health issue worldwide. The burden that this condition is likely to place on health care systems is set to increase in the coming decades. Though there is no universally accepted definition, most researchers agree that it is a distinct clinical syndrome with reduced physiologic reserve affecting multiple organ systems and associated with increased susceptibility to adverse outcomes [1, 2]. It is an aggregation of risk resulting from age or pathology-related summation of decrements affecting various organ systems that renders the individual vulnerable to functional decline.

Based on clinical consensus and research evidence, a phenotype of the clinically frail older adult was operationalized by Freid et al. [2]. The criteria include low-grip strength, self-reported exhaustion, weight loss, low physical activity, and slow walking speed. Those who satisfy three or more criteria are categorised as frail, while those who fulfil one or two criteria are categorised as intermediate or pre-frail. The above definition was tested in the Cardiovascular Health Study in a sample of 4,317 community-dwelling adults aged 65 years and older.

Consequences of Frailty

The prevalence of frailty in a cardiovascular health study was 6.9% [2]. The ultimate physical and clinical manifestations of being frail are its association with adverse health outcomes including, increased risk of falls, fractures, diminished ability to perform activities of daily living (ADL), institutionalisation, hospitalisation and death. In the cardiovascular health study [2], frail people had a sixfold higher mortality than people who are not frail for a 3-year cumulative survival. They also had a higher risk of first hospitalisation (59%), first fall (28%), worsening activities of daily living (39%) and mobility disability (51%), compared to men who are not frail over a 3-year period. People who were pre-frail had an intermediate risk of the above-mentioned adverse outcomes, as well as twice the risk of becoming frail over 3–4 years of follow-up compared to people who are not frail.

Aetiopathogenesis of Frailty

Frailty is multi-factorial in aetiology (fig. 1) with age-associated skeletal muscle loss (sarcopenia), comorbidity, hormonal dysregulation, and immune dysfunction contributing. The summative effect of the hormonal dysregulation, increased levels of catabolic cytokines and immune system dysfunction results in an accelerated loss of muscle mass [3]. This loss of muscle mass (sarcopenia) is central to the concept of physical frailty and explains its manifold manifestations. Decrease in muscle mass and muscle strength, in combination with reduced endurance contributes to reduced physical activity. Maximal oxygen uptake declines and this contributes to muscles fatigue that occurs more easily with advancing age [4].

Comorbidity is an important cause of frailty. Certain comorbid conditions such as lung disease, cancer, cerebrovasclar disease and diabetes are more likely to be associated with muscle loss. Comorbid illness act in multiple ways including via their effect on GH pulsatility, leading to a decrease in IGF-1 and the hypothalamopituitary gonadal axis leading to low testosterone (T) levels.

There is a complex physiological interaction between various anabolic hormones (GH, IGF-1 and T), inflammatory cytokines (IL-2, IL-6, TNF-α), biochemical and molecular pathways mediating catabolism of muscle protein, contributing to age related muscle loss and consequently to physical frailty. Dysregulation of the inflammatory response plays a major role in the age-related muscle loss and decline of physical performance [5]. An increase in the release of catabolic agents including, interleukin-6 (IL-6), TNF-α, and C-reactive protein are associated with reduced muscle mass, physical performance and strength. These agents promote a negative protein balance, and together with elevated markers of blood clotting (factor VIII, D-dimer) contribute to ageing-associated sarcopenia and physical frailty. This is supported by the association between high levels of inflammatory markers (IL-6 and

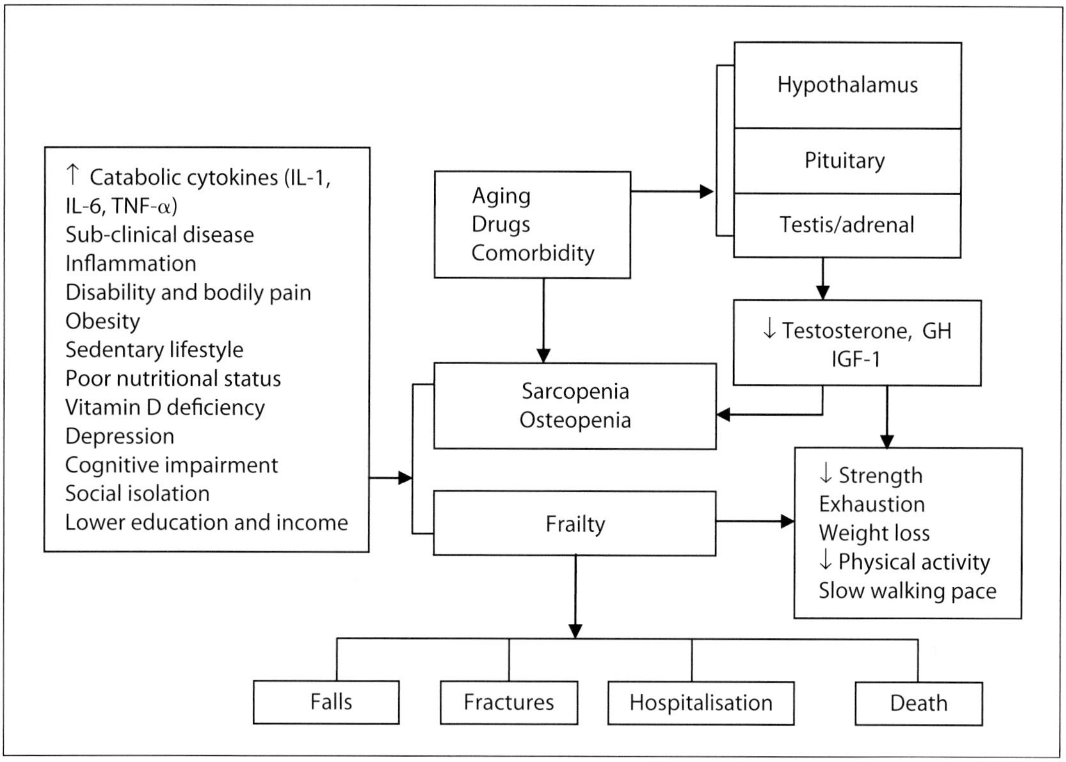

Fig. 1. Schematic diagram representing the aetiopathogensis, consequences and interaction between low testosterone and frailty.

CRP) and low-grip strength [6]. Further, inflammatory cytokines (IL-6) might inhibit the secretion of IGF-1 and adversely affect its biological activity.

Hypothalamopituitary gonadal and adrenal axis and the somatotrophic axis have been implicated in the aetiopathogenesis of frailty. A decrease in the production of anabolic hormones (testosterone, GH and IGF-1) impairs the capacity of skeletal muscle to incorporate amino acids and synthesise proteins.

It is known that DHEA and DHEAS levels decline with age. Data from the InCHIANTI study [7] suggest that DHEAS levels are related to lower extremity muscle strength and calf muscle area among men aged between 60 and 79 years. Leng et al. [8] have reported that frail people have lower levels of serum IGF-1 and DHEA-S and higher levels of IL-6 than non-frail, age-matched individuals. There is loss of pulsatile GH secretion and a decline in IGF-1 levels (including muscle IGF-1) with aging. More than a quarter of circulating IGF-1 is produced by the skeletal muscle and reduced muscle IGF-1 signalling leads to muscle atrophy. Furthermore, there is also an association between IGF-1 levels and measures of physical performance. It has been shown that frail older men have lower levels of IGF-1 levels compared to non-frail men. The association between testosterone and frailty is discussed in more detail latter in the chapter.

Testosterone and Aging

It is well known that total testosterone (TT) levels decrease with age in men from 40 years onwards. The age related decline in free testosterone (FT) and bioavailable testosterone (BT) is greater than TT due to an increase in SHBG with age. Although testosterone levels decrease with age, this decrease in TT is not invariable as a proportion of elderly men have levels in the range of normal young men. The fall in TT with age is exacerbated by comorbidity and chronic use of medication (steroids, opioid analgesia).

Association of Low Testosterone with Frailty

Hypogonadism and physical frailty are multifactorial syndromes and share common aetiologies (fig. 1). Many chronic conditions including, obesity, type 2 diabetes, chronic obstructive pulmonary disease (COPD), liver disease and rheumatoid arthritis are associated with low levels of testosterone and frailty. Some symptoms and signs associated with low testosterone levels are similar to the manifestations of frailty. Loss of muscle mass and strength, lethargy or exhaustion is common to both the conditions.

Persistently low testosterone levels are associated with chronic diseases (rheumatoid arthritis, diabetes, cancer, chronic obstructive pulmonary disease, acquired immunodeficiency syndrome (AIDS)). There is a decrease in endogenous secretion of TT by a much as 30–50% in men with AIDS [9] and a high prevalence of hypogonadism has been shown with COPD [10]. Furthermore, the treatment of several chronic conditions with drugs including steroid, chemotherapeutic agents and opioids might be associated with low testosterone levels. Low testosterone levels have been shown to be associated with decreased physical function and increased risk of 6-month mortality [11].

Relationship between Testosterone and Muscle Mass and Strength

It is well known that muscle mass and strength are related to circulating testosterone levels. Men with primary or secondary hypogonadism or those on androgen deprivation therapy show a decrease in muscle mass and strength and increase in body fat. In a cross-sectional study of 121 men aged 65–97 years, Baumgartner et al. [12] showed that grip strength and appendicular muscle mass were significantly correlated with TT and FT. Further, Perry et al. [13] among men aged 70–102 years, reported that testosterone levels correlate with upper and lower limb strength and functional status.

This relationship between testosterone and muscle mass, strength and physical performance is also seen in unhealthy cohorts. Among hypogonadal men with AIDS wasting syndrome, Grinspoon et al. [14] found that FT levels correlated with total body potassium and muscle mass. In a cross-sectional study of 370 nursing home residents with a median age of 85 years, lower sex hormone levels were significantly associated with greater dependency. Conversely, higher sex hormone levels were associated with better activities of daily living performance. Among men aged 50–85 years in the Minos study [15], an inverse association was reported between TT and the risk of falling. Further, hypogonadal men had impaired balance and inability to stand up from a chair and perform the tandem walk.

Changes in Muscle Mass, Strength and Physical Function with Aging

Aging is associated with decrease in skeletal mass and an increase in peripheral and visceral fat. Skeletal muscle mass gradually begins to decline from fourth and fifth decades of life and occurs even in healthy elderly people. The decrease in skeletal muscle mass approximates 1.9 kg/decade in men. It has been estimated that the prevalence of sarcopenia is over 50% among men older than 80 years [16]. There is a reduction in cross-sectional area of the muscles of the mid-thigh in healthy individuals from the fourth decade onwards. Limb muscles from older men are 25–35% smaller and have significantly more fat and connective tissue than limb muscles from younger individuals. The loss of skeletal muscle mass with age is greater in the lower body with greater reduction in muscle strength than in muscle mass [17]. Table 1 lists the mechanisms underlying age related changes in muscle and body fat.

Unsurprisingly muscle strength decreases with a reduction in muscle mass. Muscle strength, however, tends to decline more significantly with advancing age than does muscle mass. After the age of 50 years, muscle strength decreases at a rate of 10–15% per decade of life. Loss of skeletal muscle mass and strength below a certain threshold leads to impairment in physical function and disability. Among people aged between 65 and 89 years isometric strength and leg extensor power decrease at 1–2 and 3.5% per year, respectively. Decline in power occurs at a faster rate than the decline in knee extensor strength. Further, isometric knee extensor strength and power are significantly associated with simple physical performance tasks like chair rise time [18]. In the cardiovascular health study, severe sarcopenia was an independent risk factor for the development of physical disability.

Among elderly male (mean age >88.5 years) residents of a chronic care hospital, Bassey et al. [19] demonstrated that leg extensor power correlated with physical performance measures. Although, physical function declines with age, there is significant inter individual variation. It has been shown that older adults with sarcopenia

Table 1. Mechanisms underlying age-related changes in muscle and body fat

Changes in muscle
Decrease in muscle fibre size and number
Selective atrophy of type 2 fibre
Decreased skeletal muscle innervation and capillary density
Infiltration of muscle with fat and connective tissue
Decrease in the synthesis rates of myosin heavy chain (MHC)
Reduced area of (MHC) 2a/(MHC) 1 ratio
Loss of motor units
Reduced mitochondrial protein
Reduction in resting metabolic rate (reduced ATP stores)
Reduced protein synthesis (reduction in glycolytic and oxidative enzyme activities)
Changes in Body Fat
Alteration of fatty acid metabolism
Increased number of adipocytes
Fat accumulation in extra-adipose tissues
Differentiation of non-adipose precursor cells into adipocyte-like cells

are more likely to have disability than older adults with normal muscle mass. Further, decrease in lean body mass with age contributes to decrease in resting metabolic rate. In addition, decrease in muscle fatigability and aerobic exercise tolerance, loss of endurance and flexibility contribute to the spectrum of age related physical frailty.

Mechanism of Anabolic Effects of Testosterone

Testosterone induces skeletal muscle hypertrophy by acting at multiple sites within the muscle through several mechanisms. Testosterone facilitates muscle anabolism by promoting nitrogen retention, stimulating fractional muscle protein synthesis, inhibiting muscle protein degradation, and by augmenting the efficiency of amino acid reuse by the skeletal muscle.

Urban et al. [20] demonstrated that administration of testosterone in elderly men increases the mRNA concentrations of muscle IGF-1 and reduces the expression of IGFBP-4 (IGF-binding protein 4). IGF-1, in turn, stimulates protein synthesis and reduces protein degradation. Ferrando et al. [21] reported that testosterone replacement for 6 months maintained IGF-1 protein expression through out the period of administration. Sinha-Hikim et al. [22] demonstrated that the increases in muscle volume in healthy young men, treated with graded doses of testosterone are associated with concentration dependent increase in muscle fibre cross-sectional area. The increase in the cross-sectional areas of both type I and II muscle fibres was dependent on testosterone dose, with the relative proportion of these fibres remaining unchanged.

The muscle fiber hypertrophy induced by testosterone has been shown to be associated with a dose-dependent increase in myonuclear number and androgen receptor expression in satellite cells and myonuclei [23]. Testosterone causes these satellite cells to proliferate and fuse with the muscle fibres resulting in an increase in myonuclear number and consequent muscle fibre hypertrophy.

Singh [24] demonstrated that testosterone regulates the pluripotent stem cells by promoting their commitment to myogenic lineage to produce muscle cells while inhibiting their differentiation into adipocytes. The uncommitted pluripotent stem cells have the ability to generate new satellite cells or myoblasts. In addition, testosterone treatment is associated with ultrastructural changes in satellite cells, including a decrease in the nuclear-to-cytoplasmic ratio and an increase in cellular and mitochondrial areas.

The molecular basis of androgen action on human skeletal muscle is just beginning to be unravelled. In addition to its effects on GH/IGF-1, testosterone might exert its anabolic effects via other regulators of muscle growth like myostatin.

Myostatin, a member of the TGF-β family, is a negative regulator of skeletal muscle growth. Animal studies suggest that androgens may exert a negative effect on myostatin expression [25]. Some actions of testosterone might be mediated through nongenomic, membrane-binding sites. The effects of testosterone on the ubiquitin-proteasome pathway and apoptosis in skeletal muscle remain to be studied.

Effects of Testosterone on Muscle Mass and Strength among Healthy Older Men

Testosterone treatment increases, muscle mass, decreases fat mass (FM) and increases muscle strength in healthy young hypogonadal men [26]. Among healthy young men in a 20-week randomised double-blind placebo-controlled study of combined treatment with GnRH agonist and one of five replacement doses (25, 50, 125, 300 or 600 mg/week) of testosterone enanthate, there was a dose dependent increase in maximal voluntary strength and power, but not fatigability or specific tension [27].

Most interventional studies with testosterone among the elderly are on healthy men. Many of these studies have consistently shown an increase in lean body mass [28–32] and decrease in FM [28–31] (table 2). Although Bhasin et al. [33] reported that older men are as responsive as younger men to graded doses of testosterone with regard to gains in muscle strength, the data on the effects of testosterone in older men from randomised placebo controlled studies are contradictory. Some studies [29, 34] have reported improvements in grip strength in healthy older men. Despite significant improvements in lean body mass, several other studies have not

Table 2. Double-blind placebo-controlled studies with testosterone in healthy elderly men: effects on muscle strength and body composition

First author	Age range (mean)	Testosterone preparation, dose, duration of treatment	Baseline mean testosterone nmol/l	Treatment mean testosterone nmol/l	Body composition	Muscle strength (lower limb)	Grip strength
Snyder [28] (n = 108)	≥65 years	scrotal patch (4–6 mg/day) 36 months	12.7	21.7	↑LBM (1.9 kg) ↓FM (2.9 kg)	↔	↔
Page [29] (n = 70)	65–83 years (71)	TE, 200 mg 3 every 2 weeks 36 months	9.9	16.6 ± 1.1	↑LBM (3.8 kg) ↓Total FM	↔	↑
Emmelot-vonk [30] (n = 207)	60–80 years (67)	TU, 80 mg twice daily 6 months	11.0	11.0	↑LBM (1.1 kg) ↓FM (1.0 kg)	↔	↔
Tenover [48] (n = 13)	57–76 years (67.5)	TE, 100 mg/week 3 months	11.6	19.7	↑LBM (1.7 kg) ↔body fat	not tested	↔
Clague [35] (n = 14)	>60 years (66.5)	TE 200 mg IM 2 weekly for 3 months	11.3	19.5	↔LBM	↔	↔
Wittert [31] (n = 76)	60–86 years (68.5)	TU 80 mg/day 12 months	17.0	16.3	↑LBM (0.7 kg) ↓FM (1.07 kg)	↔	↔
Sih [34] (n =32) Hypogonadal men	≥50 years (67)	TC 200 mg /2weekly 12 months	10.1	16.4	not tested	not tested	↑

Blackman [42] (n = 21)	65–88 years (72)	TE 100 mg/2 weekly 26 weeks	14.1	20.8	↑ LBM (1.4 kg) ↔ FM	↔	↔
Nair [32] (n = 27)	66–70 years (67)	testosterone patch 5 mg/day 24 months	12.4	16.0	↑ FFM	↔	not tested
Ferrando [21] (n = 12)	>60 years 68 (3)	TE 6 months	12.6	30.6	↑ LBM (4.2 kg)	↑	not tested
Kenny [49] (n= 67)	65–87 years 76 (4)	testosterone patch two 2.5 mg/day 12 months	9.0	15.0	↑ LBM (1 kg)	↔	not tested

n = Number of men included in the study; TE = testosterone enanthate; TC = testosterone cypionate; TU = testosterone undecanoate; LBM = lean body mass; FM = fat mass; FFM = fat-free mass.

been able to demonstrate improvements in grip strength [28, 30, 31, 35]. Some of these studies [28, 29] achieved a significant rise in treatment testosterone levels over 36 months, yet were unable to show improvements in lower limb muscle strength. Even a study [29] that had a low, mean (SD) baseline testosterone concentration (9.9 ± 1.6 nmol/l) was only able to show improvements in grip strength, not lower limb muscle strength.

While several studies have been able to demonstrate improvements in upper limb muscle strength (grip strength), only one small placebo-controlled study [21] reported improvements in lower limb muscle strength among healthy older men. In this study, muscle strength was assessed using 1 repetition maximum (1-RM, maximum amount of weight that can be lifted only once). However, muscle endurance assessed using dynamometry did not improve compared to the placebo group.

There could be several possible reasons for the lack of improvement in muscle strength in the lower limb in studies listed in table 2. Most of these placebo-controlled studies used dynamometry to assess lower limb muscle strength. While dynamometry is a physiological method of muscle strength assessment, following instructions and performing dynamometry might be difficult for the elderly research participants as it involves certain amount of learning. Further, dynamometry takes considerable amount of time and effort and elderly participants might find this demanding. Since assessment of muscle strength is effort dependent, the complexity of the assessment might hinder an accurate estimation of maximal muscle function. Ideally, maximality of muscle contraction has to be ensured using twitch interpolation techniques. Only one study [35] listed in table 2 used this technique.

Incorporation of a practice session prior to baseline and follow up dynamometry assessments would allow the participant to become familiar with the procedure and offset the learning effect to some extent. It is not clear how many of the studies listed in table 2 incorporated a separate dynamometry practice session. Further, simpler dynamometry protocols might enable a more accurate estimation of muscle strength parameters. Following 12 weeks of resistance training, Frontera et al. [36] among men aged 60–72 years, reported a107% increase in 1 RM, while isokinetic leg strength improved by 11–15%. This suggests that 1 RM might be more sensitive in detecting improvements in muscle strength than dynamometry.

Measurement of grip strength using a hand held dynamometer is a simple assessment, even for the elderly research participants. This may explain why several research studies have reported improvements in grip strength but not lower limb muscle strength. In addition, heterogeneity (varying baseline muscle mass and strength, differing comorbidity profiles and wide age ranges) inherent to aging populations may account for some of the discrepancies between studies. In most of the studies listed in table 2, pre-treatment testosterone levels were not in the frankly hypogonadal range, although, many of these studies achieved a significant rise in testosterone levels with treatment. It is likely that grossly hypogonadal older men might show more significant improvements in muscle strength.

Effects of Testosterone on Muscle Mass and Strength in Older Unhealthy and Frail Men

There is paucity of data on the effects of testosterone on muscle mass and strength in unhealthy older men and no studies among frail elderly men. Studies on men with chronic obstructive pulmonary disease [33, 37], human immunodeficiency virus-infected men with abdominal obesity [38] and men on long-term steroids [39] have shown improvements in body composition (table 3). Some of these studies also reported improvements in muscle strength. In a randomised placebo-controlled study [39], middle-aged men on long term glucocorticoids treated with mixed testosterone esters for 12 months showed improvements in isokinetic peak torque in knee flexion and extension. Casaburi et al. [40] treated elderly men with COPD with 100 mg/week of testosterone enanthate for 10 weeks and reported improvements in quadriceps strength measured by one 1 RM. In another randomized, double-blind placebo-controlled study [41], elderly men receiving supraphysiological doses of testosterone enanthate, 100 mg/week showed improvements in grip strength and task-specific performance using the functional independence measure (FIM – tested the ability to stand from a bed or chair, ambulation and climb stairs) suggesting that testosterone supplementation may thus improve rehabilitation outcomes in ill older men. Evidence from the small number of studies mentioned above are encouraging and suggest that relatively unhealthy/frail older men might respond well to testosterone supplementation with regards improvements in muscle mass, strength and physical performance.

Effects of Testosterone on Physical Function in Older Men

Although several studies have reported beneficial effects of testosterone in healthy and unhealthy/frail elderly men on lean body mass and muscle strength, there is a paucity of data on effects of testosterone on physical function. Testosterone administered to healthy elderly men, in randomised double-blind placebo-controlled studies [28, 30] did not improve objective physical performance tests. Page et al. [29] in a double blind placebo controlled study, reported improvements in physical function (modified physical performance test) among healthy elderly men treated with testosterone enanthate. They attribute the improvement in physical function, despite lack of improvement in lower limb muscle strength to a significant rise in haemoglobin in the active compared to the placebo group. They further suggest that the positive effects of intervention with testosterone on mood and energy could have contributed. The improvement in physical function correlated with the change in Ttestosterone levels on treatment but not with baseline TT.

Peak aerobic capacity, measured by maximum volume of oxygen consumed per minute (VO_2) was unchanged among healthy elderly men in several randomised double blind placebo controlled studies with testosterone [32, 42, 43]. Liu et al. [44] treated 17

Table 3. Double-blind placebo-controlled studies with testosterone in unhealthy elderly men: effects on muscle strength and body composition

Study Cohort First Author	Age range (mean)	Testosterone preparation, dose, duration of treatment	Baseline mean testosterone nmol/l	Treatment mean testerone nmol/l	Body composition	Muscle strength (lower limb)	Grip strength
Men with COPD Svartberg [37] (n = 29)	54–75 years (66)	TE 250 mg/ 4 weekly 26 weeks	21.6	22.8	↓ FM (−1.5%) ↑FFM (1.1 kg)	not tested	not tested
Men with HIV Bhasin [38] (n = 88)	18–70 years (45.5)	testosterone gel 10 g/day 24 weeks	14.8	17.4	↑ LBM (1.3 kg)	not tested	not tested
Men admitted to a geriatric rehabilitation unit Bakhsi [41] (n = 15)	65–90 years (78)	TE 100 mg/week 8 weeks	not reported	not reported	not tested	not tested	↑
Men on steroids Crawford [39] (n = 18)	>20 years (60)	mixed TE 200 mg i.m. 12 months	13.8	24.2	↑ LBM (1.8 kg) ↓ FM (2.3 kg)	↑	not tested
Men with COPD Casaburi [40] (n = 12)	55–80 years (66.6)	TE 100 mg/week 10 weeks	10.5	20.8	↑ LBM (5.5%) ↓ FM (5%)	↑	not tested
Men undergoing Knee replacement Amory [45] (n = 25)	58–86 years (70)	TE 600 mg/week 4 weeks (pre-operatively)	12.5	82.5	not tested	not tested	not tested

n = Number of men included in the study; COPD= chronic obstructive pulmonary disease; HIV = human immunodeficiency virus; TE = testosterone enanthate; mixed TE = mixed testosterone esters; LBM = lean body mass; FM = fat mass; FFM = fat-free mass.

community-dwelling healthy men aged over 60 years, with parenteral testosterone esters and did not find an increase in physical activity, using accelerometry and the Physical Activity Scale in the Elderly (PASE) questionnaire. In a double-blind placebo-controlled study [30] of 237 healthy men treated with oral testosterone undecanoate for 6 months, self-assessed physical ability did not improve. Self-assessed physical performance did not improve in the testosterone-treated group, but worsened in the placebo group in a double placebo-controlled study [28] on elderly men. This suggests that treatment with testosterone might help in maintaining the subjective perception of physical function.

Only few small studies have reported improvements in physical function among unhealthy/frail older men. Amory et al. [45] in a double-blind placebo-controlled study demonstrated that pre-operative administration of supra-physiological testosterone in older men (mean age 70 years) undergoing elective knee replacement was associated with significant improvement in ability to stand on the third post-operative day. Fifteen men aged 65–90 years undergoing rehabilitation in a geriatric evaluation and management unit were randomized to receive intramuscular injections of testosterone enanthate, 100 mg/ week for a maximum of 8 weeks. Testosterone-treated men in this study improved their functional status and grip strength, but the length of stay on the in-patient unit remained unchanged [41]. Crawford et al. [39] reported significant improvements in Qualeffo-41 questionnaire scores (physical function, pain, social function, general health perception and mental function) among men on long term glucocorticoids treated were treated with mixed testosterone esters for 12 months.

There could be several possible explanations for the lack of demonstrable improvements in physical performance. The lack of tests sensitive enough to detect change could be an important factor. Using tests that have a ceiling effect prevents detection of change, pre- and post-treatment. Most of the physical function tests used in studies of testosterone intervention among elderly men did not require the individual to work at their maximal physical capacity. These tests required that the individual to do routine activities such as walking and stair climbing at a comfortable pace. In such a situation, change might be masked by day to day and intra individual variation. In addition, performance of these tests is susceptible to variability and bias introduced by factors such as mood and motivation of the research participant.

Further, healthy older men are likely to require greater increases in muscle strength, to translate into improvements in physical performance. The association between strength and physical performance is curvilinear [46]. A certain amount of strength is needed for a task of certain intensity. Further increases of strength above this threshold are unlikely to manifest as improvements in physical performance. In a study [47] on functionally impaired community dwelling men (mean age 78 years), an improvement in peak torque of around 5 N-m (9–16% improvement in strength) was associated with improvements in physical performance. Further, the impact of the intervention was greater among frailer men. Thus, unhealthy and frail men are likely to require smaller degrees of muscle strength improvement to cause an appreciable difference in physical performance.

It needs to be borne in mind that physical performance does not rely on muscle strength alone. Other variables contribute to physical function in the elderly and include, balance, joint position sense, peripheral neuropathy, peripheral vascular disease, vision, hearing, confidence, cognition, arthritis, bodily pain and the presence of cardio-respiratory comorbidity. Although, some evidence from the above-mentioned studies suggests that intervention with testosterone might lead to beneficial effects on physical performance among unhealthy and frail elderly men, currently unequivocal evidence of improvement in physical performance is lacking.

Conclusion

Intervention with testosterone produces clear benefits in terms of improvements in lean body mass among healthy and unhealthy/frail older men. There is inconsistent evidence of a beneficial effect on muscle strength and limited data on the improvement in physical performance among unhealthy/frail older men. Given the paucity of data on the effects of testosterone on unhealthy older and frail men, well-designed studies are needed to clarify the potential benefits on muscle strength and physical performance. Treatment with testosterone may prove beneficial in carefully selected subgroups of unhealthy and frail elderly men. Tests to assess muscle strength and physical performance should be tailored to the study population, keeping in mind the methodological flaws of earlier studies. Further research should clarify the duration of treatment, and subgroups of men most likely to benefit from intervention. It needs to be remembered that the management of physical frailty is multidisciplinary with all aspects contributing of the syndrome taken into account. The balance between benefits and risk would need to be established on an individual basis before treatment is initiated. There remain many unresolved issues with testosterone supplementation in unhealthy elderly and frail men. Testosterone supplementation, however, offers promise of improving muscle strength and physical performance and halting the downward spiral of immobility, institutionalisation, hospitalisation and death.

References

1 Strawbridge WJ, Shema SJ, Balfour JL, Higby HR, Kaplan GA: Antecedents of frailty over three decades in an older cohort. J Gerontol [B] 1998;53:S9–S16.

2 Fried LP, Tangen CM, Walston J, Newman AB, Hirsch C, Gottdiener J, Seeman T, Tracy R, Kop WJ, Burke G, McBurnie MA: Frailty in older adults: evidence for a phenotype. J Gerontol A Biol Sci Med Sci 2001;56:M146–M156.

3 Rosenberg IH: Sarcopenia: origins and clinical relevance. J Nutr 1997;127:990S–991S.

4 Short KR, Vittone JL, Bigelow ML, Proctor DN, Nair KS: Age and aerobic exercise training effects on whole body and muscle protein metabolism. Am J Physiol Endocrinol Metab 2004;286:E92–E101.

5 Cesari M, Penninx BW, Pahor M, Lauretani F, Corsi AM, Rhys Williams G, Guralnik JM, Ferrucci L: Inflammatory markers and physical performance in older persons: the InCHIANTI study. J Gerontol [A] 2004;59:242–248.

6 Taaffe DR, Harris TB, Ferrucci L, Rowe J, Seeman TE: Cross-sectional and prospective relationships of interleukin-6 and C-reactive protein with physical performance in elderly persons: MacArthur studies of successful aging. J Gerontol [A] 2000;55:M709–M715.
7 Valenti G, Denti L, Maggio M, Ceda G, Volpato S, Bandinelli S, Ceresini G, Cappola A, Guralnik JM, Ferrucci L: Effect of DHEAS on skeletal muscle over the life span: the InCHIANTI study. J Gerontol [A] 2004;59:466–472.
8 Leng SX, Cappola AR, Andersen RE, Blackman MR, Koenig K, Blair M, Walston JD: Serum levels of insulin-like growth factor-I (IGF-I) and dehydroepiandrosterone sulfate (DHEA-S), and their relationships with serum interleukin-6, in the geriatric syndrome of frailty. Aging Clin Exp Res 2004; 16:153–157.
9 Croxson TS, Chapman WE, Miller LK, Levit CD, Senie R, Zumoff B: Changes in the hypothalamic-pituitary-gonadal axis in human immunodeficiency virus-infected homosexual men. J Clin Endocrinol Metab 1989;68:317–321.
10 Laghi F, Antonescu-Turcu A, Collins E, Segal J, Tobin DE, Jubran A, Tobin MJ: Hypogonadism in men with chronic obstructive pulmonary disease: prevalence and quality of life. Am J Respir Crit Care Med 2005;171:728–733.
11 Shores MM, Moceri VM, Gruenewald DA, Brodkin KI, Matsumoto AM, Kivlahan DR: Low testosterone is associated with decreased function and increased mortality risk: a preliminary study of men in a geriatric rehabilitation unit. J Am Geriatr Soc 2004;52: 2077–2081.
12 Baumgartner RN, Stauber PM, McHugh D, Koehler KM, Garry PJ: Cross-sectional age differences in body composition in persons 60+ years of age. J Gerontol [A] 1995;50:M307–M316.
13 Perry HM 3rd, Miller DK, Patrick P, Morley JE: Testosterone and leptin in older African-American men: relationship to age, strength, function, and season. Metabolism 2000;49:1085–1091.
14 Grinspoon S, Corcoran C, Lee K, Burrows B, Hubbard J, Katznelson L, Walsh M, Guccione A, Cannan J, Heller H, Basgoz N, Klibanski A: Loss of lean body and muscle mass correlates with androgen levels in hypogonadal men with acquired immunodeficiency syndrome and wasting. J Clin Endocrinol Metab 1996;81:4051–4058.
15 Szulc P, Claustrat B, Marchand F, Delmas PD: Increased risk of falls and increased bone resorption in elderly men with partial androgen deficiency: the MINOS study. J Clin Endocrinol Metab 2003;88: 5240–5247.
16 Baumgartner RN, Koehler KM, Gallagher D, Romero L, Heymsfield SB, Ross RR, Garry PJ, Lindeman RD: Epidemiology of sarcopenia among the elderly in New Mexico. Am J Epidemiol 1998; 147:755–763.
17 Gallagher D, Visser M, De Meersman RE, Sepulveda D, Baumgartner RN, Pierson RN, Harris T, Heymsfield SB: Appendicular skeletal muscle mass: effects of age, gender, and ethnicity. J Appl Physiol 1997;83:229–239.
18 Skelton DA, Greig CA, Davies JM, Young A: Strength, power and related functional ability of healthy people aged 65–89 years. Age Ageing 1994;23:371–377.
19 Bassey EJ, Fiatarone MA, O'Neill EF, Kelly M, Evans WJ, Lipsitz LA: Leg extensor power and functional performance in very old men and women. Clin Sci (Lond) 1992;82:321–327.
20 Urban RJ, Bodenburg YH, Gilkison C, Foxworth J, Coggan AR, Wolfe RR, Ferrando A: Testosterone administration to elderly men increases skeletal muscle strength and protein synthesis. Am J Physiol 1995;269:E820–E826.
21 Ferrando AA, Sheffield-Moore M, Yeckel CW, Gilkison C, Jiang J, Achacosa A, Lieberman SA, Tipton K, Wolfe RR, Urban RJ: Testosterone administration to older men improves muscle function: molecular and physiological mechanisms. Am J Physiol Endocrinol Metab 2002;282:E601–E607.
22 Sinha-Hikim I, Artaza J, Woodhouse L, Gonzalez-Cadavid N, Singh AB, Lee MI, Storer TW, Casaburi R, Shen R, Bhasin S: Testosterone-induced increase in muscle size in healthy young men is associated with muscle fiber hypertrophy. Am J Physiol Endocrinol Metab 2002;283:E154–E164.
23 Sinha-Hikim I, Taylor WE, Gonzalez-Cadavid NF, Zheng W, Bhasin S: Androgen receptor in human skeletal muscle and cultured muscle satellite cells: up-regulation by androgen treatment. J Clin Endocrinol Metab 2004;89:5245–5255.
24 Singh R, Artaza JN, Taylor WE, Gonzalez-Cadavid NF, Bhasin S: Androgens stimulate myogenic differentiation and inhibit adipogenesis in C3H 10T1/2 pluripotent cells through an androgen receptor-mediated pathway. Endocrinology 2003;144:5081–5088.
25 Mendler L, Baka Z, Kovacs-Simon A, Dux L: Androgens negatively regulate myostatin expression in an androgen-dependent skeletal muscle. Biochem Biophys Res Commun 2007;361:237–242.
26 Bhasin S, Storer TW, Berman N, Yarasheski KE, Clevenger B, Phillips J, Lee WP, Bunnell TJ, Casaburi R: Testosterone replacement increases fat-free mass and muscle size in hypogonadal men. J Clin Endocrinol Metab 1997;82:407–413.

27 Storer TW, Magliano L, Woodhouse L, Lee ML, Dzekov C, Dzekov J, Casaburi R, Bhasin S: Testosterone dose-dependently increases maximal voluntary strength and leg power, but does not affect fatigability or specific tension. J Clin Endocrinol Metab 2003;88:1478–1485.

28 Snyder PJ, Peachey H, Hannoush P, Berlin JA, Loh L, Lenrow DA, Holmes JH, Dlewati A, Santanna J, Rosen CJ, Strom BL: Effect of testosterone treatment on body composition and muscle strength in men over 65 years of age. J Clin Endocrinol Metab 1999;84:2647–2653.

29 Page ST, Amory JK, Bowman FD, Anawalt BD, Matsumoto AM, Bremner WJ, Tenover JL: Exogenous testosterone (T) alone or with finasteride increases physical performance, grip strength, and lean body mass in older men with low serum T. J Clin Endocrinol Metab 2005;90:1502–1510.

30 Emmelot-Vonk MH, Verhaar HJ, Nakhai Pour HR, Aleman A, Lock TM, Bosch JL, Grobbee DE, van der Schouw YT: Effect of testosterone supplementation on functional mobility, cognition, and other parameters in older men: a randomized controlled trial. JAMA 2008;299:39–52.

31 Wittert GA, Chapman IM, Haren MT, Mackintosh S, Coates P, Morley JE: Oral testosterone supplementation increases muscle and decreases fat mass in healthy elderly males with low-normal gonadal status. J Gerontol [A] 2003;58:618–625.

32 Nair KS, Rizza RA, O'Brien P, Dhatariya K, Short KR, Nehra A, Vittone JL, Klee GG, Basu A, Basu R, Cobelli C, Toffolo G, Dalla Man C, Tindall DJ, Melton LJ 3rd, Smith GE, Khosla S, Jensen MD: DHEA in elderly women and DHEA or testosterone in elderly men. N Engl J Med 2006;355:1647–1659.

33 Bhasin S, Woodhouse L, Casaburi R, Singh AB, Mac RP, Lee M, Yarasheski KE, Sinha-Hikim I, Dzekov C, Dzekov J, Magliano L, Storer TW: Older men are as responsive as young men to the anabolic effects of graded doses of testosterone on the skeletal muscle. J Clin Endocrinol Metab 2005;90:678–688.

34 Sih R, Morley JE, Kaiser FE, Perry HM 3rd, Patrick P, Ross C: Testosterone replacement in older hypogonadal men: a 12-month randomized controlled trial. J Clin Endocrinol Metab 1997;82:1661–1667.

35 Clague JE, Wu FC, Horan MA: Difficulties in measuring the effect of testosterone replacement therapy on muscle function in older men. Int J Androl 1999;22:261–265.

36 Frontera WR, Meredith CN, O'Reilly KP, Knuttgen HG, Evans WJ: Strength conditioning in older men: skeletal muscle hypertrophy and improved function. J Appl Physiol 1988;64:1038–1044.

37 Svartberg J, Aasebo U, Hjalmarsen A, Sundsfjord J, Jorde R: Testosterone treatment improves body composition and sexual function in men with COPD, in a 6-month randomized controlled trial. Respir Med 2004;98:906–913.

38 Bhasin S, Parker RA, Sattler F, Haubrich R, Alston B, Umbleja T, Shikuma CM: Effects of testosterone supplementation on whole body and regional fat mass and distribution in human immunodeficiency virus-infected men with abdominal obesity. J Clin Endocrinol Metab 2007;92:1049–1057.

39 Crawford BA, Liu PY, Kean MT, Bleasel JF, Handelsman DJ: Randomized placebo-controlled trial of androgen effects on muscle and bone in men requiring long-term systemic glucocorticoid treatment. J Clin Endocrinol Metab 2003;88:3167–3176.

40 Casaburi R, Bhasin S, Cosentino L, Porszasz J, Somfay A, Lewis MI, Fournier M, Storer TW: Effects of testosterone and resistance training in men with chronic obstructive pulmonary disease. Am J Respir Crit Care Med 2004;170:870–878.

41 Bakhshi V, Elliott M, Gentili A, Godschalk M, Mulligan T: Testosterone improves rehabilitation outcomes in ill older men. J Am Geriatr Soc 2000;48: 550–553.

42 Blackman MR, Sorkin JD, Munzer T, Bellantoni MF, Busby-Whitehead J, Stevens TE, Jayme J, O'Connor KG, Christmas C, Tobin JD, Stewart KJ, Cottrell E, St Clair C, Pabst KM, Harman SM: Growth hormone and sex steroid administration in healthy aged women and men: a randomized controlled trial. JAMA 2002;288:2282–2292.

43 Giannoulis MG, Sonksen PH, Umpleby M, Breen L, Pentecost C, Whyte M, McMillan CV, Bradley C, Martin FC: The effects of growth hormone and/or testosterone in healthy elderly men: a randomized controlled trial. J Clin Endocrinol Metab 2006;91: 477–484.

44 Liu PY, Yee B, Wishart SM, Jimenez M, Jung DG, Grunstein RR, Handelsman DJ: The short-term effects of high-dose testosterone on sleep, breathing, and function in older men. J Clin Endocrinol Metab 2003;88:3605–3613.

45 Amory JK, Chansky HA, Chansky KL, Camuso MR, Hoey CT, Anawalt BD, Matsumoto AM, Bremner WJ: Preoperative supraphysiological testosterone in older men undergoing knee replacement surgery. J Am Geriatr Soc 2002;50:1698–1701.

46 Buchner DM, Beresford SA, Larson EB, LaCroix AZ, Wagner EH: Effects of physical activity on health status in older adults. II. Intervention studies. Annu Rev Publ Health 1992;13:469–488.

47 Chandler JM, Duncan PW, Kochersberger G, Studenski S: Is lower extremity strength gain associated with improvement in physical performance and disability in frail, community-dwelling elders? Arch Phys Med Rehabil 1998;79:24–30.
48 Tenover JS: Effects of testosterone supplementation in the aging male. J Clin Endocrinol Metab 1992;75: 1092–1098.
49 Kenny AM, Prestwood KM, Gruman CA, Marcello KM, Raisz LG: Effects of transdermal testosterone on bone and muscle in older men with low bioavailable testosterone levels. J Gerontol [A] 2001;56: M266–M272.

Prof. Frederick C.W. Wu
Department of Endocrinology, University of Manchester
Manchester Royal Infirmary, Oxford Road
Manchester M13 9WL (UK)
Tel. +44 161 276 6330, Fax +44 161 276 8019, E-Mail frederick.wu@manchester.ac.uk

Jones TH (ed): Advances in the Management of Testosterone Deficiency.
Front Horm Res. Basel, Karger, 2009, vol 37, pp 150–162

Testosterone Effects on Cognition in Health and Disease

Monique M. Cherrier

Department of Psychiatry and Behavioral Sciences, University of Washington School of Medicine and Veterans Administration Puget Sound Health Care System S-182 GRECC, Seattle, Wash., USA

Abstract

Low testosterone is associated with many physical complaints as well as cognitive complaints. This article reviews the neurobiologic connection between gonadal steroids and cognitive functions, and mechanisms by which T may be considered neuroprotective. Studies of hormone replacement therapy in hypogonadal men as well as older men with late-onset hypogonadism (LOH) are reviewed as well as epidemiological studies of endogenous hormones and cognition. Studies examining T treatment in men with memory disorders such as Alzheimer's disease (AD) will also be reviewed. Some but not all studies of androgen replacement therapy in hypogonadal younger men, older men with LOH and AD patients suggest a potential beneficial effect on cognition, however a recent study indicated a negative effect. Most studies to date have been small and need further replication with randomized controlled studies using larger sample sizes with specific consideration of treatment risk factors.

Hormonal Mechanisms of Action in the Central Nervous System

Several central nervous system functions are regulated by gonadal steroids and in particular testosterone. Examples include prenatal sexual differentiation of the brain, adult sexual behavior, gonadotropin secretion and cognition. The effects of testosterone are mediated through the androgen receptor (AR) that is widely but selectively distributed throughout the brain [1]. Castration rapidly decreases AR expression in brain and testosterone upregulates neural AR in a dose-dependent manner in both male and female mice. Testosterone also acts via rapid, nongenomic methods of action through G-protein-coupled, agonist-sequestrable testosterone membrane receptors that initiate a transcription-independent signaling pathway affecting calcium channels. Thus androgen effects on brain may occur rapidly through nongenomic mechanisms or within the traditional longer time frame of genomic/protein transformation mechanisms.

Another important aspect of testosterone action is its active metabolism in vivo. In the body, testosterone is converted to estradiol (E_2) by the enzyme cytochrome P450 aromatase, and to di-hydrotestosterone (DHT) by the enzymes 5α-reductase (5α-R) types 1 and 2. E_2 formed from testosterone may then act on target organs via intracellular estrogen receptors alpha (α) and beta (β). DHT binds to ARs with greater affinity than testosterone and is a more potent androgen. Both E_2 and DHT are also widely distributed throughout the male brain, therefore, androgen effects on cognition may occur through testosterone directly or via its active metabolites, E_2 and DHT.

Androgen receptors and aromatase activity (AA) in mice, rats and monkeys have been shown to be widely distributed throughout the hypothalamus and limbic system in hormone-sensitive brain circuitry structures that serve essential roles in the central regulation of both reproductive function and cognition. For example, castration in male rats produces androgen-sensitive increases in dopamine axon density in pre-frontal cortex and significant decreases in cholinergic neurons in the anterior cingulate, posterior parietal cortex and medial septum compared to sham operated animals or gonadectomized (GDX) with testosterone replacement. Testosterone supplementation to the hippocampus, increases neuronal spine density in GDX animals [2]. The pre-frontal cortices are involved in cognitive, affective and memory functions and gonadectomized rats demonstrate impairments in learning a maze that is restored with testosterone administration. These effects appear to be selective for the memory aspects of maze performance as gonadectomy did not effect performance on a motor task [3].

Studies of testosterone replacement in mice and rats have generally supported a positive relationship between testosterone manipulation and cognitive task performance. Studies of age-accelerated mice and young rats have found beneficial effects of testosterone on avoidance learning and memory tasks with other studies failing to find beneficial effects of testosterone on learning and memory. Differences in these studies may be due to the dose level of testosterone, as a recent study found a beneficial effect of testosterone on spatial memory at a modest dose with detrimental effects on spatial memory at higher doses. In addition, the type of memory assessed may also contribute to differences between studies. Recent development of a working memory water maze task, which separates working memory – a form of scratch pad or temporary memory from reference memory a form of declarative or 'long-term' memory, found older male rats given testosterone demonstrate a beneficial increase in working memory capacity compared to older sham-operated and DHT-treated rats [4]. This finding suggests that changes in cognition from androgen supplementation or replacement may be selective frontal brain regions which underlie working memory and other executive functions.

The effects of DHT on cognition are less well known. However, once formed, DHT is a potent steroid in the CNS. The affinity of DHT for the AR is approximately four times that of testosterone. Like testosterone, DHT upregulates neural AR following castration. Although both testosterone and DHT upregulate AR after castration, only

DHT appears to sustain this effect for a prolonged period. There is also evidence that DHT may effect hippocampally mediated memory tasks as gonadectomized (GDX) animals given DHT replacement learn an inhibitory avoidance task more quickly compared to control or GDX vehicle-replaced animals [5].

Endogenous Testosterone Studies in Humans

Studies examining the relationship between endogenous androgen levels and cognitive performance in humans have produced inconsistent results. Correlations between endogenous testosterone levels and spatial abilities in men range from near zero to 0.53 [6]. In healthy young men, positive relationships have been found between circulating or endogenous testosterone levels and visuospatial orientation, spatial form comparison, and composite visuospatial scores. Positive relationships have also been found for tactual spatial tasks. Other studies examining endogenous testosterone levels have failed to find such a relationship between circulating androgen levels and visuospatial abilities. Low testosterone levels in men have also been found to be associated with better performance on spatial ability tasks and high levels of estradiol with better visual memory in men. In contrast, Gouchie and Kimura [7] divided men and women into groups according to endogenous testosterone levels (high versus low), and found that women with high testosterone and men with low testosterone levels demonstrated better spatial abilities compared to women with low testosterone and men with high testosterone levels. Young men examined during periods of high versus low testosterone levels from natural diurnal variation revealed a significant positive association with performance on a mental rotation test and average testosterone levels but not with changes in testosterone levels (i.e. high versus low), and there were no significant relationships between other tests (e.g. anagrams and an attention task) and testosterone levels [8]. These findings have led some to suggest that the beneficial effects of testosterone may be described by a curvilinear relationship such that low-to-moderate testosterone levels improve cognitive abilities but higher levels result in no further improvements or even decrements in some abilities (e.g. verbal).

In a comprehensive review of the literature, Kimura [9] found large sex differences favoring males on spatial tasks sometimes approaching one standard deviation for targeting (e.g. throwing darts or catching a ball) and spatial orientation (e.g. imagined spatial rotation). Modest effect sizes were found for spatial visualization (e.g. imagining the result of folding paper in a pre-cut shape), disembedding (finding a simple figure located in a more complex one) and spatial perception (e.g. determining the true vertical among distracting cues). Although some have suggested that experience with spatial tasks (e.g. driving, throwing and catching) may account for these sex differences, studies controlling for experience continue to find sex differences, and these differences may be present as early as 5 years of age.

Variability of results in the literature may be due to wide variability in the selection of cognitive tests and their unique task demands. This includes use of the term 'spatial' to describe numerous tests that may tap different cognitive processes or rely upon different brain structures and networks. For example, men tend to outperform women on tasks that require spatial rotation or manipulation. Robust gender differences have been found for performance spatial rotation tasks which require mental or imagined rotation of an object and performance of this task correlates with circulating testosterone levels [10] in men. It does not appear that this difference is due to the three-dimensional aspect of the task as these differences are also apparent on a test of two dimensional rotation. Interestingly, with a virtual reality adaptation of the mental rotation task, in which participants could manipulate a virtual reality version of the complex design with their hands, these gender differences disappeared. This latest result indicates a lack of gender differences on nonimagined spatial rotation tasks.

Memory for the location of objects is also considered a spatial task. Although recalling the location of objects clearly has a spatial component to it, several studies have demonstrated that women outperform men at recalling the location and spatial relationship between objects to be remembered in a spatial array. Interestingly, this demonstrated difference between men and women on spatial tasks such as mental rotation and memory for spatial array is consistent with findings of gender differences on spatial navigation tasks. For example, men on average tend to use a Euclidean (distance) or cardinal direction (N, S, E, W) approach to spatial navigation whereas women on average tend to use landmark references. Galea and Kimura [11] found that when young men and women were required to learn a route on a table-top map, men were able to learn the route in fewer trials but women remembered more of the landmarks located along the route. Studies comparing men and women on their ability to learn virtual reality environments tend to support the findings of male advantage in landmark-free or landmark-limited environments. A tendency to use a non-landmark or cardinal-direction-based route finding strategy has been found to be positively associated with endogenous testosterone levels. Although there is some debate regarding the neural structures that underlie spatial navigation, most studies of humans and animals support a direct role for the hippocampus in spatial navigation or representation of large-scale space and the parahippocampal gyrus in recall of landmarks [12]. As noted previously, the hippocampus along with hypothalamus and other limbic structures are target areas for gonadal steroids. Male and female rats treated with testosterone demonstrate a larger or 'more masculine'-like hippocampus characterized by the size and assymetric shape of the dentate gyrus. Thus, these behavioral tendencies or cognitive styles may reflect differential effects of gonadal hormones on place and landmark systems in the hippocampus.

Recent evidence from functional magnetic resonance imaging (fMRI) studies provides further evidence that cognitive processing, and in particular processing of spatial information activates specific brain regions and neural networks that are unique to the particular task demands. For example, healthy control participants demonstrate activation or use of unique brain regions according to their use of a spatial or nonspatial method to solving a radial arm maze [13]. These results along with several other recent behavioral and neuroimaging studies indicate that specific cognitive task demands will activate unique corresponding brain regions or neural networks. These neural networks have been shown to be gender specific for certain tasks [14]. Navigation of a virtual environment in men and women demonstrates common areas of activation between men and women (e.g. hippocampus, parahippocampus) [14]. However, there is some evidence that women demonstrate unique activation of right parietal and right prefrontal cortices. Thus, evidence from human studies suggests that both developmental and dynamic aspects of hormones interact with task demands and underlying neural networks associated with those cognitive tasks to produce the outcome of human behavioral performance.

Cognitive Changes from Androgen Supplementation

Cognitive changes from exogenously manipulated androgen levels have been examined in healthy young men, women, transsexuals and hypogonadal males (see section below). For example, Gordon and Lee [15] examined cognitive performance in a group of healthy young men in response to the administration of testosterone enanthate. They administered a low dose of testosterone enanthate (10 mg) to young men followed by a battery of cognitive tests immediately after injection and 4 h later. They reported no appreciable effects from hormone administration as participants demonstrated the same improvement from baseline to the second test session during the placebo condition as in the testosterone condition. However, no hormone values were reported. Therefore, the relationship between cognition and hormone levels is unknown. In contrast, a group of female to male transsexuals (FMs) administered testosterone, demonstrated improved spatial abilities but with decreased verbal abilities [16]. In a subsequent study by the same research group, beneficial effects of androgen treatment on spatial abilities were again confirmed in female-to-male transsexuals (FMs) and remained over a period of one and a half years [17]. As expected, untreated male-to-female transsexuals (MFs) had higher scores on visuospatial tasks than untreated FMs and after 3 months of cross-sex hormone treatment, the group differences disappeared. The Slabbekoorn et al. [17] study indicates that testosterone had an enhancing and not quickly reversible effect on spatial ability performance, but no deleterious effect on verbal fluency in FMs. In contrast, MFs demonstrated improved verbal memory in response to estrogen treatment with no differences between the treatment and control groups on tests of attention, mental rotation or verbal fluency [18]. Although it has been suggested that results from transsexual studies may be affected by co-morbid psychiatric or mood conditions, there were no appreciable differences between the hormone-treated and waiting list groups on mood measures in the Miles et al. [18] study. Further, in a population of healthy non-transsexual young women, Postma et al. [19] found that short term testosterone administration (0.5 mg testosterone cyclodextrine) resulted in improved spatial memory compared to placebo on some measures but not others.

Overall, the results from exogenous manipulation of androgens in healthy young men and women suggest that androgens may exert beneficial effects on spatial abilities. However, due to study design and lack of documented change in hormone levels, the findings to date remain inconclusive.

Aging Effects on Androgens

Serum levels of total testosterone and bioavailable testosterone (i.e. testosterone that is not bound to sex hormone-binding globulin) decrease with age in men. Although this decrease is gradual, it can result in decreased muscle mass, osteoporosis, decreased sexual activity, increased incidence of depression, decreased functional ability and changes in cognition. Androgen replacement therapy in normal older men has demonstrated benefits on bone mass, muscle strength, sexual functioning, and physical functioning [20].

In addition to peripheral physiological effects, age-related declines in testosterone levels may affect cognitive abilities. Several epidemiological, cross-sectional studies involving large groups of healthy older males, found bioavailable or free testosterone to be significantly and positively correlated with tests of global cognitive functioning, measures of attention and measures of visuospatial ability, semantic and episodic memory. In a large cohort, longitudinal study, the Baltimore Longitudinal Study of Aging (BLSA) which used a battery of sensitive neuropsychological rather than global measures to assess specific areas of cognitive functioning, high levels of free testosterone were associated with better performance on visual memory, verbal memory, divided attention, and visuospatial rotation [21]. Further, when this large cohort of elderly men was divided into eugonadal and hypogonadal status, hypogonadal men evidenced significantly poorer performance for visual memory, verbal memory, divided attention and visuospatial rotation compared to eugonadal men. In a subset of the BLSA men, assessment of regional cerebral blood flow (rCBF) changes over time as measured by ^{15}O-radiolabeld water positron emission tomography (PET) revealed an association between higher free testosterone and increased brain metabolism in the hippocampus bilaterally, suggesting that endogenous testosterone plays a role in brain regions important for memory [22].

However, not all studies have found a positive relationship between cognitive abilities and endogenous testosterone levels. Several large cohort studies have reported either no association or a negative association between endogenous testosterone levels and cognitive abilities. It is possible that modulating factors such as genetic risk factors and age may play a role. For example, testosterone has been found to have a beneficial relationship with cognition in men for young-old (average 60 years) [23] as well as older subjects (71–80 years) [24], but with more studies with older subjects (68–72 years average) failing to find a relationship between testosterone and cognition. An interaction between carriers of the apolipoprotein E4 (APOE) allele, a known risk factor for Alzheimer's disease (AD), has been reported, such that higher levels of free testosterone were associated with better general cognition, executive functions, working memory and attention only for non-APOE-4 carriers [25].

Testosterone Replacement in Older, Eugonadal Men

Studies examining exogenous testosterone administration in older men have produced mixed results. Studies utilizing testosterone undecanoate are not included in this section as circulating testosterone levels do not appear to be robustly or reliably increased from baseline in these studies. Sih et al. [26], using a double-blind, placebo-controlled design, gave older, hypogonadal men bi-weekly injections of 200 mg testosterone cypionate for 12 months. Fifteen men were randomly assigned to receive placebo and 17 to receive testosterone. The men were in good general health with a mean age of 68 years. Tests of verbal and visual memory were administered prior to treatment and again after 6 months. Although grip strength improved, memory measures remained unchanged. Lack of significant findings in this study may be due to the nonsignificant change in testosterone levels from baseline and/or assessment of cognition during nadir periods of testosterone levels. In a double-blind study using daily 15 mg testosterone skin patches, Janowsky et al. [27] found improvements in spatial abilities. In this study, 56 healthy older men, mean age 67 years participated and were randomized to placebo or testosterone for 3 months of treatment. Participants were administered a battery of tests measuring semantic knowledge, constructional ability, verbal memory, fine motor coordination and divided attention prior to and after 3 months of treatment. The treatment group demonstrated improvement on a measure of visuoconstructional ability. In a second study, Janowsky et al. [28] found that weekly injections of testosterone enanthate 150 mg improved spatial working memory in a group of healthy older males. These improvements were evident compared to an age-matched placebo group and exceeded practice effects demonstrated by young men (without testosterone treatment). Working memory refers to one's ability to maintain information in mind while simultaneously manipulating or updating the information as needed. It is the mind's scratchpad and therefore improvements in working memory can affect a number of cognitive and day-to-day tasks.

Consistent with these results, we have reported significant improvements in spatial and verbal memory in a group of healthy older men in response to short-term administration of testosterone enanthate [29]. Twenty-five healthy older men, mean age 68 years, were randomized to 100 mg testosterone enanthate or placebo and received treatment for 6 weeks followed by 6 weeks of washout. Participants were administered a comprehensive battery of tests including verbal and spatial memory, spatial abilities, verbal fluency, and selective attention. Testosterone-treated participants demonstrated significant improvements on spatial memory (recall of a walking route), spatial ability (block construction) and verbal memory (recall of a short story). Improvements in spatial memory for a task that utilizes navigation in three-dimensional space, and verbal memory have not been reported previously. Although improvements were not found for all cognitive measures, we did not expect changes on measures of verbal fluency or selective attention. In a subsequent study, we examined the relative role of increased testosterone alone (testosterone plus an aromatase inhibitor) versus increased testosterone and estradiol (testosterone supplementation alone) [30] and found beneficial improvements in spatial memory for both groups whereas verbal memory only improved in the group with increased estradiol as well as increased testosterone.

A more recent neuroimaging study by Maki et al. [31], reported a decline in short delay verbal memory with 6 months of testosterone treatment in eugondal, older men and a decrease in relative, task-associated brain activation in the temporal cortex – the region associated with memory functions. Other areas of cognitive function remained stable and there were also areas of increased, task-associated activation such as bilateral pre-frontal cortex which is associated with executive functions.

Testosterone Replacement in Older Hypogonadal Men

Several studies have examined androgen supplementation in older, hypogondal men. Kenny et al. [32] assessed a group of 44 older (65–87 years) hypogonadal men randomized to placebo or testosterone patches for 1 year. Significant improvement associated with testosterone levels was observed on a measure of divided attention (Trail Making Test Part B) in the treatment group. Both the treatment and placebo group demonstrated improvement on a measure of complex attention. We have also observed improvement in cognition in a group of older hypogonadal men given testosterone or DHT gel [33]. Twelve older (mean age 57 years) hypogonadal men were given testosterone gel and a battery of cognitive tests assessing verbal and spatial memory, language and attention at baseline (prior to medication) and again at day 90 and 180 of treatment. In addition to robustly raised testosterone and estradiol levels, a significant improvement in verbal memory compared to baseline was evident at day 180 of treatment. A beneficial increase in spatial memory was also evident, however, this increase did not reach statistical significance. In a separate study, 9 older hypogonadal men (mean age 74) were randomized to receive dihydrotestosterone (DHT) or placebo gel. Participants were given a comprehensive cognitive battery at baseline and days 30 and 90 of treatment. DHT gel significantly increased DHT and decreased testosterone levels significantly compared to baseline, and a significant improvement in spatial memory was observed. Results from these two studies suggest that aromatization of testosterone to estradiol may regulate verbal memory in men whereas non-aromatizable androgens may regulate spatial memory [33].

A recent study of testosterone supplementation in older (65–80 years) hypogonadal men given testosterone or testosterone combined with finasteride found improved working memory (digits backwards) in the testosterone only group compared to the testosterone and finasteride and placebo groups and improved verbal memory in the testosterone and finasteride group after 36 months of treatment [34]. However, the authors concluded that testosterone replacement does not improve cognition as no improvements were seen on the other cognitive measures.

In addition to cognitive changes measured by psychometric tests, two recent studies provide some evidence that androgen supplementation may change or optimize brain metabolism. Assessment of cerebral perfusion as measured by single-photon emission-computed tomography (SPECT) increased in the superior frontal gyrus and midbrain of 7 older (aged 58–72) hypogonadal men treated with testosterone at weeks 3–5 of treatment with further increases in midbrain perfusion at weeks 12–14 [35]. Although objective assessment of cognitive function was not included, responses to a questionnaire indicated that the increases in brain perfusion were coincident with self reported increases in cognitive function. These findings are consistent with increases in brain metabolism assessed with positron emission tomography (PET) in a small group (n = 4) of young hypogonadal men given testosterone replacement [36].

Low Testosterone Is a Risk Factor for Alzheimer's Disease

Recent evidence, indicates that low testosterone levels, due to aging are a risk factor for the development of AD. Findings from the Baltimore Longitudinal Study of Aging (BLSA), a longitudinal study, found that low testosterone levels over time was a significant risk factor for the development of AD [37]. Although it has been suggested that declines in testosterone levels may be coincident with disease or health decline, these findings remained significant when controlling for variables known to effect cognitive status such as age, education and health status and have been replicated in other large cohorts [38].

AD patients demonstrate lower serum testosterone levels compared to age matched controls [38] as well as lower testosterone levels in brain tissue [39]. In brain, lower testosterone levels from aging result in a compensatory upregulation of the AR which fails to occur in AD.

The two major pathological hallmarks for AD are the accumulation of senile plaques and neurofibrillary tangles (NFTs) in vulnerable brain regions. Senile plaques (SP) are thought to be related to the deposition of beta-amyloid (abeta) 40/42 peptides and NFTs are related to abnormally hyperphosphorylated tau protein. In humans, abeta 40/42 and total tau (T-tau) and phosphorylated-tau-181 and 231 (pT-181, pT-231) can be reliably measured and are associated with diagnostic differentiation, disease progression and neuropathology in both AD and MCI patients. Both testosterone and estradiol have been shown to reduce or prevent hyperphosphorylation of tau in neuronal cell cultures [40]. Testosterone has been shown to reduce beta-amyloid in neuronal cell cultures, as well as intraneuronal accumulation of beta-amyloid [41]. Induced, complete hypogonadism for treatment of prostate cancer results in a dramatic increase in serum beta-amyloid levels [42] and estradiol supplementation in women with AD reduces serum abeta 40 levels [43].

Androgens may also modulate disease onset and progression due to interactions with the apolipoprotein E*4 (APOE*4), a known risk factor in the onset and progression of cognitive deficits and AD in older adults. In a study by Hogervorst et al. [44], healthy, cognitively normal men with APOE*4 demonstrated significantly lower serum testosterone levels than men without the APOE*4 allele. In animal studies, male transgenic mice expressing human apolipoprotein E*4 (APOE*4) fail to demonstrate cognitive deficits comparable to females. This appears to be an AR-mediated effect as blocking the AR results in the expected cognitive impairments that occur with female mice [45]. These studies suggest mechanisms by which low testosterone and other known AD risk factors such as APOE*4 may interact in promoting AD pathogenesis.

Testosterone Replacement in Men with Alzheimer's Disease or Mild Cognitive Impairment

Although observational studies suggest that lower testosterone levels may confer a risk for developing AD, there are few studies that have examined whether testosterone supplementation may be beneficial in AD patients, and findings to date are mixed. Tan and Pu [46] treated 10 male patients with AD who also met the criteria for hypogonadism. Participants were given 200 mg testosterone every 2 weeks. A comprehensive cognitive test battery was administered at baseline and 3, 6 and 9 months of treatment. AD patients demonstrated a significant improvement at months 3, 6 and 9 compared to baseline and compared to the placebo group. A study of testosterone supplementation in 16 eugondal AD patients treated with 75 mg daily of testosterone gel, found no changes in cognition but improved on a quality-of-life measure [47].

Older adults who experience age-associated decrements in memory but do not meet criteria for AD are now defined with a new diagnostic category termed mild-cognitive impairment (MCI). Approximately, 50–70% of these individuals progress to develop AD, and therefore MCI is often considered a pro-dromal condition to AD. A study of older hypogonadal men who also met the criteria for MCI, found no significant changes on mood or cognitive measures in response to testosterone supplementation for 12 weeks [48]. A study of eugondal, mixed MCI and AD patients given

100 mg testosterone enanthate weekly for 6 weeks found an improvement in spatial memory compared to baseline but no changes in other cognitive domains [49]. Thus, it is difficult to determine whether testosterone supplementation is beneficial for cognition in AD or MCI patients. As with the studies of older and hypogonadal men, the findings in AD and MCI patients are mixed and have generally been from small sample sizes. However, it does not yet appear that testosterone supplementation worsens cognition as was reported in a study of estradiol supplementation in women with AD.

Conclusions

In conclusion, previous studies suggest that testosterone administration may have beneficial effects on spatial and verbal memory, although findings across studies are inconsistent with a recent study indicating a potential adverse effect on cognition. Potential beneficial effects of androgen supplementation on cognition may be particularly important for older males who may have age-related decreases in endogenous testosterone levels which are predictive of cognitive loss and increased risk for the development of AD. More studies of testosterone supplementation are needed to better evaluate the balance between benefits and risk. This is further emphasized by a recent Institute of Medicine Report which concluded that additional studies of testosterone supplementation in older men are needed and noted that cognition should be included among study outcomes.

References

1 Roselli CE, Klosterman S, Resko JA: Anatomic relationships between aromatase and androgen receptor mRNA expression in the hypothalamus and amygdala of adult male cynomolgus monkeys. J Comp Neurol 2001;439:208–223.
2 Leranth C, Hajszan T, MacLusky NJ: Androgens increase spine synapse density in the CA1 hippocampal subfield of ovariectomized female rats. J Neurosci 2004;24:495–499.
3 Kritzer MF, McLaughlin PJ, Smirlis T, Robinson JK: Gonadectomy impairs T-maze acquisition in adult male rats. Horm Behav 2001;39:167–174.
4 Bimonte-Nelson HA, Singleton RS, Nelson ME, Eckman CB, Barber J, Scott TY, Granholm AC: Testosterone, but not nonaromatizable dihydrotestosterone, improves working memory and alters nerve growth factor levels in aged male rats. Exp Neurol 2003;181:301–312.
5 Edinger KL, Lee B, Frye CA: Mnemonic effects of testosterone and its 5alpha-reduced metabolites in the conditioned fear and inhibitory avoidance tasks. Pharmacol Biochem Behav 2004;78:559–568.
6 McKeever WF, Deyo RA: Testosterone, dihydrotestosterone, and spatial task performances of males. Bull Psychonomic Soc 1990;28:305–308.
7 Gouchie C, Kimura D: The relationship between testosterone levels and cognitive ability patterns. Psychoneuroendocrinology 1991;16:323–334.
8 Silverman JM, Keefe RSE, Mohs RC, Davis KL: A study of the reliability of the family history method in genetic studies of Alzheimer disease. Alzheim Dis Assoc Disord 1989;3:218–223.
9 Kimura D: Sex and Cognition. Cambridge, MA: The MIT Press, 1999.
10 Hooven CK, Chabris CF, Ellison PT, Kosslyn SM: The relationship of male testosterone to components of mental rotation. Neuropsychologia 2004;42:782–790.
11 Galea LA, Kimura D: Sex differences in route learning. Pers Individ Diff 1993;14:53–65.
12 Aguirre GK, Zarahn E, D'Esposito M: An area within human ventral cortex sensitive to 'building' stimuli: evidence and implications. Neuron 1998;21:373–383.

13 Iaria G, Petrides M, Dagher A, Pike B, Bohbot VD: Cognitive strategies dependent on the hippocampus and caudate nucleus in human navigation: variability and change with practice. J Neurosci 2003;23: 5945–5952.
14 Gron G, Wunderlich AP, Spitzer M, Tomczak R, Riepe MW: Brain activation during human navigation: gender-different neural networks as substrate of performance. Nat Neurosci 2000;3:404–408.
15 Gordon HW, Lee PA: A relationship between gonadotropins and visuospatial function. Neuropsychologia 1986;24:563–576.
16 Van Goozen SHM, Cohen-Kettenis PT, Gooren LJG, Frijda NH, Van De Poll NE: Activating effects of androgens on cognitive performance: causal evidence in a group of female-to-male transsexuals. Neuropsychologia 1994;32:1153–1157.
17 Slabbekoorn D, van Goozen SH, Megens J, Gooren LJ, Cohen-Kettenis PT: Activating effects of cross-sex hormones on cognitive functioning: a study of short-term and long-term hormone effects in transsexuals. Psychoneuroendocrinology 1999;24:423–447.
18 Miles C, Green R, Sanders G, Hines M: Estrogen and memory in a transsexual population. Horm Behav 1998;34:199–208.
19 Postma A, Meyer G, Tuiten A, van Honk J, Kessels RP, Thijssen J: Effects of testosterone administration on selective aspects of object- location memory in healthy young women. Psychoneuroendocrinology 2000;25:563–575.
20 Matsumoto AM: 'Andropause': are reduced androgen levels in aging men physiologically important? West J Med 1993;159:618–620.
21 Moffat SD, Zonderman AB, Metter EJ, Blackman MR, Harman SM, Resnick SM: Longitudinal assessment of serum free testosterone concentration predicts memory performance and cognitive status in elderly men. J Clin Endocrinol Metab 2002;87:5001–5007.
22 Moffat SD, Resnick SM: Long-term measures of free testosterone predict regional cerebral blood flow patterns in elderly men. Neurobiol Aging 2007;28: 914–920.
23 Hogervorst E, De Jager C, Budge M, Smith AD: Serum levels of estradiol and testosterone and performance in different cognitive domains in healthy elderly men and women. Psychoneuroendocrinology 2004;29:405–421.
24 Muller M, Aleman A, Grobbee DE, de Haan EH, van der Schouw YT: Endogenous sex hormone levels and cognitive function in aging men. Neurology 2005;64:866–871.
25 Burkhardt MS, Foster JK, Clarnette RM, Chubb SA, Bruce DG, Drummond PD, Martins RN, Yeap BB: Interaction between testosterone and apolipoprotein E epsilon4 status on cognition in healthy older men. J Clin Endocrinol Metab 2006;91:1168–1172.
26 Sih R, Morley JE, Kaiser FE, Perry HM, Patrick P, Ross C: Testosterone replacement in older hypogonadal men: a 12 month randomized controlled trial. J Clin Endocrinol Metab 1997;82:1661–1667.
27 Janowsky JS, Oviatt SK, Orwoll ES: Testosterone influences spatial cognition in older men. Behav Neurosci 1994;108:325–332.
28 Janowsky JS, Chavez B, Orowoll E: Sex steroids modify working memory. J Cogn Neurosci 2000;12: 407–414.
29 Cherrier MM, Asthana S, Baker LD, Plymate S, Matsumoto A, Peskind E, Raskind MA, Brodkin K, Bremner W, Petrova A, Latendresse S, Craft S: Testosterone supplementation improves spatial and verbal memory in healthy older men. Neurology 2001;57:80–88.
30 Cherrier MM, Matsumoto AM, Amory JK, Ahmed S, Bremner W, Peskind ER, Raskind MA, Johnson M, Craft S: The role of aromatization in testosterone supplementation: effects on cognition in older men. Neurology 2005;64:290–296.
31 Maki PM, Ernst M, London ED, Mordecai KL, Perschler P, Durso SC, Brandt J, Dobs A, Resnick SM: Intramuscular testosterone treatment in elderly men: evidence of memory decline and altered brain function. J Clin Endocrinol Metab 2007;92:4107–4114.
32 Kenny AM, Bellantonio S, Gruman CA, Acosta RD, Prestwood KM: Effects of transdermal testosterone on cognitive function and health perception in older men with low bioavailable testosterone levels. J Gerontol [A] 2002;57:M321–M325.
33 Cherrier MM, Craft S, Matsumoto AH: Cognitive changes associated with supplementation of testosterone or dihydrotestosterone in mildly hypogonadal men: a preliminary report. J Androl 2003; 24: 568–576.
34 Vaughan C, Goldstein FC, Tenover JL: Exogenous testosterone alone or with finasteride does not improve measurements of cognition in healthy older men with low serum testosterone. J Androl 2007;28: 878–882.
35 Azad N, Pitale S, Barnes WE, Friedman N: Testosterone treatment enhances regional brain perfusion in hypogonadal men. J Clin Endocrinol Metab 2003;88:3064–3068.
36 Zitzmann M, Weckesser M, Schober O, Nieschlag E: Changes in cerebral glucose metabolism and visuospatial capability in hypogonadal males under testosterone substitution therapy. Exp Clin Endocrinol Diabetes 2001;109:302–304.
37 Moffat SD, Zonderman AB, Metter EJ, Kawas C, Blackman MR, Harman SM, Resnick SM: Free testosterone and risk for Alzheimer disease in older men. Neurology 2004;62:188–193.

38 Hogervorst E, Bandelow S, Combrinck M, Smith AD: Low free testosterone is an independent risk factor for Alzheimer's disease. Exp Gerontol 2004;39: 1633–1639.
39 Rosario ER, Chang L, Stanczyk FZ, Pike CJ: Age-related testosterone depletion and the development of Alzheimer disease. JAMA 2004;292:1431–1432.
40 Alvarez-de-la-Rosa M, Silva I, Nilsen J, Perez MM, Garcia-Segura LM, Avila J, Naftolin F: Estradiol prevents neural tau hyperphosphorylation characteristic of Alzheimer's disease. Ann NY Acad Sci 2005;1052:210–224.
41 Zhang Y, Champagne N, Beitel LK, Goodyer CG, Trifiro M, LeBlanc A: Estrogen and androgen protection of human neurons against intracellular amyloid beta1–42 toxicity through heat shock protein 70. J Neurosci 2004;24:5315–5321.
42 Almeida OP, Waterreus A, Spry N, Flicker L, Martins RN: One year follow-up study of the association between chemical castration, sex hormones, beta-amyloid, memory and depression in men. Psychoneuroendocrinology 2004;29:1071–1081.
43 Baker LD, Sambamurti K, Craft S, Cherrier M, Raskind MA, Stanczyk FZ, Plymate SR, Asthana S: 17beta-Estradiol reduces plasma Abeta40 for HRT-naive postmenopausal women with Alzheimer disease: a preliminary study. Am J Geriatr Psychiatry 2003;11:239–244.
44 Hogervorst E, Lehmann DJ, Warden DR, McBroom J, Smith AD: Apolipoprotein E epsilon4 and testosterone interact in the risk of Alzheimer's disease in men. Int J Geriatr Psychiatry 2002;17:938–940.
45 Raber J, Wong D, Yu GQ, Buttini M, Mahley RW, Pitas RE, Mucke L: Apolipoprotein E and cognitive performance. Nature 2000;404:352–354.
46 Tan RS, Pu SJ: A pilot study on the effects of testosterone in hypogonadal aging male patients with Alzheimer's disease. Aging Male 2003;6:13–17.
47 Lu PH, Masterman DA, Mulnard R, Cotman C, Miller B, Yaffe K, Reback E, Porter V, Swerdloff R, Cummings JL: Effects of testosterone on cognition and mood in male patients with mild Alzheimer disease and healthy elderly men. Arch Neurol 2006;63:177–185.
48 Kenny AM, Fabregas G, Song C, Biskup B, Bellantonio S: Effects of testosterone on behavior, depression, and cognitive function in older men with mild cognitive loss. J Gerontol [A] 2004;59:75–78.
49 Cherrier MM, Matsumoto AH, Asthana S, Amory JK, Bremner W, Peskind E, Raskind M, Craft S: Testosterone improves spatial memory in men with alzheimer disease and mild cognitive impairment. Neurology 2005;64:2063–2068.

Dr. Monique M. Cherrier
Department of Psychiatry and Behavioral Sciences
University of Washington School of Medicine and Veterans Administration Puget Sound
Health Care System S-182 GRECC, Seattle, WA 98108 (USA)
Tel. +1 206 277 3594, Fax +1 206 764 2476, E-Mail cherrier@u.washington.edu

Jones TH (ed): Advances in the Management of Testosterone Deficiency.
Front Horm Res. Basel, Karger, 2009, vol 37, pp 163–182

Anabolic Applications of Androgens for Functional Limitations Associated with Aging and Chronic Illness

Shalender Bhasin · Thomas W. Storer

Boston University School of Medicine, Section of Endocrinology, Diabetes, and Nutrition,
Boston Medical Center, Boston, Mass., USA

Abstract

Total and free testosterone concentrations decline progressively with advancing age because of defects at all levels of the hypothalamic-pituitary-testicular axis. Low total and bioavailable testosterone levels have been associated with decreased skeletal muscle mass, muscle strength, physical function, bone mineral density, and fracture risk, although these associations are weak. The risks and health benefits of long-term testosterone remain poorly understood. Physiologic testosterone replacement of young, androgen-deficient men and older men with low testosterone levels is associated with an increase in fat-free mass, grip strength, and fractional muscle protein synthesis, but we do not know whether testosterone replacement improves quadriceps strength, power, muscle fatigability, and physical function in older men, and whether it can reduce the risk of disability and falls. Testosterone replacement increases vertebral bone mineral density in young hypogonadal men and older men with low testosterone levels, but we do not know whether testosterone reduces fracture risk. Concerns about the potential adverse effects of testosterone on the prostate have encouraged the development of selective androgen receptor modulators that increase muscle mass while sparing the prostate.

Androgens are the front runners in the growing efforts to develop function-promoting anabolic therapies (FPATs) for the prevention and treatment of functional limitations and disability associated with aging and chronic illnesses. Functional limitations refer to restrictions in an individual's ability to perform specific tasks or actions such as walking, while disability represents a person's inability or limitation in performing socially accepted activities and roles, such as personal care. As men and women grow older, their skeletal muscle mass, muscle strength, and leg power decline [1, 2]. The age-related decline in skeletal muscle mass, strength, and power predispose individuals to increased risk of functional limitations, falls, fractures, dependency and poor quality of life [1]. Physical function has been described as the mirror to an individual's health [3]. Limitations in physical function are associated with adverse health outcomes: increased risk of incident disability, mortality, hospitalization, and poor quality of life [3]. For people over age 65, 35–40% experience activity limitations or disability [4]. Although the actual prevalence and incidence rates of disability vary in different countries, the human populations are aging on all continents except Africa, and the percentage of population aged 65 years or over will increase in the coming decades. In the developed world, the oldest old – men and women 85 years of age or older – constitute the fastest-growing segment of the population. The majority of individuals who reach this age will experience some limitation in function. The costs of support services and lost productivity associated with disabling conditions have consequences for the entire population [4]. Currently, the practicing physicians have few therapeutic choices for the treatment of older individuals with functional limitations and physical disability. Exercise and behavioral interventions have proven difficult to implement at a population level and have had limited impact. Therefore, there is growing interest in developing pharmacological therapies for the treatment of functional limitations.

Although a number of molecular pathways are being explored, including myostatin antagonists, androgens, muscle growth factor, and inhibitors of proteolytic and apoptotic pathways, the androgens are the farthest along in the drug development process and the focus of this review. The rationale for the use of androgens as function promoting anabolic therapies in the treatment of functional limitations associated with aging and chronic illness is based on several hypotheses: aging and chronic illness are associated with high prevalence of low testosterone levels; low testosterone levels are associated with adverse outcomes; testosterone therapy by increasing skeletal muscle mass and strength would improve physical function and health-related outcomes, and testosterone therapy is safe. Each of these hypotheses is discussed below.

Age-Related Changes in Testosterone Production

Over 40 cross-sectional studies and several longitudinal studies are in agreement that serum testosterone levels decline in men with advancing age [5]. As sex hormone-binding globulin (SHBG) concentrations are higher in older than in young men [5], the age-related decline in free and bioavailable testosterone concentrations is greater than the decline in total testosterone concentrations. Unlike women in whom estradiol levels decrease abruptly at menopause, there is no discrete inflection point in men; the age-related decline in testosterone concentrations begins in the third decade of life and continues inexorably throughout life. In the Baltimore Longitudinal Study of Aging (BLSA) [6], 30% of men over the age of 60 and 50% of men over the age of 70 had total testosterone concentration below the lower limit of normal range for healthy young men (325 ng/dl, 11.3 nmol/l). The prevalence rates were even higher when these investigators used a free testosterone index to define androgen deficiency [6]. Other studies such as the European Male Aging Study have reported lower prevalence (less than 10%) of low testosterone levels in older men than those observed in the BLSA and the Massachusetts Male Aging Study (MMAS) [7].

Travison et al. [8] using data from the Massachusetts Male Aging Study (MMAS) have reported that circulating testosterone concentrations in men are in an age-independent, secular decline. This population level decline in testosterone concentrations in men could not be explained by increasing body mass index and prevalence of obesity, other co-morbid conditions, or decreasing incidence of smoking [8]. These provocative findings need further confirmation.

The rate of age-related decline is affected by co-morbid conditions, medications, and adiposity. Thus, individuals with chronic disorders such as diabetes mellitus, cardiovascular disease, chronic obstructive pulmonary disease, and chronic kidney disease are likely to experience a more accelerated decline in testosterone levels than healthy individuals [9]. Similarly, the degree of adiposity and weight gain affect the trajectory of age-related decline in testosterone levels; men who gain weight experience a greater decrease in testosterone levels than men who do not.

The age-related decline in testosterone levels is the result of decreased testosterone production rates [5, 10]; the plasma clearance of testosterone is lower in older men than in young men. The decreased testosterone production rates in older men result from abnormalities at all levels of the hypothalamic-pituitary-testicular axis. Leydig cell response to human chorionic gonadotropin (hCG) is attenuated in older men [5, 10]. Serum luteinizing hormone (LH) and follicle-stimulating hormone (FSH) concentrations are higher in older than young men [10]. However, the increase in serum LH concentrations is less than that expected from the age-related decline in circulating testosterone levels, probably due to the impairment of gonadotropin-releasing hormone (GnRH) secretion and alterations in gonadal steroid feed-back and feed-forward relationships [11]; both of these mechanisms are operative in older men.

Aging-associated changes at the hypothalamic-pituitary sites result in attenuated pulsatile GnRH secretion in older men [12]. In addition, the orderliness of LH pulses and the synchrony between LH and testosterone pulses are decreased in older men [13]. Thus, LH pulse frequency, amplitude, and secretory mass show greater variability in older than in younger men [13]. The diurnal changes in testosterone secretion that are observed in young men are also less pronounced in older men than in young men [5].

In the Brown Norway rat, a widely used model of reproductive aging, the prepro-GnRH mRNA content, the number of neurons expressing prepro GnRH mRNA, and the GnRH content of several hypothalamic areas are lower in older male rats in comparison to young rats [14]. Significant reductions in glutamate and γ-aminobutyric acid levels also have been reported in the hypothalamus of older rats compared to young rats [14], leading to speculation that the decreased hypothalamic excitatory amino acid expression and the reduced responsiveness of GnRH neurons to N-methyl-D-aspartate (NMDA) contribute to decreased GnRH secretion and the altered LH pulsatile secretion observed in old rats [14].

Older men are more sensitive to the feedback inhibitory effects of testosterone on LH than young men; thus, older men receiving DHT infusion or transdermal testosterone therapy experience greater inhibition of LH than young men [11]. The data on age-related changes in LH response to GnRH are conflicting; some studies have reported decreased LH response to GnRH, but other studies have not confirmed these findings.

Associations of Low Testosterone Levels with Health Outcomes in Older Men

In epidemiologic studies of older men, lower bioavailable testosterone concentrations are associated with less lean body mass and strength of upper and lower extremity muscles [2]. Low testosterone levels are also associated with worse physical function, both self-reported and performance-based, and increased risk of falls in older men, although the associations are weak [15, 16]. In the Longitudinal Aging Study of Amsterdam, serum testosterone concentrations were positively correlated with muscle strength and physical performance [17]. In the Massachusetts Male Aging Study, performance on a physical function test was positively correlated with the serum testosterone concentration up to a threshold level of 461 ng/dl [16]. Testosterone levels were also positively correlated with self-reported physical function, as assessed by SF-36 questionnaire [16].

Low Testosterone Levels in Chronic Illness

The longevity of patients with many chronic illnesses, such as those associated with HIV-infection, chronic obstructive lung disease, end-stage renal disease, congestive heart failure, untreated diabetes, and many types of cancers has improved substantially. However, the clinical course of these illnesses is often complicated by loss of skeletal muscle mass, physical dysfunction, and a high prevalence of low testosterone levels. The loss of muscle mass in chronic illnesses is associated with increased risk of functional limitations, loss of independence, impaired quality of life, and mortality.

High prevalence of low testosterone levels has been reported in men with many chronic disorders. In early days of the HIV epidemic before the advent of effective anti-retroviral therapy, 40–50% of HIV-infected men had testosterone levels in the hypogonadal range [18]. Surprisingly, even recent surveys have reported low testosterone levels in 20–30% of HIV-infected men on highly effective anti-retroviral drug therapy [19]. The pathophysiology of low testosterone levels in HIV-infected men is complex; 80% of HIV-infected men have low or low normal LH levels and 20% have elevated LH levels suggesting primary testicular dysfunction [19]. Histologic studies of testes of HIV-infected men have shown loss of tubular architecture, hyalinization, fibrosis, mononuclear cell infiltration, and loss of germ cells [20]. Low testosterone levels in HIV-infected men are associated with low lean body mass, decreased exercise capacity, wasting and more accelerated disease progression to AIDS [19, 20].

Fifty percent of men with chronic obstructive lung disease and 50–70% of men with end-stage renal disease have testosterone levels in the hypogonadal range [21]. Thus, a high frequency of low testosterone levels has been found in all the chronic illnesses that have been investigated.

Data from Intervention Trials of Testosterone and Other Androgens

The anabolic effects of androgens had been the subject of contentious debate for many years [22]. The widespread abuse of androgenic steroids by competitive athletes and recreational body builders was based on the belief that these drugs enhance muscle mass and strength. However, the published data were inconclusive because of well known flaws in the design of earlier studies. Some of these studies were neither randomized nor placebo-controlled [23]. The energy and protein intake was not controlled; in some studies, the participants continue to ingest protein supplements ad lib [22]. The exercise stimulus was not standardized; thus, the effects of resistance exercise training could not be separated from those of androgen [22, 23]. The doses of androgens used in earlier trials were considerably smaller than those used by athletes and body builders. However, a large body of clinical trials data generated in the past decade has established that testosterone supplementation increases whole body and appendicular skeletal muscle mass, maximal voluntary muscle strength, and leg power [24].

Studies in Healthy Hypogonadal Men

Androgen-deficient men have lower fat-free mass and higher fat mass than age-matched, eugonadal controls [25]. Suppression of endogenous testosterone production by administration of a GnRH agonist in young men is associated with decreased fat-free mass and fractional muscle protein synthesis [26].

Systematic review of testosterone trials in hypogonadal men reveal that testosterone therapy of healthy, hypogonadal men increases fat-free mass by an average of 2.8 kg [24, 27]. Some studies have reported significant improvements in maximal voluntary strength [28]. Testosterone administration increases fractional muscle protein synthesis and fatty acid oxidation in healthy hypogonadal men [29].

Studies in Healthy, Eugonadal Men

To overcome the problems that had plagued earlier trials, we conducted a placebo-controlled, randomized trial of a supraphysiologic dose of testosterone enanthate in healthy eugonadal men [30]. In a 2×2 factorial design, we randomly assigned subjects to receive either weekly intramuscular injections of placebo or 600 mg testosterone enanthate with or without a program of standardized resistance exercise training. Treatment duration was 10 weeks [30]. Energy and protein intake were standardized. The exercise stimulus was also standardized based on the subject's baseline muscle strength. The administration of supraphysiologic doses of testosterone was associated with greater increments in fat-free mass, muscle size, and maximal voluntary strength than placebo [30]. The effects of combined administration of resistance exercise training and testosterone on fat-free mass and muscle strength gains were greater than those of testosterone administration alone (fig. 1) [30]. These data demonstrated unequivocally that when nutritional intake and exercise stimulus are controlled, raising testosterone levels above the physiologic range in eugonadal men leads to substantial gains in fat-free mass and muscle strength [30].

The gains in fat-free mass, muscle size, and maximal voluntary strength in response to testosterone administration are highly correlated with testosterone dose and circulating testosterone concentrations, which account for 40–67% of the variance in the change in fat-free mass and muscle size [31, 32]. Polymorphisms in polyglutamine and polyglycine tract length in exon 1 of androgen receptor account for a small fraction of the variance in anabolic response [32].

The effects of testosterone on muscle performance are domain-specific: testosterone increases maximal voluntary strength and leg power, but does not affect fatigability or specific force [33]. Thus, the gains in muscle strength during testosterone administration are proportional to the gains in muscle mass; testosterone does not improve the contractile properties of the skeletal muscle [33]. Androgens do not affect endurance measures, such as $VO_{2\,max}$ or lactate threshold.

The anabolic effects of testosterone are augmented by resistance exercise training [30]. Combined administration of testosterone and rhGH also enhances the anabolic response to androgen administration.

Studies in Older Men with Low or Low Normal Testosterone Levels

A number of studies have examined the effects of testosterone therapy in older men with low or low normal testosterone levels [5, 24, 27]. The men included in these first generation testosterone trials were generally healthy, community dwelling individuals without functional limitations. These studies have reported consistent increases in fat-free mass and a decrease in fat mass. In a meta-analysis of randomized testosterone trials in middle-aged and older men (fig. 2), testosterone therapy was associated with a greater improvement in fat-free mass (+2.5 kg, 95% CI 1.5–3.4 kg), grip strength (3.3 kg, 95% CI 0.7–5.8 kg) and self-reported physical function (0.5 SD, 95% CI, 0.3, 0.7 SDs) than placebo [24]. Only a few studies examined the effects of testosterone on muscle strength and physical function. Some studies have observed increases in the strength of lower extremity muscles, while others found no significant change [24]. Changes in performance-based measures of physical function have been inconsistent across trials [34, 35]. However, testosterone administration is associated with significant improvements in self-reported physical function, as assessed by the physical function domain of the SF-36 questionnaire [34].

Why did the first-generation studies fail to demonstrate improvements in physical function in spite of a significant increase in fat-free mass? Most studies recruited men with low normal testosterone levels. The testosterone doses used in these studies were

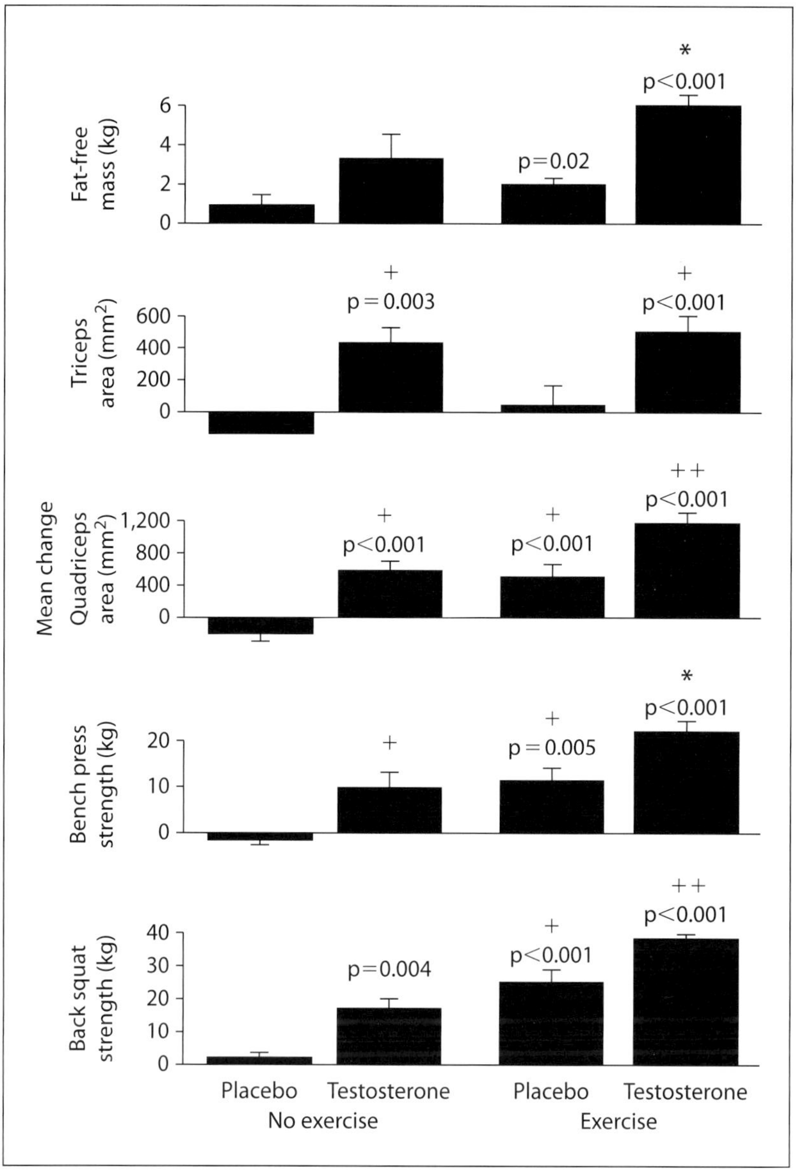

Fig. 1. Effects of a supraphysiologic dose of testosterone with or without a program of resistance exercise training on change from baseline in fat-free mass, triceps cross-sectional area, quadriceps cross-sectional area, and strength (1-RM) in the bench press and back squat exercises. Healthy young men were randomly assigned to receive either placebo or 600 mg testosterone enanthate intramuscularly weekly with or without a standardized program of resistance exercise training. The p values shown are for the comparison with a zero change. $^*p < 0.05$ for the comparison between the change indicated and that in either no-exercise group; $^+p < 0.05$ for the comparison between the change indicated and that in the group assigned to placebo with no exercise; $^{++}p < 0.05$ for the comparison against the changes in all three other groups. Reproduced with permission from Bhasin et al. [30].

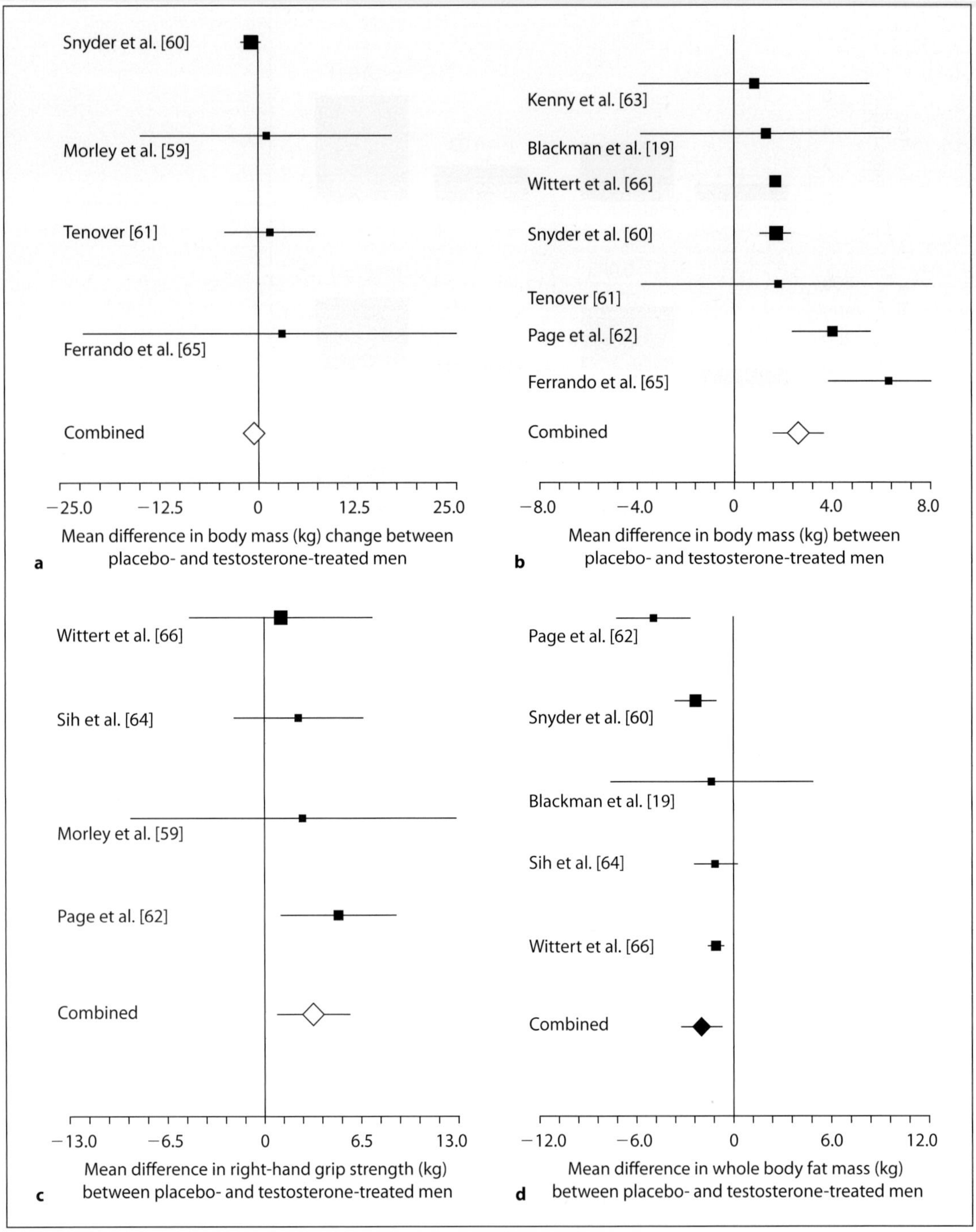

Fig. 2. Effects of testosterone therapy in healthy, middle-aged and older men. Shown below are meta-analysis plots of contrasts between testosterone-treated and placebo-treated men for change (kg) in whole body mass (**a**), lean body mass change (**b**), right-hand grip strength (**c**), and whole body fat mass (**d**) in men more than 45 years of age. A positive difference is a favorable testosterone effect on body mass, lean body mass, fat-free mass, and grip strength; a negative difference is a

relatively small and were associated with relatively small gains in muscle mass. The studies generally lacked adequate power to detect small but clinically important changes in physical function measures. Because of the considerable test-to-test variability in tests of physical function, previous studies may have had inadequate power to detect meaningful differences in measures of physical function between the treatment groups. The measures of physical function used in these studies had low ceiling, requiring only a small fraction of an individual's maximal voluntary strength. Most of the studies performed to date were performed in asymptomatic, healthy, older men, whose baseline maximal voluntary strength is far higher than the threshold below which these measures would detect impairment. Given the low intensity of the tasks used, relatively healthy older men show neither impairment in these measures of physical function at baseline nor an improvement during testosterone administration.

The effects of testosterone administration on health-related outcomes have not been investigated. Furthermore, none of the first generation studies included men with symptomatic functional limitations. Further studies are needed to determine whether testosterone therapy can improve physical function and health-related outcomes in older men with functional limitations.

Studies in HIV-Infected Men with Weight Loss

A number of trials have examined the effects of androgen therapy in HIV-infected men with weight loss [24, 36]. A variety of androgens including testosterone, nandrolone decanoate, oxandrolone, and oxymetholone, have been used in these trials. In systematic reviews [24, 36] of randomized, placebo-controlled trials of testosterone therapy in HIV-infected men with weight loss, 3–6 months of testosterone supplementation was associated with greater gains in lean body mass than placebo administration (difference in lean body mass change between placebo and testosterone therapy 1.22 kg, 95% CI 0.23–2.22 for the random effect model) (fig. 3) [24]. In 2 [37, 38] of 3 trials that measured muscle strength [37–39], testosterone administration was associated with significantly greater improvements in maximal voluntary strength than placebo.

In the four trials that reported effects on depression in HIV-infected men [24], overall, testosterone therapy had a moderate effect on depression indices. There were no significant testosterone effects on any domain of quality of life [24].

The placebo and testosterone groups did not differ significantly in the frequency of adverse events [36]. There were no significant changes in CD4+ T lymphocyte counts, HIV copy number, PSA, and plasma HDL cholesterol. Overall, short-term (3–6 months) testosterone use in HIV-infected men with low testosterone levels and

favorable testosterone effect on fat mass. Confidence intervals that do not overlap with zero represent significant differences between placebo and testosterone groups. Reproduced with permission from Bhasin et al. [24].

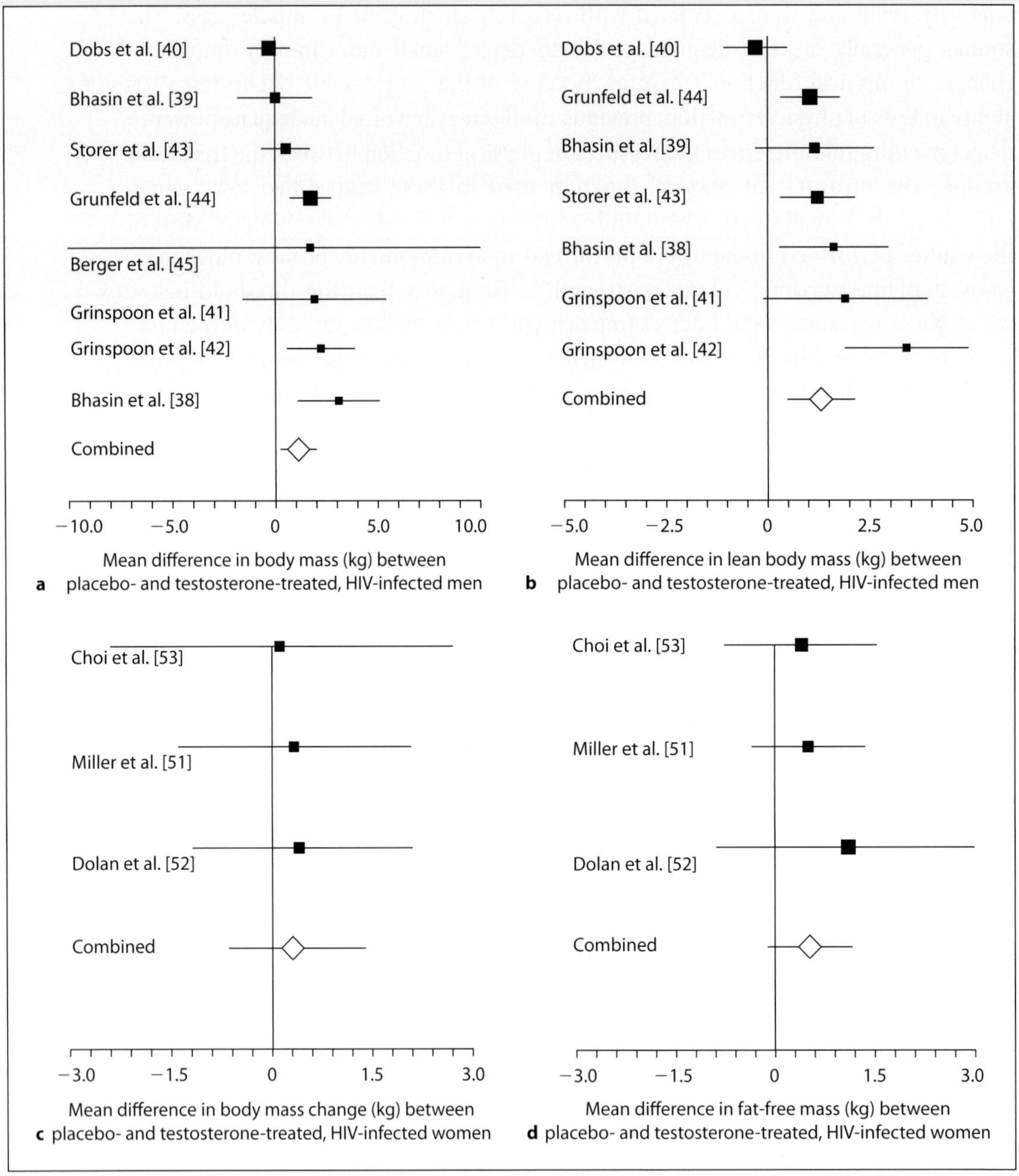

Fig. 3. Effects of testosterone therapy in HIV-infected men and women. Shown are meta-analysis plots of contrasts between androgen-treated and placebo-treated HIV-infected men with weight loss, showing the change (kg) in whole body mass (**a**), and lean body mass (**b**) and HIV-infected women with weight loss, showing the change in whole body mass (**c**) and fat-free mass (**d**). Confidence intervals that do not overlap with zero represent significant differences between placebo and testosterone groups. Reproduced with permission from Bhasin et al. [24].

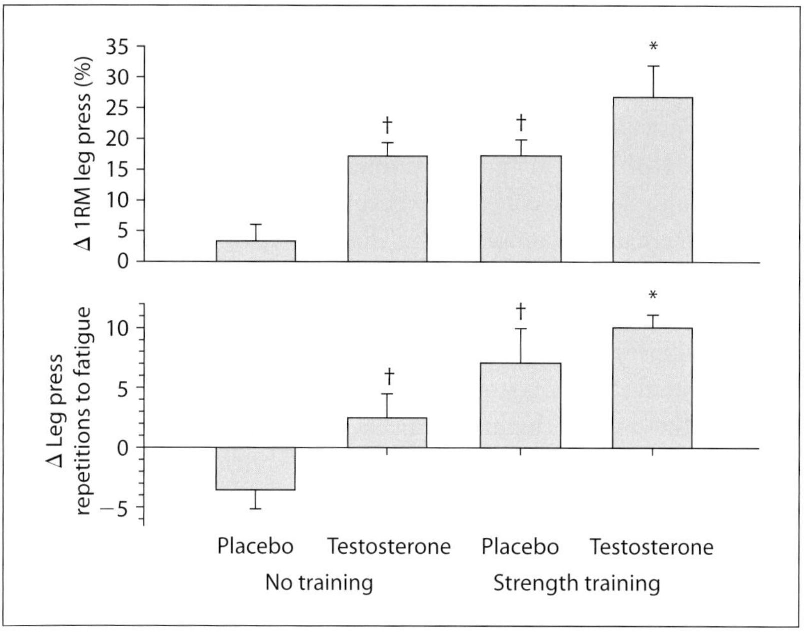

Fig. 4. Effects of testosterone with or without resistance exercise training on maximal voluntary strength and fatigability in the leg press exercise in men with COPD and low testosterone levels. Data for the four study groups are percentage changes in one-repetition maximum (1RM) of the leg press and in the number of repetitions of the leg press exercise completed at a weight equal to 80% of the subject's preintervention one-repetition maximum. The treatment assignments are shown below. *Response to intervention significantly different from nontraining groups. Response to intevention significantly different from placebo + no training group. Reproduced with permission from Casaburi et al. [44].

weight loss can induce modest gains in body weight and lean body mass with minimal change in quality of life and mood. These data led an Expert Panel of the Endocrine Society [27] to suggest that 'clinicians consider short-term testosterone therapy as an adjunctive therapy in HIV-infected men with low testosterone levels and weight loss to promote weight maintenance and gains in lean body mass (LBM) and muscle strength'. The Expert Panel recognized that its inferences were weakened by inconsistent results across trials, and heterogeneity among trials in inclusion criteria, disease status, testosterone formulations and doses, treatment duration, and methods of body composition analysis. There are no data on testosterone effects on physical function, risk of disability, disease progression, or long term safety.

Effects of Testosterone Supplementation in Glucocorticoid-Treated Men

Skeletal muscle atrophy, osteoporosis, and the suppression of endogenous testosterone production are well known complications of glucocorticoid administration in pharmacologic doses. Both increased protein catabolism and reduced protein synthesis contribute to glucocorticoid-induced loss of muscle mass [40]. Glucocorticoids inhibit ribosomal protein translation by inhibiting mTOR signaling by reduced phosphorylation of the downstream targets S6K1 and 4E-BP1 [40]. Dexamethasone upregulates the expression of REDD1 (a stress-induced gene that represses mTOR signaling) in rat skeletal muscle in vivo and in L6 myoblasts in culture and attenuates the assembly of mTOR regulatory complex, thus downregulating mTOR signaling [40]. Glucocorticoids also upregulate myostatin (an inhibitor of muscle growth) expression in the skeletal muscle cells in vivo and in vitro. Glucocorticoids lower testosterone levels by suppressing all components of the hypothalamic-pituitary-testicular axis [41]. In animal studies, testosterone has been shown to antagonize glucocorticoid effects on the muscle by mechanisms that are poorly understood. Testosterone down regulates glucocorticoid receptor in the skeletal muscle cells, and may also act downstream of glucocorticoid receptor to attenuate glucocorticoid signaling.

In two randomized, placebo-controlled trials [42, 43], testosterone supplementation of men receiving glucocorticoid treatment for bronchial asthma or chronic obstructive pulmonary disease was associated with greater gain (contrast with placebo 2.3 kg, 95% CI 2.0, 3.6) in lean body mass and a greater decrease in fat mass (contrast −3.1 kg, 95% CI, −3.5, −2.8) than placebo. These two trials found an increase in bone mineral density in the lumbar spine (+4%, 95% CI 2–7%); the effect on femoral bone density was inconsistent and not significant [42, 43]. The effects of testosterone supplementation on bone fractures in glucocorticoid-treated men have not been investigated. The frequency of testosterone-related adverse events was low [42, 43]. However, the small size of these studies, high drop-out rates in one study, and heterogeneity of inclusion criteria weaken these inferences.

Effects of Testosterone Therapy in Men with Chronic Obstructive Lung Disease

Exercise intolerance is a common symptom among patients with chronic obstructive pulmonary disease, and muscle wasting and dysfunction are recognized as correctable causes of functional limitations and disability in patients with COPD. In a randomized trial that used a 2 × 2 factorial design, Casaburi et al. [44] compared the effects of a replacement dose of testosterone enanthate (100 mg weekly) against placebo with or without a standardized program of resistance exercise training in men with COPD who have low testosterone levels. Testosterone therapy was associated with greater gains in fat free mass, muscle size, and muscle strength than placebo [44]. Testosterone and resistance exercise training when administered together were associated with greater gains in fat-free mass and strength than either intervention alone. In another randomized trial, a low dose of nandrolone was compared with placebo in 217 men and women with COPD; these authors reported modest increases in lean body mass and respiratory muscle strength [45]. Other studies, using nandrolone or oxandrolone, have reported variable results.

Testosterone Effects in Patients with End-Stage Renal Disease

There are over 350,000 patients receiving dialysis therapy for end-stage renal disease in the USA; this number has been steadily rising. Dialysis patients have reduced muscle size and strength and are severely limited in their physical performance as well as self-reported physical function [46]. Reduced muscle mass and functional limitations are associated with low overall quality of life, increased need for institutionalization, and higher mortality. Multiple metabolic perturbations – low levels of anabolic hormones testosterone, GH, and IGF-1, decreased physical activity, oxidative stress, chronic inflammation, endothelial dysfunction, malnutrition, and abnormalities in the cardiovascular, hematological, and neuromuscular systems – contribute to the multifactorial etiology of muscle loss and physical dysfunction [46].

Almost two thirds of men with end-stage renal disease have low testosterone levels because of multiple pathophysiologic factors that suppress all components of the hypothalamic-pituitary-testicular axis. The decrease in testosterone levels is a potentially correctable cause of muscle loss and dysfunction and has been the subject of a number of investigations.

In a randomized trial, nandrolone administration was associated with significant improvements in lean body mass, walking speed and stair climbing time [47]; the improvements in lean body mass were greater than those in the placebo group [47]. In a more recent randomized, placebo-controlled trial of nandrolone decanoate and resistance exercise training, Johansen et al. [48] demonstrated that patients receiving nandrolone decanoate (100 mg/week for women, 200 mg/week for men) showed a significant (+3.1 kg) increase in LBM and that combined administration of nandrolone and resistance exercise training increased quadriceps cross-sectional area in an additive manner. Androgens have been used for over three decades for the treatment of anemia in patients with end stage renal disease. Adequately powered studies are needed to determine the effects of androgen therapy on physical function, quality of life, erythropoietin use, and other clinically relevant outcomes.

Androgen Studies in Women

Undeniably, supraphysiologic doses of testosterone would be expected to increase muscle mass and strength in women. Improvements in nitrogen retention in healthy young women have been demonstrated with large doses of testosterone propionate. Anecdotal experience in female athletes who abuse large doses of androgenic steroids also supports this premise. However, the clinically relevant issue is whether meaningful improvements in physical function and patient-important outcomes are achievable with testosterone doses that do not induce virilizing side effects. We do not know whether testosterone dose-response relationships are different in women than they are in men.

A small number of trials have examined the effects of raising testosterone levels in to the high normal or slightly above the normal range in menstruating women. Testosterone supplementation in HIV-infected women in doses that raise serum testosterone levels into the high normal range was not associated with significant weight gain, LBM gain, or HRQOL indices between placebo and testosterone-treated women in any of the three randomized controlled trials [49–51]. No significant difference in muscle strength change between placebo and testosterone-treated women in one study [51]; another study [49] reported statistically significantly greater gains in muscle strength in testosterone-treated women than in placebo-treated women, but the magnitude of change was not clinically significant.

Another randomized trial evaluated the effects of esterified estrogen plus 2.5 mg methyltestosterone daily in postmenopausal women [52]. Combined therapy with methyltestosterone and estrogen increased total lean body mass and lower body strength, and reduced their percentage fat to a greater extent than placebo [52]. Methyltestosterone administration was also associated with small increments in sexual function and quality of life measures [52].

The long-term safety of testosterone therapy in women is unknown and the data are too limited to make a general recommendation about the usefulness of testosterone in women.

Testosterone Effects on Fat Mass and Distribution, and Insulin Sensitivity

Spontaneous as well as experimentally induced androgen deficiency is associated with gains in fat mass [53]. Conversely testosterone administration reduces whole body fat mass [24, 27]. The loss of fat mass during testosterone administration is distributed evenly between the truck and the appendices and between the superficial subcutaneous and deep imtamuscular and intrabdominal compartments [54]. Although some earlier studies had reported that testosterone therapy preferentially decreases visceral fat [55], other studies have not confirmed these findings.

Androgen deficiency has been linked to insulin resistance [56, 57], although other studies have reported conflicting results [58]. The effects of testosterone on insulin sensitivity are biphasic; for instance, in the male rat, lowering of testosterone levels by surgical orchidectomy worsened insulin sensitivity [59]. Replacement doses of testosterone in orchidectomized rats normalized insulin sensitivity [59]. However, administration of supraphysiologic doses of testosterone induced insulin resistance [59]. The effects of testosterone on insulin sensitivity in older men need further investigation.

Mechanisms of the Anabolic Effects of Androgen on the Skeletal Muscle

Although the mechanisms by which testosterone increases skeletal muscle mass are not fully understood, emerging data have implicated an interplay of several pathways. Testosterone-induced increase in muscle mass is associated with dose-dependent hypertrophy of both type I and type II fibers and an increase in the number of satellite cells [60, 61]. Neither the absolute number nor the relative proportion of type I and type II fibers changes during testosterone therapy.

Testosterone promotes the differentiation of mesenchymal, multipotent cells into myogenic lineage and inhibits their differentiation into adipogenic lineage [62]. Thus, in multipotent C3H10T1/2 cells, testosterone and DHT, two prototypical androgens, upregulate myogenic markers MyoD, and myosin heavy chain II, and downregulate adipogenic markers, such as PPAR-γ and C/EBP-α [62]. The effects of testosterone on mesenchymal stem cells could provide a unifying explanation for observed reciprocal changes in muscle and fat mass during testosterone therapy. Testosterone has also been reported to activate and promote satellite cell entry into the cell cycle under some experimental conditions; these data need confirmation.

Testosterone and DHT regulate mesenchymal multipotent cell differentiation by promoting the association of AR with β-catenin and translocation of the AR-β-catenin complex into the nucleus, resulting in activation of TCF-4 [63]. The activation of TCF-4 modulates a number of Wnt-regulated genes that promote myogenic differentiation and inhibit adipogenic differentiation. The effects of testosterone on myogenic differentiation are blocked by concomitant treatment with bicalutamide, and AR antagonist. These data suggest that these effects are mediated through an AR pathway.

It has been know for over 70 years that injections of testosterone propionate promote nitrogen retention in castrated males of many mammalian species, eunuchoidal men, and in women. More recently, in elegant stable isotope studies, testosterone has also been shown to increase fractional muscle protein synthesis and improve the reutilization of amino acids by the muscle [29]. The effects of testosterone on muscle protein degradation have not been well studied.

Role of 5α-Reductase and CYP19 Aromatase in Mediating Testosterone's Effects on the Skeletal Muscle

Testosterone is converted in the body to two active metabolites: 5α-DHT and 17β-estradiol. We do not know whether 5-alpha reduction of testosterone to DHT is required for mediating androgen effects on the muscle. The steroid 5α-reductase gene is expressed at low levels in the skeletal muscle. Individuals with congenital 5α-reductase deficiency undergo normal muscle development at puberty [64]; furthermore, patients treated with 5α-reductase inhibitors for the treatment of benign prostatic hypertrophy do not experience skeletal muscle loss.

The role of aromatization in mediating the effects of testosterone on body composition is also unclear. Aromatase knockout mice have lower muscle mass and higher fat mass than wild-type controls [65]. Similarly, men with congenital CYP19 mutations have decreased muscle mass and higher fat mass. The role of aromatization of testosterone to estradiol in mediating its anabolic effects on the muscle needs further investigation.

Selective Androgen Receptor Modulators

The concerns about the long-term risks of prostate and cardiovascular disorders in older men treated with testosterone have encouraged efforts to develop selective androgen receptor modulators that have the desired anabolic effects on the muscle, but that do not have adverse effects on prostate and cardiovascular outcomes [24, 66, 67]. These nonsteroidal SARMs do not serve as substrates for CYP19 aromatase or 5α-reductase, act as full agonists in muscle and bone and as partial agonists in prostate and seminal vesicles [24, 67]. The differing interactions of steroidal and nonsteroidal compounds with the AR may at least partially contribute to their unique pharmacologic actions [24, 68]. Bicalutamide adapts a greatly bent conformation in the AR [68]. Although A-ring and amide bond of the bicalutamide molecule overlaps the steroidal plane, the B-ring of the molecule folds away from the plane, pointing to the top of the ligand-binding pocket (LBP), which forms a unique structural feature of this class of ligands [68]. These H-bonding interactions are believed to be critical for high binding affinity.

Structural modifications of aryl propionamide analogs bicalutamide and hydroxyflutamide led to the discovery of the first generation of SARMs [24]. SARM pharmacophores can be classified into four categories: aryl-propionamide, bicyclic hydantoin, quinoline, and tetrahydroquinoline analogs [24]. A number of first-generation SARMs in these four structural classes are in phase I or early II trials.

The mechanistic basis of the tissue selective actions of SARMs is poorly understood, although several mechanisms have been proposed. Ligand binding induces specific conformational changes in the ligand- binding domain, which could modulate surface topology and subsequent protein-protein interactions between AR and other coregulators involved in genomic transcriptional activation or cytosolic proteins involved in nongenomic signaling [24, 66, 67]. Differences in ligand-specific receptor conformation and protein-protein interactions could result in tissue-specific gene regulation, due to potential changes in interactions with ARE, coregulators or transcription factors.

The first generation SARMs do not undergo aromatization or 5α reduction. Because a number of physiologic effects of testosterone require its conversion to DHT or estradiol, the failure of these compounds to undergo conversion to estradiol or DHT may pose unknown healthy risks.

Conceptual and Regulatory Hurdles in the Approval of Androgens and SARMs as Function-Promoting Therapies

There is strong evidence that testosterone supplementation increases skeletal muscle mass and maximal voluntary strength. There is weak evidence that testosterone therapy improves self-reported physical function. However, the effects of testosterone therapy on performance-based measures of physical function and health-related outcomes in patients with functional limitations have not been investigated. The long-term risks and benefits of testosterone administration remain unknown. Although there is a great deal of excitement about the potential applications of novel function promoting anabolic therapies, a number of conceptual and regulatory issues have retarded clinical development of these candidate molecules. There is considerable debate about the types of indications for which initial trails should be conducted and the outcome measures that should constitute evidence of efficacy. The minimal clinically important differences in important outcomes measures that should guide power and sample size estimates are unknown. A resolution of these vexing issues would greatly accelerate the translation of these promising candidate molecules into approved function promoting therapies.

References

1 Baumgartner RN, Koehler KM, Gallagher D, Romero L, Heymsfield SB, Ross RR, Garry PJ, Lindeman RD: Epidemiology of sarcopenia among the elderly in New Mexico. Am J Epidemiol 1998;147:755–763.

2 Roy TA, Blackman MR, Harman SM, Tobin JD, Schrager M, Metter EJ: Interrelationships of serum testosterone and free testosterone index with FFM and strength in aging men. Am J Physiol Endocrinol Metab 2002;283:E284–E294.

3 Guralnik JM, Ferrucci L, Simonsick EM, Salive ME, Wallace RB: Lower-extremity function in persons over the age of 70 years as a predictor of subsequent disability. N Engl J Med 1995;332:556–561.

4 Spillman BC: Changes in elderly disability rates and the implications for health care utilization and cost. Milbank Q 2004;82:157–194.

5 Kaufman JM, Vermeulen A: The decline of androgen levels in elderly men and its clinical and therapeutic implications. Endocr Rev 2005;26:833–876.

6 Harman SM, Metter EJ, Tobin JD, Pearson J, Blackman MR: Longitudinal effects of aging on serum total and free testosterone levels in healthy men. Baltimore Longitudinal Study of Aging. J Clin Endocrinol Metab 2001;86:724–731.

7 Wu FCW: Subclinical hypogonadism. Endocrine Society Meetings, Philadelphia, 2003, abstr S22–23.

8 Travison TG, Araujo AB, O'Donnell AB, Kupelian V, McKinlay JB: A population-level decline in serum testosterone levels in American men. J Clin Endocrinol Metab 2007;92:196–202.

9 Gray A, Feldman HA, McKinlay JB, Longcope C: Age, disease, and changing sex hormone levels in middle-aged men: results of the Massachusetts Male Aging Study. J Clin Endocrinol Metab 1991;73:1016–1025.

10 Bhasin S, Buckwalter JG: Testosterone supplementation in older men: a rational idea whose time has not yet come. J Androl 2001;22:718–731.

11 Winters SJ, Sherins RJ, Troen P: The gonadotropin-suppressive activity of androgen is increased in elderly men. Metabolism 1984;33:1052–1059.

12 Veldhuis JD, Zwart A, Mulligan T, Iranmanesh A: Muting of androgen negative feedback unveils impoverished gonadotropin-releasing hormone/luteinizing hormone secretory reactivity in healthy older men. J Clin Endocrinol Metab 2001;86: 529–535.

13 Pincus SM, Mulligan T, Iranmanesh A, Gheorghiu S, Godschalk M, Veldhuis JD: Older males secrete luteinizing hormone and testosterone more irregularly, and jointly more asynchronously, than younger males. Proc Natl Acad Sci USA 1996;93: 14100–14105.

14 Bonavera JJ, Swerdloff RS, Sinha Hakim AP, Lue YH, Wang C: Aging results in attenuated gonadotropin releasing hormone-luteinizing hormone axis responsiveness to glutamate receptor agonist N-methyl-D-aspartate. J Neuroendocrinol 1998;10: 93–99.

15 Orwoll E, Lambert LC, Marshall LM, Blank J, Barrett-Connor E, Cauley J, Ensrud K, Cummings SR: Endogenous testosterone levels, physical performance, and fall risk in older men. Arch Intern Med 2006;166:2124–2131.

16 O'Donnell AB, Travison TG, Harris SS, Tenover JL, McKinlay JB: Testosterone, dehydroepiandrosterone and physical performance in older men: results from the Massachusetts Male Aging Study. J Clin Endocrinol Metab 2005;91:425–431.

17 Schaap LA, Pluijm SM, Smit JH, van Schoor NM, Visser M, Gooren LJ, Lips P: The association of sex hormone levels with poor mobility, low muscle strength and incidence of falls among older men and women. Clin Endocrinol (Oxf) 2005;63:152–160.

18 Dobs AS, Dempsey MA, Ladenson PW, Polk BF: Endocrine disorders in men infected with human immunodeficiency virus. Am J Med 1988;84: 611–616.

19 Arver S, Sinha-Hikim I, Beall G, Guerrero M, Shen R, Bhasin S: Serum dihydrotestosterone and testosterone concentrations in human immunodeficiency virus-infected men with and without weight loss. J Androl 1999;20:611–618.

20 Salehian B, Jacobson D, Swerdloff RS, Grafe MR, Sinha-Hikim I, McCutchan JA: Testicular pathologic changes and the pituitary-testicular axis during human immunodeficiency virus infection. Endocr Pract 1999;5:1–9.

21 Handelsman DJ: Hypothalamic-pituitary gonadal dysfunction in renal failure, dialysis and renal transplantation. Endocr Rev 1985;6:151–182.

22 Wilson J: Androgen abuse by athletes. Endocr Rev 1988;9:181–191.

23 Bhasin S, Woodhouse L, Storer TW: Proof of the effect of testosterone on skeletal muscle. J Endocrinol 2001;170:27–38.

24 Bhasin S, Calof OM, Storer TW, Lee ML, Mazer NA, Jasuja R, Montori VM, Gao W, Dalton JT: Drug insight: testosterone and selective androgen receptor modulators as anabolic therapies for chronic illness and aging. Nature Clin Pract 2006;2:146–159.

25 Katznelson L, Finkelstein JS, Schoenfeld DA, Rosenthal DI, Anderson EJ, Klibanski A: Increase in bone density and lean body mass during testosterone administration in men with acquired hypogonadism. J Clin Endocrinol Metab 1996;81:4358–4365.

26 Mauras N, Hayes V, Welch S, Rini A, Helgeson K, Dokler M, Veldhuis JD, Urban RJ: Testosterone deficiency in young men: marked alterations in whole body protein kinetics, strength, and adiposity. J Clin Endocrinol Metab 1998;83:1886–1892.

27 Bhasin S, Cunningham GR, Hayes FJ, Matsumoto AM, Snyder PJ, Swerdloff RS, Montori VM: Testosterone therapy in adult men with androgen deficiency syndromes: an endocrine society clinical practice guideline. J Clin Endocrinol Metab 2006; 91:1995–2010.

28 Bhasin S, Storer TW, Berman N, Yarasheski KE, Clevenger B, Phillips J, Lee WP, Bunnell TJ, Casaburi R: Testosterone replacement increases fat-free mass and muscle size in hypogonadal men. J Clin Endocrinol Metab 1997;82:407–413.

29 Brodsky IG, Balagopal P, Nair KS: Effects of testosterone replacement on muscle mass and muscle protein synthesis in hypogonadal men: a clinical research center study. J Clin Endocrinol Metab 1996;81:3469–3475.

30 Bhasin S, Storer TW, Berman N, Callegari C, Clevenger B, Phillips J, Bunnell TJ, Tricker R, Shirazi A, Casaburi R: The effects of supraphysiologic doses of testosterone on muscle size and strength in normal men. N Engl J Med 1996;335:1–7.

31 Bhasin S, Woodhouse L, Casaburi R, Singh AB, Bhasin D, Berman N, Chen X, Yarasheski KE, Magliano L, Dzekov C, Dzekov J, Bross R, Phillips J, Sinha-Hikim I, Shen R, Storer TW: Testosterone dose-response relationships in healthy young men. Am J Physiol Endocrinol Metab 2001;281: E1172–E1181.

32 Woodhouse LJ, Reisz-Porszasz S, Javanbakht M, Storer TW, Lee M, Zerounian H, Bhasin S: Development of models to predict anabolic response to testosterone administration in healthy young men. Am J Physiol Endocrinol Metab 2003;284: E1009–E1017.

33 Storer TW, Magliano L, Woodhouse L, Lee ML, Dzekov C, Dzekov J, Casaburi R, Bhasin S: Testosterone dose-dependently increases maximal voluntary strength and leg power, but does not affect fatigability or specific tension. J Clin Endocrinol Metab 2003;88:1478–1485.

34 Snyder PJ, Peachey H, Hannoush P, Berlin JA, Loh L, Lenrow DA, Holmes JH, Dlewati A, Santanna J, Rosen CJ, Strom BL: Effect of testosterone treatment on body composition and muscle strength in men over 65 years of age. J Clin Endocrinol Metab 1999;84:2647–2653.

35 Page ST, Amory JK, Bowman FD, Anawalt BD, Matsumoto AM, Bremner WJ, Tenover JL: Exogenous testosterone (T) alone or with finasteride increases physical performance, grip strength, and lean body mass in older men with low serum T. J Clin Endocrinol Metab 2005;90:1502–1510.

36 Kong A, Edmonds P: Testosterone therapy in HIV wasting syndrome: systematic review and meta-analysis. Lancet Infect Dis 2002;2:692–699.

37 Bhasin S, Storer TW, Javanbakht M, Berman N, Yarasheski KE, Phillips J, Dike M, Sinha-Hikim I, Shen R, Hays RD, Beall G: Testosterone replacement and resistance exercise in HIV-infected men with weight loss and low testosterone levels. JAMA 2000;283:763–770.

38 Grinspoon S, Corcoran C, Parlman K, Costello M, Rosenthal D, Anderson E, Stanley T, Schoenfeld D, Burrows B, Hayden D, Basgoz N, Klibanski A: Effects of testosterone and progressive resistance training in eugonadal men with AIDS wasting: a randomized, controlled trial. Ann Intern Med 2000; 133:348–355.

39 Bhasin S, Storer TW, Asbel-Sethi N, Kilbourne A, Hays R, Sinha-Hikim I, Shen R, Arver S, Beall G: Effects of testosterone replacement with a nongenital, transdermal system, Androderm, in human immunodeficiency virus-infected men with low testosterone levels. J Clin Endocrinol Metab 1998;83: 3155–3162.

40 Wang H, Kubica N, Ellisen LW, Jefferson LS, Kimball SR: Dexamethasone represses signaling through the mammalian target of rapamycin in muscle cells by enhancing expression of REDD1. J Biol Chem 2006;281:39128–39134.

41 Kamischke A, Kemper DE, Castel MA, Luthke M, Rolf C, Behre HM, Magnussen H, Nieschlag E: Testosterone levels in men with chronic obstructive pulmonary disease with or without glucocorticoid therapy. Eur Respir J 1998;11:41–45.

42 Crawford BA, Liu PY, Kean MT, Bleasel JF, Handelsman DJ: Randomized placebo-controlled trial of androgen effects on muscle and bone in men requiring long-term systemic glucocorticoid treatment. J Clin Endocrinol Metab 2003;88:3167–3176.

43 Reid IR, Wattie DJ, Evans MC, Stapleton JP: Testosterone therapy in glucocorticoid-treated men. Arch Intern Med 1996;156:1173–1177.

44 Casaburi R, Bhasin S, Cosentino L, Porszasz J, Somfay A, Lewis MI, Fournier M, Storer TW: Effects of testosterone and resistance training in men with chronic obstructive pulmonary disease. Am J Respir Crit Care Med 2004;170:870–878.

45 Schols AM, Soeters PB, Mostert R, Pluymers RJ, Wouters EF: Physiologic effects of nutritional support and anabolic steroids in patients with chronic obstructive pulmonary disease: a placebo-controlled randomized trial. Am J Respir Crit Care Med 1995;152:1268–1274.

46 Johansen KL, Shubert T, Doyle J, Soher B, Sakkas GK, Kent-Braun JA: Muscle atrophy in patients receiving hemodialysis: effects on muscle strength, muscle quality, and physical function. Kidney Int 2003;63:291–297.

47 Johansen KL, Mulligan K, Schambelan M: Anabolic effects of nandrolone decanoate in patients receiving dialysis: a randomized controlled trial. JAMA 1999;281:1275–1281.

48 Johansen KL, Painter PL, Sakkas GK, Gordon P, Doyle J, Shubert T: Effects of resistance exercise training and nandrolone decanoate on body composition and muscle function among patients who receive hemodialysis: a randomized, controlled trial. J Am Soc Nephrol 2006;17:2307–2314.

49 Dolan S, Wilkie S, Aliabadi N, Sullivan MP, Basgoz N, Davis B, Grinspoon S: Effects of testosterone administration in human immunodeficiency virus-infected women with low weight: a randomized placebo-controlled study. Arch Intern Med 2004; 164:897–904.

50 Miller K, Corcoran C, Armstrong C, Caramelli K, Anderson E, Cotton D, Basgoz N, Hirschhorn L, Tuomala R, Schoenfeld D, Daugherty C, Mazer N, Grinspoon S: Transdermal testosterone administration in women with acquired immunodeficiency syndrome wasting: a pilot study. J Clin Endocrinol Metab 1998;83:2717–2725.

51 Choi HH, Gray PB, Storer TW, Calof OM, Woodhouse L, Singh AB, Padero C, Mac RP, Sinha-Hikim I, Shen R, Dzekov J, Dzekov C, Kushnir MM, Rockwood AL, Meikle AW, Lee ML, Hays RD, Bhasin S: Effects of testosterone replacement in human immunodeficiency virus-infected women with weight loss. J Clin Endocrinol Metab 2005;90: 1531–1541.

52 Dobs AS, Nguyen T, Pace C, Roberts CP: Differential effects of oral estrogen versus oral estrogen-androgen replacement therapy on body composition in postmenopausal women. J Clin Endocrinol Metab 2002;87:1509–1516.

53 Katznelson L, Rosenthal DI, Rosol MS, Anderson EJ, Hayden DL, Schoenfeld DA, Klibanski A: Using quantitative CT to assess adipose distribution in adult men with acquired hypogonadism. AJR Am J Roentgenol 1998;170:423–427.

54 Woodhouse LJ, Gupta N, Bhasin M, Singh AB, Ross R, Phillips J, Bhasin S: Dose-dependent effects of testosterone on regional adipose tissue distribution in healthy young men. J Clin Endocrinol Metab 2004;89:718–726.

55 Marin P, Holmang S, Jonsson L, Sjostrom L, Kvist H, Holm G, Lindstedt G, Bjorntorp P: The effects of testosterone treatment on body composition and metabolism in middle-aged obese men. Int J Obes Relat Metab Disord 1992;16:991–997.

56 Pitteloud N, Mootha VK, Dwyer AA, Hardin M, Lee H, Eriksson KF, Tripathy D, Yialamas M, Groop L, Elahi D, Hayes FJ: Relationship between testosterone levels, insulin sensitivity, and mitochondrial function in men. Diabetes Care 2005;28:1636–1642.

57 Kapoor D, Goodwin E, Channer KS, Jones TH: Testosterone replacement therapy improves insulin resistance, glycaemic control, visceral adiposity and hypercholesterolaemia in hypogonadal men with type 2 diabetes. Eur J Endocrinol 2006;154:899–906.

58 Singh AB, Hsia S, Alaupovic P, Sinha-Hikim I, Woodhouse L, Buchanan TA, Shen R, Bross R, Berman N, Bhasin S: The effects of varying doses of T on insulin sensitivity, plasma lipids, apolipoproteins, and C-reactive protein in healthy young men. J Clin Endocrinol Metab 2002;87:136–143.

59 Holmang A, Bjorntorp P: The effects of testosterone on insulin sensitivity in male rats. Acta Physiol Scand 1992;146:505–510.

60 Sinha-Hikim I, Artaza J, Woodhouse L, Gonzalez-Cadavid N, Singh AB, Lee MI, Storer TW, Casaburi R, Shen R, Bhasin S: Testosterone-induced increase in muscle size in healthy young men is associated with muscle fiber hypertrophy. Am J Physiol Endocrinol Metab 2002;283:E154–E164.

61 Sinha-Hikim I, Roth SM, Lee MI, Bhasin S: Testosterone-induced muscle hypertrophy is associated with an increase in satellite cell number in healthy, young men. Am J Physiol Endocrinol Metab 2003; 285:E197–E205.

62 Singh R, Artaza JN, Taylor WE, Gonzalez-Cadavid NF, Bhasin S: Androgens stimulate myogenic differentiation and inhibit adipogenesis in C3H 10T1/2 pluripotent cells through an androgen receptor-mediated pathway. Endocrinology 2003;44:5081–5088.

63 Singh R, Artaza JN, Taylor WE, Braga M, Yuan X, Gonzalez-Cadavid NF, Bhasin S: Testosterone inhibits adipogenic differentiation in 3T3-L1 cells: nuclear translocation of androgen receptor complex with beta-catenin and T-cell factor 4 may bypass canonical Wnt signaling to down-regulate adipogenic transcription factors. Endocrinology 2006;147:141–154.

64 Wilson JD, Griffin JE, Russell DW: Steroid 5 alpha-reductase 2 deficiency. Endocr Rev 1993;14:577–593.

65 Jones ME, Thorburn AW, Britt KL, Hewitt KN, Wreford NG, Proietto J, Oz OK, Leury BJ, Robertson KM, Yao S, Simpson ER: Aromatase-deficient (ArKO) mice have a phenotype of increased adiposity. Proc Natl Acad Sci USA 2000;97:12735–12740.

66 Negro-Vilar A: Selective androgen receptor modulators (SARMs): a novel approach to androgen therapy for the new millennium. J Clin Endocrinol Metab 1999;84:3459–3462.

67 Dalton JT, Mukherjee A, Zhu Z, Kirkovsky L, Miller DD: Discovery of nonsteroidal androgens. Biochem Biophys Res Commun 1998;244:1–4.

68 Bohl CE, Miller DD, Chen J, Bell CE, Dalton JT: Structural basis for accommodation of nonsteroidal ligands in the androgen receptor. J Biol Chem 2005; 280:37747–37754.

Prof. Shalender Bhasin
Boston University School of Medicine
Section of Endocrinology, Diabetes, and Nutrition
Boston Medical Center, Boston, MA 02118 (USA)
Tel. +1 617 414 2951, Fax +1 617 638 8217, E-Mail Shalender.Bhasin@bmc.org

Jones TH (ed): Advances in the Management of Testosterone Deficiency.
Front Horm Res. Basel, Karger, 2009, vol 37, pp 183–196

Testosterone in Chronic Heart Failure

Chris J. Malkin[a] · T. Hugh Jones[b,d] · Kevin S. Channer[a,c]

[a]Department of Cardiology, Royal Hallamshire Hospital, [b]Academic Unit of Diabetes, Endocrinology and Metabolism, Division of Genomic Medicine, University of Sheffield and [c]Faculty of Health and Well-being, Sheffield Hallam University, Sheffield, and [d]Centre for Diabetes and Endocrinology, Barnsley District General Hospital, Barnsley, UK

Abstract

Chronic heart failure is common and can be described as a syndrome characterized by impairment of cardiac function associated with a maladaptive metabolic and neurohormonal axis. The thesis that testosterone replacement therapy may be helpful as a treatment for chronic heart failure may seem at first to be unlikely. Testosterone therapy is widely believed to be deleterious to the cardiovascular system and there is a common misconception that the excess of ischaemic heart disease in young and middle-aged males compared to females is a direct effect of endogenous serum testosterone levels. In this chapter we will present the published evidence of the effects of endogenous and therapeutic testosterone on the heart and the human cardiovascular system with an emphasis on the pathologic syndrome of chronic heart failure. There is developing evidence that of all morbid populations, patients with chronic heart failure in particular are likely to benefit from testosterone treatment since the natural history is that of progressive disordered metabolism with catabolic excess and androgen imbalance.

Introduction

Chronic heart failure (CHF) is a common clinical problem and a major public health issue. The prevalence of CHF in the UK is 1% and in Europe alone it is thought that around 10 million people are affected by CHF [1]. The financial burden required to support this patient group is enormous and in the UK accounts for 4–5% of the NHS budget. Numerous treatment modalities exist – these can be conveniently divided into medical therapies and surgical and device treatments (table 1). Corrective surgery for valvular or congenital disease is rarely curative. Coronary revascularization either by coronary artery bypass surgery or percutaneous angioplasty may also be helpful for a minority. Cardiac transplantation may be offered to selected patients but this modality is limited due to the availability of donor organs. Modern device therapy includes cardiac resynchronization therapy, a technique using multisite pacing to improve cardiac performance and efficiency or implantable cardiac defibrillators designed to prevent sudden

Table 1. Medical therapies and surgical and device treatments

	Treatment modality	Target population	Frequency of use	Effect on symptoms	Effect on mortality
Surgical	Corrective surgery	Valvular pathology Congenital disease	Infrequent Rare	Improve	Improve
	Cardiac transplant	Severe heart failure, unresponsive to other modalities	Rare	Improve	Improve
	Revascularization CABG PCI	Proportion of patients with coronary disease	Infrequent	Improve	Improve
Device	Cardiac resynchronization	Moderate severity heart failure fulfilling stringent criteria	Rare	Improve	Improve
	Cardiac defibrillators	Moderate severity heart failure	Rare	None	Improve
Medical therapy	ACE-I ARBs	All	High	Improve	Improve
	β-Blockers	All	High	Improve	Improve
	Aldosterone antagonists	Moderate severity heart failure	Moderate	Improve	Improve
	Diuretics	Heart failure with fluid retention	High	Improve	None
	Digoxin	Heart failure with AF	Moderate	Improve	None

Guide to frequency terms: high: >50% CHF population; moderate: 10–50% CHF population; infrequent: <10% CHF population; rare: <1.5% CHF population. CABG = Coronary artery bypass grafting; PCI = percutaneous coronary intervention; ARB = angiotensin receptor blockers; AF = atrial fibrillation.

death due to malignant ventricular arrhythmias. Most patients however are ineligible for surgical or device therapy and are faced with a clinical condition characterized primarily by breathlessness, poor exercise tolerance and fatigue that is relentlessly progressive. Modern medical therapy for heart failure using combinations of angiotensin-converting enzyme inhibitors (ACE-I), β-adrenergic receptor blockers (β-blockers) and direct aldosterone antagonists improve symptoms and prolong life but do not prevent eventual decompensation to progressive heart failure. Other widely used therapies such as loop diuretics, digoxin and other anti-arrhythmics may improve symptoms and keep patients from unwanted hospital admission but have no demonstrable effect on mortality [1].

Despite modern advances in the detection, diagnosis and treatment of CHF the prognosis of this condition is still poor and is no better than the prognosis of most malignancies. Severe heart failure characterized by breathlessness at rest or minimal exertion has an annualized mortality of 50% and even selected heart failure patients managed aggressively within the confines of clinical trials have an annual mortality of around 10% [1].

Pathophysiology

CHF is a unique metabolic syndrome characterized by perturbation of numerous endocrine and inflammatory parameters. These changes are important since they relate to the severity of heart failure and directly contribute to deterioration and prognosis. A summary of the heart failure metabolic syndrome is displayed in table 2.

Many of these adaptive parameters are ultimately detrimental and cause worsening of cardiac function and eventually deterioration in severity of heart failure. The natural history of untreated heart failure is very poor with worsening cardiac function, symptoms and death. Strategies to simply increase cardiac muscle contraction with inotropes, for example, merely accelerate the natural history and are associated with a poorer prognosis. In the absence of surgically remedial lesions, modification of these neuro-endocrine responses in heart failure has been explored as potential therapies, with varying efficacy. As discussed above and summarized in table 1, inhibition of the renin-angiotensin-aldosterone axis and blockade of catecholamine receptors are the mainstay of heart failure therapy and will be offered to all patients. Disordered and excess immune activation has been explored with small trials of immunoglobulin and also pentoxyphylline with varying benefit. The possibility of reducing pro-inflammatory cytokines has been intensively investigated and although initial studies of anti-tumour necrosis factor (TNF) 'biological' drugs were promising, definitive benefit has not been borne out in major clinical trials [2].

Androgen Status in Heart Failure

It is notable that there is a clear anabolic-catabolic imbalance with an excess of catabolic hormones and a deficiency of many anabolic hormones. This aberration has until relatively recently been ignored, yet there is no doubt that this hormone derangement is a poor prognostic sign and contributes to significant symptoms [3]. Testosterone levels in heart failure in particular are low and this finding alone is a poor prognostic marker [4]. About a quarter of men with moderate severity heart failure have biochemical evidence of testosterone deficiency [5, 6]. One of the most feared clinical signs and a marker of very severe anabolic-catabolic imbalance in heart failure is cachexia [3], defined clinically as the non-intentional loss of 6 kg lean mass over a 6-month period. Cachexia is the most extreme symptom of heart failure and most subjects experience a more gradual catabolic decline. However the fact that severe heart failure can cause muscular wasting and weakness illustrates that the

Table 2. The metabolic syndrome of heart failure

Metabolic axis	Specific compounds	Relationship with CHF	Clinical effect in heart failure	Effect of pharmacologic modification	Available therapies
Renin-angiotensin	Angiotensin-2	Relate to severity of CHF and predict deterioration and mortality	Vasoconstriction, fluid retention, myocardial fibrosis	Improve symptoms and mortality	ACE-I ARBs
	Aldosterone		Myocardial fibrosis	Improve symptoms and mortality	Spironolactone, eplenerone
Catecholamines	Adrenaline Noradrenaline	Relate to severity of CHF and predict deterioration mortality and sudden death	Risk of sudden death, worsening cardiac function	Improve symptoms and mortality	β-Blockers
Glucocorticoid	Cortisol	Elevated	Catabolic	Unknown	None
Insulin		Resistance to insulin action in proportion to severity of CHF	Impaired glucose delivery, catabolic	Unknown	
Growth hormone		Reduced in heart failure, resistance at receptor level	Catabolic		Recombinant growth hormone
Androgens	Testosterone	Reduced in heart failure	Catabolic	Improve endurance	Testosterone
	Dehydroepiandrosterone	Reduced in heart failure	Catabolic	Unknown	
Immune/cytokine	TNF	Elevated	Catabolic	None	Monoconal antibodies
	IL-1	Elevated	Catabolic	None	Monoconal antibodies

ARB = Angiotensin receptor blockers.

condition is not simply a disease of the heart: there are multisystem effects and many of the cardinal symptoms of heart failure such as breathlessness and fatigue are due to abnormal muscle function, impaired mobilization of energy and ultimately loss of lean muscle mass [7]. It is these features of heart failure, intuitively similar to a state of frank androgen deficiency, where the hypothesis of testosterone treatment as an adjunct to heart failure therapy was first described.

Endogenous Testosterone and the Heart

Male sex is a risk factor for the premature development for coronary disease, with a relative risk ratio of 2.5:1, which is consistent throughout the world despite a widespread variation in the background incidence of coronary disease. This consistent epidemiological ratio infers that for any given genetic profile or exposure to risk factors there is an inherent advantage of being female or a disadvantage of being male [8]. This fact is difficult to explain and currently remains somewhat controversial. There is a widespread belief that higher serum testosterone levels in men compared with women are responsible. The concept stems partly from numerous case reports of adverse cardiovascular events in subjects who abuse high-dose anabolic steroids and partly from the simple association of male status and higher endogenous testosterone levels. Were this to be true then it follows that the higher the testosterone blood level the worse the cardiovascular effect. In fact there is a considerable volume of published data examining this issue, with approximately 40 cross-sectional studies and 8 prospective long-term follow-up studies and there does not appear to be any relationship with the levels of serum testosterone and the risk of atherosclerotic vascular disease. Indeed in many of the cross-sectional studies an inverse relationship is observed, with lower levels of testosterone associated with vascular disease [8]. Similarly in women, endogenous oestrogens appear to be protective and although the recent mega-trials of hormone replacement therapy in postmenopausal women have found hormone replacement therapy to cause an excess of vascular events, most of these effects are driven primarily by prothrombotic mechanisms. In summary, there appear to be sex-specific effects of endogenous sex hormones; in both sexes there is evidence that endogenous sex hormones, testosterone in males and oestrogens in women, are protective against atherosclerotic vascular disease. The clinical challenge is delivering effective therapeutic preparations of hormone replacement. In women for example this has been hampered by prothrombotic and procancerous effects of oestrogen. In men hormone replacement therapy in partial androgen deficiency is a relatively untested field. The prothrombotic effects of oestrogen therapy are not a problem with testosterone treatment since testosterone is a weak activator of fibrinolysis [9]. The risks of malignancy, particularly prostate cancer, are uncertain and require further evaluation.

Testosterone as a Treatment for Heart Failure

Testosterone is in many ways a logical choice as a treatment for heart failure. Heart failure is a characterized by anabolic deficiency, low-grade inflammation and a loss of muscle mass and strength; these are effects that testosterone treatment even at physiological doses may improve. In addition heart failure is a condition of disordered vascular behaviour specifically peripheral vasoconstriction and increased systemic vascular resistance, testosterone has effects on both the systemic and the coronary vasculature that increase both coronary perfusion and cardiac output.

Cardiac Effects of Testosterone Treatment

Within the boundaries of the normal physiological range testosterone therapy seems to have relatively little effect on myocardial morphology and function. There is animal data that profound testosterone depletion due to castration in early life regulates the expression of certain calcium ion channels and protein synthesis. In these studies castration was associated with reduced left ventricular (LV) mass, reduced cardiac output and reduced ejection fraction [10]. There is considerably more data on the effects of supraphysiological testosterone treatment on the myocardium. There is general uniformity in cell culture studies, animal treatment studies and observational studies of power athletes known to abuse anabolic androgens that a very high dose is detrimental to the myocardium. The important specific findings from the human observational studies included increased LV mass and hypertrophy, smaller LV cavity dimensions and evidence of early diastolic dysfunction due to stiffening and loss of LV compliance [11].

Non-Cardiac Effects of Testosterone Treatment

The non-cardiac effects of testosterone therapy are important. Analogous to many of the current pharmacological heart failure treatments, testosterone acts in a positive manner on the maladaptive heart failure metabolic syndrome and the direct effects on the myocardium appear to be less important.

Body Composition and Physical Strength

Numerous clinical trials of androgen therapy on the effects of body composition and voluntary physical strength exist within the literature. The trials can be broadly divided into those using physiological or non-physiological testosterone therapy and those testing the effects in morbid populations, androgen-deficient males and normal subjects. There is general consistency within the literature, with well-conducted prospective randomized controlled trials finding that testosterone improves anabolic function. This improvement in function is characterized by increased voluntary muscle strength, increased lean (muscle) mass and reduced fat mass [12]. These effects are seen in all patient groups and with testosterone preparations within the physiological replacement range. The morbid populations studied include patients with weight loss and cachexia due to malignancy, HIV infection and inflammatory autoimmune disease.

Insulin Resistance

One of the major hormonal derangements in heart failure is resistance to insulin. Insulin resistance is another example of a maladaptive hormone system in the complex syndrome of heart failure. The severity of heart failure is related to the severity of the insulin resistance and impaired insulin-mediated glucose uptake is a powerful independent prognostic marker [3]. The mechanism underlying insulin resistance in heart failure is obscure, though it appears functionally different than insulin resistance in other morbid populations which in general are characterized by reduced phosphorylation of intracellular postinsulin receptor proteins. It is likely that the cause is multifactorial and involves impaired postreceptor signalling and other neurohormonal and immune alterations present in severe heart failure [13]. It is notable that insulin resistance can be improved; by both conventional heart failure treatments such as ACE-I and β-blockers as well as novel non-pharmacological treatments such as graded exercise. Testosterone treatment has a positive effect on insulin sensitivity both in normal subjects and morbid populations such as obese men and diabetics [14]. A single study has examined the effect of testosterone treatment on insulin sensitivity in CHF. In this small crossover study compared to placebo, testosterone improved fasting glucose and insulin, insulin resistance as measured by HOMA (homeostatic model assessment) index and this was associated with increased lean mass and reduced fat mass [15].

Inflammation

CHF is a condition of low-grade subclinical inflammation. Inflammatory mediators such as TNF-α and interleukins (IL) such as IL-1 and IL-6 are elevated in heart failure and are mediators of the heart failure syndrome contributing to cachexia and insulin resistance [3]. Testosterone therapy is reported to have positive effects on inflammatory cytokines in hypogonadal men with co-morbid disease such as diabetes and coronary disease [16]. However significant clinical effects in men with heart failure have not been detected in vivo [17], although clinical trials at present are limited and underpowered.

Endurance and Functional Capacity

The general anabolic actions of androgen therapy are widely accepted. The evidence is less clear regarding the effect of androgens on functional capacity, exercise endurance and effort fatigue. This property is important in patients with chronic catabolic conditions and particularly in patients with congestive heart failure. The cardinal symptoms of CHF are poor exercise tolerance and fatigue. The restriction of exercise varies widely and bears little relation to the level of cardiac dysfunction, abnormal central pressures or haemodynamics. There appears to be a closer relationship with peripheral energy handling and delivery to the skeletal muscles – the so-called 'muscle hypothesis' [7]. These pathophysiological changes include subnormal peripheral blood flow response (impaired vasodilatation), early anaerobic metabolism, early depletion of high energy phosphates, deficient oxidative and lipolytic enzymes and histological changes consistent with muscle fibre loss and de-conditioning. In short many of these 'muscle' changes are consistent with an anabolic deficiency, and studies of exercise treatment in heart failure have found a degree of reversibility and improvement. The hypothesis that testosterone supplementation may augment this is clearly an important issue. There is relatively little published evidence to reliably answer this question. The limited animal data is consistent, with testosterone therapy, albeit sometimes at supraphysiological doses improving endurance and exercise capacity whereas clinical trials in normal subjects and morbid populations (HIV-infected patients and chronic respiratory failure patients) have yielded inconsistent results. To date two trials have explored the effects of testosterone on endurance capacity in heart failure and both have reported improvements in objective assessments of functional endurance capacity [6, 18]; these trials are explored in more detail in later sections.

Haemodynamic Effects of Testosterone Therapy

Testosterone has widespread effects on vascular tone and reactivity. There is substantial evidence within the literature that testosterone is a dilator of the systemic, pulmonary, mesenteric and coronary vascular beds [19]. Although testosterone is a steroid hormone it also has non-steroidal effects and interacts with a cell membrane-bound L-type calcium ion channel, permitting calcium cellular influx and vasodilatation [20, 21]. The vasodilatator properties of testosterone offer therapeutic properties in heart failure and also in related conditions such as angina pectoris caused by coronary heart disease.

Haemodynamics in Heart Failure

Heart failure is a condition of systemic vasoconstriction, a physiological adaptation to impaired cardiac function and reduced cardiac output. The increase in systemic vascular resistance is maladaptive and contributes to progressive symptoms and deterioration in patients with CHF. Testosterone therapy has beneficial effects on the haemodynamics of heart failure. Experimental data have confirmed that testosterone in vitro is a dilator of preconstricted systemic vessels (isolated from subcutaneous fat) [22]. Furthermore an important in vivo crossover study using invasive haemodynamic monitoring in 12 patients with CHF randomized to 6 h of acute testosterone therapy or placebo in random order has confirmed the thesis that testosterone reduces systemic vascular resistance and consequently increases cardiac output/index (fig. 1) [23]. The levels of testosterone in the treatment phase of this study were in the high physiological range and show that in the short term at least testosterone increases cardiac output as a result of reducing vascular resistance and increasing myocardial stroke volume. Further analysis of these data demonstrates that the patients with the lowest baseline testosterone levels (patients below the median) derived a greater haemodynamic effect. This finding suggests biological plausibility and potentially a dose-response relationship; the observation that patients with a lower baseline serum testosterone derive a greater benefit is a consistent finding and is also found when testosterone is used to treat angina pectoris.

Haemodynamics in Angina Pectoris

Angina pectoris is a symptom of coronary ischaemia. The most frequent cause of coronary ischaemia is obstructive atheroma in the coronary artery causing blood

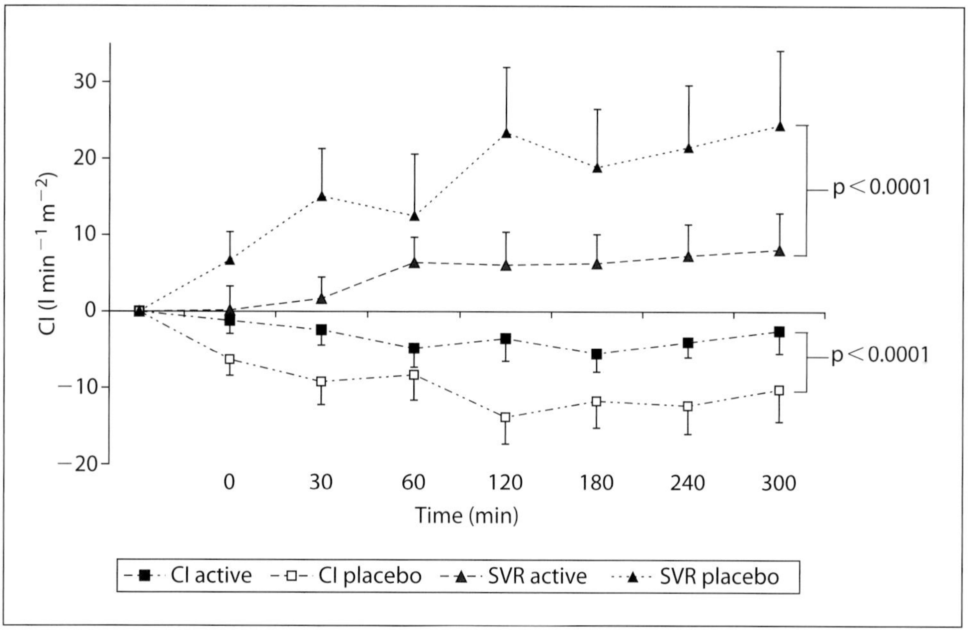

Fig. 1. Acute haemodynamic effect of testosterone vs. placebo. Data is change from baseline cardiac index (CI; cardiac output/mass). SVR = Systemic vascular resistance (dyn s cm^{-5}). n = 12 patients. Analysis in all cases by ANOVA.

flow limitation. Stable angina is common but unlike CHF has a relatively benign prognosis. Chronic angina can cause restricting symptoms and despite modern therapies including anti-anginal drugs and physical treatments such as coronary artery bypass surgery and coronary angioplasty may severely affect quality of life. Historically testosterone had been used as a therapy for angina and there are several trials from the 1940s attesting to this. Modern trials performed with more scientific methods have found testosterone to be a coronary vasodilator both in vitro and vivo, at physiological doses of therapy [24]. Low-dose testosterone treatment raises the threshold to coronary ischaemia as measured by exercise electrocardiography in an unselected male population with angina. The lower the baseline testosterone level is the greater is the improvement in ischaemic threshold [25]. If a sample of patients with low baseline testosterone levels (androgen deficient) is examined, these subjects derive greater improvement in ischaemic threshold than an unselected sample [26].

Clinical Trials of Testosterone Therapy in Heart Failure

There are few trials of androgen treatment in heart failure. A single animal study using a low dose of nandrolone decanoate improved survival in male hamsters with an inherited cardiomyopathy. An unblinded descriptive study of 12 male patients

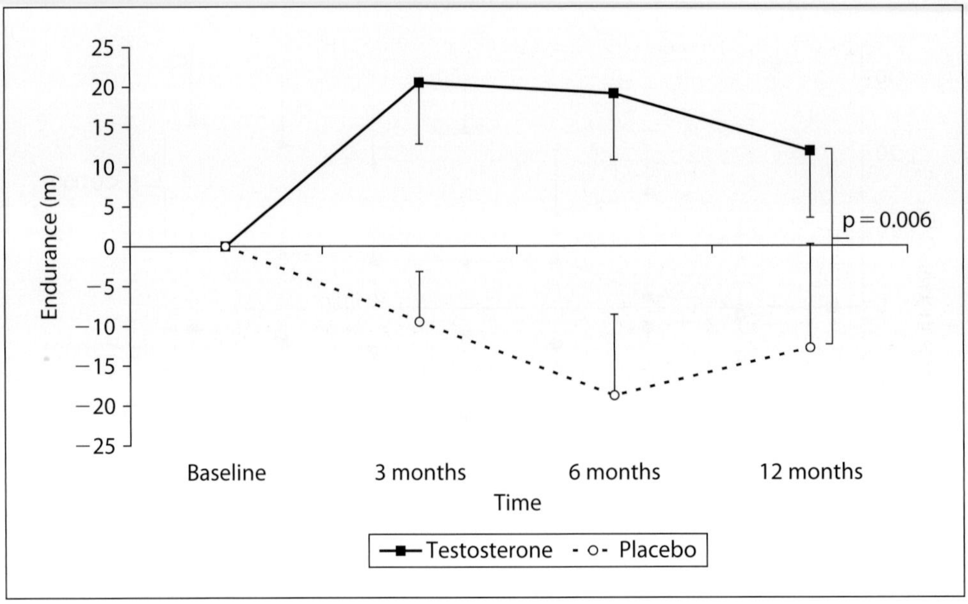

Fig. 2. Effect of testosterone on endurance in patients with CHF. Change of endurance from baseline as measured by the incremental shuttle walk test.

found improvements in echocardiographic parameters (reduced LV diameter, reduced LV mass) and reductions in brain natriuretic peptide (a serum marker of heart failure severity) [27]. The only prospective double-blind studies of testosterone treatment in heart failure are from the same scientific research group. Initially designed as a pilot study Pugh et al. [18] using fortnightly intramuscular testosterone (Sustanon 100®) found testosterone to improve mood, symptom scores and endurance (using an incremental shuttle walk test). In the larger follow-up study to this pilot [6], this time using daily testosterone patches (Androderm 5 mg vs. placebo) the effect on endurance was confirmed. Testosterone was found to increase exercise capacity as measured with an incremental shuttle walk test (fig. 2) and improve symptoms as determined by NYHA class. The improvement in exercise capacity in this study was less than observed in the pilot, in which larger doses of testosterone were administered; this suggests that there may be a dose-response relationship. Examination of the pooled data (fig. 3) confirms that the patients treated with intramuscular testosterone in the pilot study achieved higher serum levels of testosterone and greater increases in functional capacity than patients in the patch-treated study. These data suggest that the biological effects of testosterone on functional exercise capacity are related to the serum levels reached in vivo. Furthermore consistent with this notion was that there was a positive correlation with the increase in exercise capacity and serum bio-available testosterone at 3 and 6 months [6].

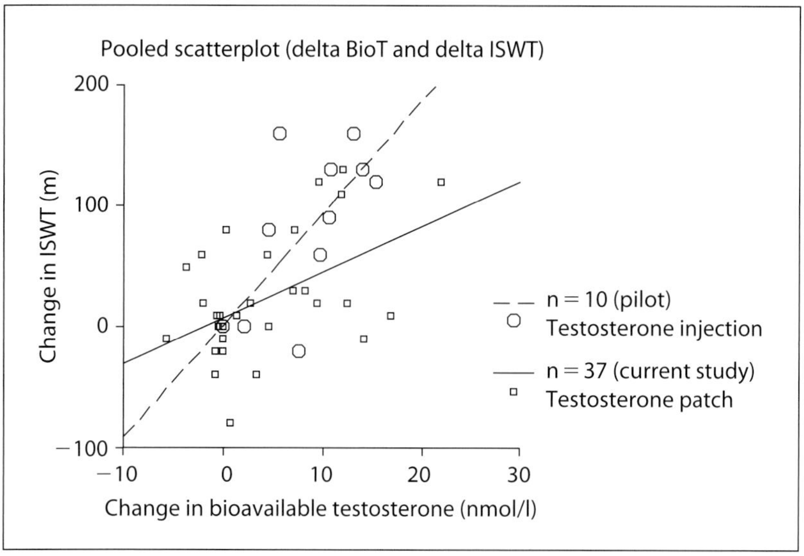

Fig. 3. Posttreatment testosterone level and shuttle walk distance. Increase in serum bioavailable testosterone after 3 months' treatment and change in endurance. Studies: pilot (n = 10) Pugh et al. [18]; current (n = 37) Malkin et al. [6] (adapted with permission from the *European Heart Journal*). ISWT = Incremental shuttle walking test.

Other secondary outcomes from this study included improved physician-assigned symptom scores, increased voluntary muscle strength, maintenance of systolic blood pressure, increased LV cavity length by echocardiography and a trend to a reduction in LV mass. There were no significant changes in 'hard' clinical outcomes such as unplanned hospitalizations or mortality. The secondary outcomes were interesting; the echo data suggest LV remodelling – a potential benefit in CHF. Systolic blood pressure decreased in the placebo group over the 12 months' follow-up. This is a part of the natural history of heart failure and is an adverse prognostic sign; however, the systolic blood pressure in the testosterone group was maintained (fig. 4).

Safety Issues

Testosterone replacement therapy appears to be safe. Long-term concerns that testosterone treatment may promote coronary disease of impaired cardiac function are not apparent within the boundaries of physiological replacement and in fact there is substantial evidence that this may be beneficial. Fluid retention, listed as an acknowledged side effect of testosterone treatment, is very rarely seen. There are realistic concerns over the risk of prostate malignancy. Prostatic malignancy should be excluded prior to commencing testosterone therapy by measurement of prostate-specific antigen and digital examination [see chapter by Morgentaler and Schulman, pp. 197–203].

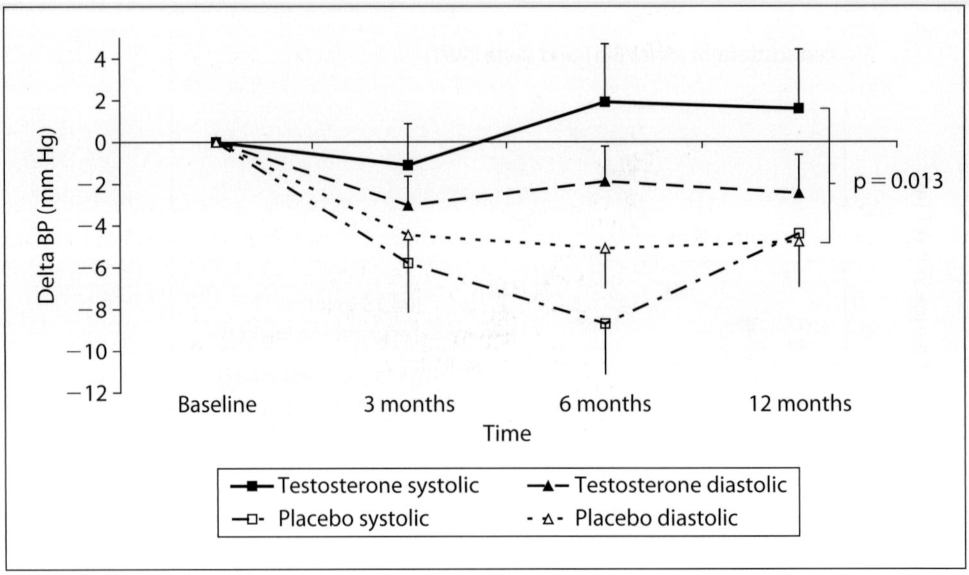

Fig. 4. Change in blood pressure from baseline (delta BP). Analysis by ANOVA in each case: change in systolic BP (p = 0.013), change in diastolic BP (p = 0.1).

Conclusions

Heart failure is a condition of high mortality, chronic debilitating symptoms and recurrent hospitalization. Novel therapies should either improve morbidity or survival or both; ideally therapy should be widely applicable, inexpensive and show benefit in the presence of co-existing heart failure therapies. Although testosterone replacement therapy cannot be advocated for women, testosterone treatment could be used cheaply in a high proportion of men in whom prostate malignancy had been excluded. It is estimated that the prevalence of biochemical androgen deficiency in males with heart failure is 25%; even in those men with testosterone levels within the normal range it can be argued that within the context of the hormonal imbalance of heart failure this represents a relative androgen deficiency. The effect on survival in heart failure is unknown; clinical trials have not yet been powered to detect any difference. The current evidence base of testosterone treatment in heart failure is small but consistent in reporting positive outcomes. At present, the use of testosterone for heart failure has not filtered into widespread clinical practice. This reflects the limited evidence base but there is also considerable anxiety and suspicion from cardiac specialists in particular to prescribe a male sex hormone to treat a cardiac condition. In this area endocrinologists may need to take a lead. Initially CHF patients with biochemical testosterone deficiency should be treated and followed up to provide registry data. However, larger clinical trials are urgently needed to reduce perceived anxieties about testosterone treatment within the cardiology community who advise and write guidelines on the management of CHF.

References

1 Swedberg K, Cleland J, Dargie H, Drexler H, Follath F, Komajda M, et al: Guidelines for the diagnosis and treatment of chronic heart failure: executive summary (update 2005): The Task Force for the Diagnosis and Treatment of Chronic Heart Failure of the European Society of Cardiology. Eur Heart J 2005;26:1115–1140.

2 Anker SD, Coats AJ: How to RECOVER from RENAISSANCE? The significance of the results of RECOVER, RENAISSANCE, RENEWAL and ATTACH. Int J Cardiol 2002;86:123–130.

3 Anker SD, Chua TP, Ponikowski P, Harrington D, Swan JW, Kox WJ, et al: Hormonal changes and catabolic/anabolic imbalance in chronic heart failure and their importance for cardiac cachexia. Circulation 1997;96:526–534.

4 Jankowska EA, Biel B, Majda J, Szklarska A, Lopuszanska M, Medras M, et al: Anabolic deficiency in men with chronic heart failure: prevalence and detrimental impact on survival. Circulation 2006;114: 1829–1837.

5 Kontoleon PE, Anastasiou-Nana MI, Papapetrou PD, Alexopoulos G, Ktenas V, Rapti AC, et al: Hormonal profile in patients with congestive heart failure. Int J Cardiol 2003;87:179–183.

6 Malkin CJ, Pugh PJ, West JN, van Beek EJ, Jones TH, Channer KS: Testosterone therapy in men with moderate severity heart failure: a double-blind randomized placebo controlled trial. Eur Heart J 2006; 27:57–64.

7 Coats AJ: Heart failure: what causes the symptoms of heart failure? Heart 2001;86:574–578.

8 Wu FC, von Eckardstein A: Androgens and coronary artery disease. Endocr Rev 2003;24:183–217.

9 Malkin CJ, Pugh PJ, Jones TH, Channer KS: Testosterone for secondary prevention in men with ischaemic heart disease? QJM 2003;96:521–529.

10 Scheuer J, Malhotra A, Schaible TF, Capasso J: Effects of gonadectomy and hormonal replacement on rat hearts. Circ Res 1987;61:12–19.

11 Urhausen A, Albers T, Kindermann W: Are the cardiac effects of anabolic steroid abuse in strength athletes reversible? Heart 2004;90:496–501.

12 Isidori AM, Giannetta E, Greco EA, Gianfrilli D, Bonifacio V, Isidori A, et al: Effects of testosterone on body composition, bone metabolism and serum lipid profile in middle-aged men: a meta-analysis. Clin Endocrinol (Oxf) 2005;63:280–293.

13 Kemppainen J, Tsuchida H, Stolen K, Karlsson H, Bjornholm M, Heinonen OJ, et al: Insulin signalling and resistance in patients with chronic heart failure. J Physiol 2003;550:305–315.

14 Kapoor D, Goodwin E, Channer KS, Jones TH: Testosterone replacement therapy improves insulin resistance, glycaemic control, visceral adiposity and hypercholesterolaemia in hypogonadal men with type 2 diabetes. Eur J Endocrinol 2006;154: 899–906.

15 Malkin CJ, Jones TH, Channer KS: The effect of testosterone on insulin sensitivity in men with heart failure. Eur J Heart Fail 2007;9:44–50.

16 Malkin CJ, Pugh PJ, Jones RD, Kapoor D, Channer KS, Jones TH: The effect of testosterone replacement on endogenous inflammatory cytokines and lipid profiles in hypogonadal men. J Clin Endocrinol Metab 2004;89:3313–3318.

17 Pugh PJ, Jones RD, Malkin CJ, Hall J, Nettleship JE, Kerry KE, et al: Physiologic testosterone therapy has no effect on serum levels of tumour necrosis factor-alpha in men with chronic heart failure. Endocr Res 2005;31:271–283.

18 Pugh PJ, Jones RD, West JN, Jones TH, Channer KS: Testosterone treatment for men with chronic heart failure. Heart 2004;90:446–447.

19 Jones RD, Pugh PJ, Jones TH, Channer KS: The vasodilatory action of testosterone: a potassium-channel opening or a calcium antagonistic action? Br J Pharmacol 2003;138:733–744.

20 Scragg JL, Jones RD, Channer KS, Jones TH, Peers C: Testosterone is a potent inhibitor of L-type Ca(2+) channels. Biochem Biophys Res Commun 2004;318:503–506.

21 Hall J, Jones RD, Jones TH, Channer KS, Peers C: Selective inhibition of L-type Ca^{2+} channels in A7r5 cells by physiological levels of testosterone. Endocrinology 2006;147:2675–2680.

22 Malkin CJ, Jones RD, Jones TH, Channer KS: Effect of testosterone on ex vivo vascular reactivity in man. Clin Sci (Lond) 2006;111:265–274.

23 Pugh PJ, Jones TH, Channer KS: Acute haemodynamic effects of testosterone in men with chronic heart failure. Eur Heart J 2003;24:909–915.

24 Webb CM, McNeill JG, Hayward CS, de Zeigler D, Collins P: Effects of testosterone on coronary vasomotor regulation in men with coronary heart disease. Circulation 1999;100:1690–1696.
25 English KM, Steeds RP, Jones TH, Diver MJ, Channer KS: Low-dose transdermal testosterone therapy improves angina threshold in men with chronic stable angina: a randomized, double-blind, placebo-controlled study. Circulation 2000;102: 1906–1911.
26 Malkin CJ, Pugh PJ, Morris PD, Kerry KE, Jones RD, Jones TH, et al: Testosterone replacement in hypogonadal men with angina improves ischaemic threshold and quality of life. Heart 2004;90: 871–876.
27 Tomoda H: Effect of oxymetholone on left ventricular dimensions in heart failure secondary to idiopathic dilated cardiomyopathy or to mitral or aortic regurgitation. Am J Cardiol 1999;83:123–125, A9.

Dr. Chris J. Malkin
Department of Cardiology
Royal Hallamshire Hospital, M Floor, Room M131
Glossop Road, Sheffield S10 2JF (UK)
Tel. +44 114 2713445, Fax +44 114 2712042, E-Mail Chris.malkin@sth.nhs.uk

Jones TH (ed): Advances in the Management of Testosterone Deficiency.
Front Horm Res. Basel, Karger, 2009, vol 37, pp 197–203

Testosterone and Prostate Safety

Abraham Morgentaler[a] · Claude Schulman[b]

[a]Division of Urology, Beth Israel Deaconess Medical Center, Harvard Medical School, Boston, Mass., USA; [b]Department of Urology, University Clinics of Brussels, Erasme Hospital, Brussels, Belgium

Abstract

For several decades it has been assumed that higher testosterone (T) leads to greater growth of benign and malignant prostate tissue, but this view has come under greater scrutiny over the last several years. Although there are as yet no large-scale, long-term controlled studies of T therapy to provide a definitive assessment of risk, numerous smaller clinical trials as well as population-based longitudinal studies consistently fail to support the historical idea that T therapy poses an increased risk of prostate cancer or exacerbation of symptoms due to benign prostatic hyperplasia. This lack of prostate risk despite increased serum T appears to be explained by data showing that exogenous T does not raise intraprostatic concentrations of T or dihydrotestosterone, suggesting a saturation model. In contrast, there is mounting evidence that low serum T is associated with greater prostate cancer risk, and more worrisome features of prostate cancer. In conclusion, the available evidence strongly suggests that T therapy is safe for the prostate. Given that the population at risk for T deficiency overlaps with the population at risk for prostate cancer, it is strongly recommended that men undergoing T therapy undergo regular monitoring for prostate cancer.

> The conventional views protect us from the principal job of thinking.
> *J.K. Galbraith,* Nobel Prize in Economy

One of the greatest impediments to treating men with testosterone (T) therapy is the fear that raising serum T concentrations will result in an increased risk of prostate cancer (PCa) or will convert an occult cancer into a clinical one [1]. This fear stems from the original work by Huggins and Hodges [2], who showed in 1941 that severe lowering of T by castration or estrogen therapy resulted in regression of advanced PCa, and who reported also that T administration caused 'enhanced growth' of PCa. This work by Huggins established the androgen dependence of PCa, and later earned him the Nobel Prize.

To this day, androgen deprivation therapy (ADT) remains a mainstay of treatment for men with advanced PCa, with rapid observable reductions in the serum marker, and prostate-specific antigen (PSA). In addition, it is well-recognized that restoration of T concentrations, such as by discontinuation of ADT, results in a rise in PSA in a substantial number of men. From these two current, clinical observations it is easy to understand why clinicians would be concerned that T therapy might pose an increased risk of PCa. Curiously, clinical experience and scientific research fail to demonstrate an increased risk.

In this chapter, we will review the available evidence regarding the relationship of T and the prostate, with special attention to safety issues regarding PCa. Although there are as yet no large-scale, long-term controlled studies of T therapy to document its safety, there does exist a substantial literature examining this relationship, and providing a rationale for why ADT causes PCa to regress but T therapy does not appear to cause PCa to progress.

T Trials

In the absence of any single large study on T therapy, one must examine the results from smaller studies, many of which have examined PSA changes and PCa detection rates in trials of 12 months to 3.5 years.

One of these was a 12-month study of 371 men on T gel therapy [3]. Over the course of 1 year three cancers were detected, all due to a rise in PSA. One of these increases in PSA was transient and resolved; however, a biopsy was performed and revealed cancer. In this study the mean rise in PSA was 0.4 ng/ml. This increase was noted at 3 months, and PSA remained unchanged over the next 9 months.

Other studies have revealed a similar rate of cancer detection in T therapy trials. In a review of nine separate T therapy trials involving 579 men and ranging from 3 to 36 months, seven cancers were identified, representing a cancer detection rate of 1.2% [4].

Wang et al. [5] performed one of the longest T therapy trials. In this study 163 men with a mean age of 51 years received T gel for 42 months. Over this time the mean PSA increased from 0.85 ng/ml at baseline to 1.1 ng/ml at 6 months, and then did not change significantly over the next 3 years of the study. Three men were diagnosed with PCa, representing a cancer rate of less than 1% per year of treatment.

Finally, PCa rates were investigated among men with and without the prostatic precancerous lesion known as high-grade prostatic intraepithelial neoplasia (PIN). In this 12-month study 75 men with hypogonadism received T therapy, including 55 men with benign pretreatment prostate biopsy, and 20 men with biopsy revealing PIN [6]. A similar 12 month increase in PSA of 0.3 ng/ml was seen in both groups, corresponding to a 15% rise. A single cancer was detected, in the PIN group, representing an overall cancer rate of 1.3%. The 5% cancer rate among men with PIN compares to a 25% risk over 3 years in this population, suggesting no significantly increased cancer risk.

One study that examined the effect of T therapy on PSA found that the overall change was mild, and the individual response varied considerably. Among 58 men who underwent T therapy for 1 year, the majority (32 men) demonstrated a mild PSA increase of 0.5 ng/ml or less [4]. There were also 14 men with a PSA increase greater than 0.5 ng/ml, but 12 men with a decline in PSA. No apparent differences in age, baseline T concentrations, or baseline PSA were noted between men with a PSA increase >0.5 ng/ml and men whose PSA declined.

To put these studies and their results in perspective, it is important to note that the observed PSA changes in multiple studies of approximately 15–20% is not much greater than the 13% increase noted over 1 year in 50- to 60-year-old men participating in the placebo arm of an unrelated study [7]. In addition, the annual cancer rate of approximately 1% that shows up repeatedly in T therapy trials compares favorably to cancer detection rates in men undergoing PCa screening [8].

Perhaps most importantly, two studies involving more than 500 men in total have shown that hypogonadal men with PSA of 4.0 ng/ml or less have a biopsy-detectable cancer rate of approximately 14% [9, 10]. If 1 in 7 men with low T has PCA, and if raising T truly caused PCa to grow more rapidly, logic would suggest that T therapy trials should be associated with a much higher rate of PCa.

Longitudinal Studies

The relationship of T and other sex hormones to subsequent development of PCa has been extensively studied in at least 16 population-based longitudinal studies [11–16]. In these studies, a health history is obtained, and blood samples at baseline are then frozen for the duration of the study, in some cases up to 20 years or longer. At the end of the study, men who have developed PCa are identified, and a matched set of men without PCa serve as controls.

A total of greater than 430,000 men have been included in these studies, including 1,400 men with PCa, and 4,400 men identified as controls. Not one study has shown a direct correlation between total T levels and PCa. Isolated associations have been reported with some measures and PCa: minor androgens in one [14], calculated free T in another [15], and with quartile analysis of hormone ratios or controlling for multiple variables in a third [16]. None of these positive associations have been supported by later studies. It is worth noting that the largest study of this type actually noted *reduced* PCa risk in men with higher T levels [13].

The importance of these studies is that they provide a sophisticated method of investigation to determine the long-term effects of endogenous hormone levels, especially T, on the subsequent risk of development of PCa. Although such studies cannot entirely replace the value of a prospective long-term controlled study of T therapy, they do address the question as to whether high levels of T (or other hormones) predispose men to a greater risk of later development of PCa. On this question these prospective longitudinal studies provide two uniform and convincing answers: first, that men who develop PCa do not have higher baseline T levels, and second, men with higher T levels are at no greater risk of developing PCa than men with lower T concentrations.

Resolving the Paradox

How is it possible that androgen deprivation and its discontinuation can have such a powerful effect on advanced PCa growth, yet T therapy trials appear to have little impact on PCa risk or even PSA?

The answer is provided by a recent landmark study by Marks et al. [17]. In this randomized, placebo-controlled, double-blind trial, 40 men with hypogonadism underwent prostate biopsy and comprehensive evaluation at baseline and after 6 months of injections of T or placebo every 2 weeks. Despite large changes in serum T concentrations, the intraprostatic concentrations of both T and dihydrotestosterone did not change significantly. Furthermore, no changes were noted in expression of androgen-related genes or genes associated with prostatic proliferation. These results indicate that substantial changes in serum androgens are not reflected within the prostate, and do not appear to induce biological changes within prostate tissue.

This study provides scientific evidence supporting the concept of saturation of the prostate androgen receptors with regard to T, as proposed recently [18]. In this saturation model, at the extreme low end of T concentrations there is a profound influence of T on prostate growth, yet at higher T concentrations this influence appears to be marginal, if present at all. Fowler and Whitmore [19] laid the groundwork for this model in their 1981 report detailing the effect of T administration in men with metastatic PCa. They noted that T administration resulted in rapid and near-universal PCa progression in men who had undergone prior androgen ablation, but not in men without prior hormonal manipulation of metastatic PCa. The authors concluded that naturally occurring endogenous T concentrations may be sufficient to produce 'near maximal stimulation' of PCa. This concept is supported by the study of Marks et al. [17], and describes the essence of the saturation model.

Low T and PCa

As clinicians have begun to let go of the old belief that raising T would necessarily increase PCa risk, there has been a coincidental recognition that low T may itself represent a risk factor for PCa. There is now emerging data that T deficiency is associated with greater risk of PCa, high Gleason scores, worse stage at presentation, and worse survival [20].

A study of 345 men with hypogonadism and PSA levels of 4.0 ng/ml or less found that the group of men in the lowest tertile of total T had more than double the risk of cancer on biopsy compared with men in the highest tertile (OR 2.15; 95% CI 1.01–4.55) [10]. In another study of 326 men who underwent radical prostatectomy, pretreatment T concentrations correlated with the likelihood of organ-confined disease [21]. In addition, there is now evidence correlating high Gleason scores with low T [22]. What these findings mean is that there is growing evidence that men with low T diagnosed with PCa are more likely to have positive margins in their prostate specimens and higher Gleason grades, and men with higher T were more likely to have negative margins and less aggressive disease.

T Therapy after Diagnosis of PCa

The growing number of men who appear to be cured from PCa after definitive therapy has created pressure to consider T therapy in those men who are symptomatic from T deficiency. Although this has been a longstanding taboo, clinical experience with T therapy together with the scientific evidence reviewed in this chapter suggests this may be far less risky than had previously been assumed. Preliminary results from 3 small studies suggest that T therapy may be used, with caution and in a carefully selected population, after PCa has been successfully treated.

The first of these was a small series of 7 cases in which T therapy was provided to symptomatic hypogonadal men who had undergone radical prostatectomy and who had an undetectable postoperative PSA [23]. No recurrences were noted in these men despite 1–12 years of T therapy.

A second study reported similar reassuring results in 10 men who had also undergone radical prostatectomy with undetectable PSA [24]. Mean total T increased from 197 to 591 ng/dl, and symptoms of hypogonadism improved. Most importantly, no PCa recurrences were noted with a median follow-up of 19 months.

A third study reported results in 31 men who received T therapy after PCa treatment with brachytherapy [25]. In this group the median duration of treatment was 4.5 years with a range of 0.5–8.5 years. Total T concentrations rose from a median of 188 to 498 ng/dl. No recurrences or PCa progression was noted, and all men remained with PSA less than 1.0 ng/ml at the end of the study.

These small clinical series provide some reassurance to physicians who wish to relieve the symptoms of hypogonadal men with T therapy following definitive treatment of localized PCa. However, determination of the true safety of this approach will require time and much larger studies.

Effects of T Therapy on the Benign Prostate

In addition to concerns regarding PCa, there have also been concerns that T therapy may cause exacerbation of lower urinary tract symptoms due to growth of the benign prostate, since the benign prostate is also under androgenic control. However, all available data indicates that any negative clinical impact on the benign prostate is minor and infrequent [5, 8]. Multiple studies have shown that T therapy is associated with only a mild increase in prostate volume as measured by transrectal ultrasound. Behre et al. [26] showed that T therapy in hypogonadal men raised prostate volume and PSA to levels seen in eugonadal controls, but no higher. In addition, studies consistently show no changes in uroflow rate, postvoid residual urine, and no changes in mean voiding symptoms as measured by the International Prostate Symptom Score [5, 8].

Monitoring for PCa

Although there is little, if any, compelling evidence that T therapy poses an increased risk of PCa, it must also be recognized that there is great overlap between the population at risk for T deficiency and the population at risk for PCa, and it is thus highly recommended that men receiving T therapy be monitored at regular intervals for PCa. Monitoring should consist of PSA determination and digital rectal examination, with biopsy performed for the development of an abnormal prostate examination, elevated PSA, or rapid increase in PSA (PSA velocity) [8].

Conclusion

Although we still lack a large-scale controlled study to definitively assess the safety of T therapy, it is becoming increasingly clear that this treatment poses little clinical risk of PCa in the short to mid-term. The reasons for the historical concern that T therapy may cause PCa progression are easy to understand given the androgen dependence of PCa and the dramatic effect of ADT in advanced metastatic PCa, yet this concern is belied by clinical experience and scientific investigations. Specifically, T therapy trials of up to 42 months as well as more than a dozen longitudinal population-based studies have consistently shown no increased PCa risk associated with higher T levels.

The explanation for the lack of PCa progression with higher T appears to be that prostate tissue is saturated with regard to T at a relatively low serum T concentration, and additional T beyond this saturation point is not reflected by intraprostatic concentrations of androgens. Recent small studies suggest that T therapy may even be a reasonable treatment for men who have undergone definitive treatment for localized PCa, a group for whom such treatment was considered taboo only a few short years ago.

On the other hand, there is now growing awareness that low T may itself be a risk for PCa, and may portend worrisome consequences once PCa is diagnosed. It will be fascinating to see what other changes come to pass over the next few years in this rapidly changing field.

References

1 Morgentaler A: Testosterone and prostate cancer: an historical perspective on a modern myth. Eur Urol 2006;50:935–939.

2 Huggins C, Hodges CV: Studies on prostatic cancer. I. The effect of castration, of estrogen and of androgen injection on serum phosphatases in metastatic carcinoma of the prostate. Cancer Res 1941;1:293–297.

3 Dean JD, Carnegie C, Rodzvilla J, Smith T: Long-term effects of Testim 1% testosterone gel in hypogonadal men. Rev Urol 2004;6:S22–S29.
4 Rhoden EL, Morgentaler A: Influence of demographic factors and biochemical characteristics on the prostate-specific antigen (PSA) response to testosterone replacement therapy. Int J Impot Res 2006;18:201–205.
5 Wang C, Cunningham G, Dobs A, et al: Long-term testosterone gel (AndroGel) treatment maintains beneficial effects on sexual function and mood, lean and fat mass, and bone density in hypogonadal men. J Clin Endocrinol Metab 2004;89:2085–2098.
6 Rhoden EL, Morgentaler A: Testosterone replacement therapy in hypogonadal men at high risk for prostate cancer: results of 1 year of treatment in men with prostatic intraepithelial neoplasia. J Urol 2003;170:2348–2351.
7 D'Amico AV, Roehrborn CG: Effect of 1 mg/day finasteride on concentrations of serum prostate-specific antigen in men with androgenic alopecia: a randomised controlled trial. Lancet Oncol 2007;8: 21–25.
8 Rhoden EL, Morgentaler A: Risks of testosterone-replacement therapy and recommendations for monitoring. N Engl J Med 2004;350:482–492.
9 Morgentaler A, Bruning CO 3rd, DeWolf WC: Incidence of occult prostate cancer among men with low total or free serum testosterone. JAMA 1996;276:1904–1906.
10 Morgentaler A, Rhoden EL: Prevalence of prostate cancer among hypogonadal men with prostate-specific antigen of 4.0 ng/ml or less. Urology 2006;68: 1263–1267.
11 Hsing AW: Hormones and prostate cancer: what's next? Epidemiol Rev 2001;23:42–58.
12 Eaton NE, Reeves GK, Appleby PN, Key TJ: Endogenous sex hormones and prostate cancer: a quantitative review of prospective studies. Br J Cancer 1999;80:930–934.
13 Stattin P, Lumme S, Tenkanen L, et al: High levels of circulating testosterone are not associated with increased prostate cancer risk: a pooled prospective study. Int J Cancer 2004;108:418–424.
14 Barrett-Connor E, Garland C, McPhillips JB, Khaw KT, Wingard DL: A prospective, population-based study of androstenedione, estrogens, and prostatic cancer. Cancer Res 1990;50:169–173.
15 Parsons JK, Carter HB, Platz EA, Wright EJ, Landis P, Metter EJ: Serum testosterone and the risk of prostate cancer: potential implications for testosterone therapy. Cancer Epidemiol Biomarkers Prev 2005;14: 2257–2260.
16 Gann PH, Hennekens CH, Ma J, Longcope C, Stampfer MJ: Prospective study of sex hormone levels and risk of prostate cancer. J Natl Cancer Inst 1996;88:1118–1126.
17 Marks LS, Mazer NA, Mostaghel E, et al: Effect of testosterone replacement therapy on prostate tissue in men with late-onset hypogonadism: a randomized controlled trial. JAMA 2006;296:2351–2361.
18 Morgentaler A: Testosterone replacement therapy and prostate cancer. Urol Clin North Am 2007;34: 555–363.
19 Fowler JE, Whitmore WF Jr: The response of metastatic adenocarcinoma of the prostate to exogenous testosterone. J Urol 1981;126:372–375.
20 Morgentaler A: Testosterone deficiency and prostate cancer: emerging recognition of an important and troubling relationship. Eur Urol 2007;52: 623–625.
21 Isom-Batz G, Bianco FJ Jr, Kattan MW, Mulhall JP, Lilja H, Eastham JA: Testosterone as a predictor of pathological stage in clinically localized prostate cancer. J Urol 2005;173:1935–1937.
22 Hoffman MA, DeWolf WC, Morgentaler A: Is low serum free testosterone a marker for high grade prostate cancer? J Urol 2000;163:824–827.
23 Kaufman JM, Graydon RJ: Androgen replacement after curative radical prostatectomy for prostate cancer in hypogonadal men. J Urol 2004;172:920–922.
24 Agarwal PK, Oefelein MG: Testosterone replacement therapy after primary treatment for prostate cancer. J Urol 2005;173:533–536.
25 Sarosdy MF: Testosterone replacement for hypogonadism after treatment of early prostate cancer with brachytherapy. Cancer 2007;109:536–541.
26 Behre HM, Bohmeyer J, Nieschlag E: Prostate volume in testosterone treated and untreated hypogonadal men in comparison to age-matched normal controls. Clin Endocrinol 1994;40:341–349.

Prof. Abraham Morgentaler
Division of Urology, Beth Israel Deaconess Medical Center
Harvard Medical School Boston, One Brookline Place, #624
Brookline, MA 02445 (USA)
Tel. +1 617 277 5000, Fax +1 617 277 5444, E-Mail amorgent@bidmc.harvard.edu

Author Index

Subject Index